2012
YEAR BOOK OF
ORTHOPEDICS®

The 2012 Year Book Series

Year Book of Anesthesiology and Pain Management™: Drs Chestnut, Abram, Black, Gravlee, Lien, Mathru, and Roizen

Year Book of Cardiology®: Drs Gersh, Cheitlin, Elliott, Gold, Graham, and Thourani

Year Book of Critical Care Medicine®: Drs Dries, Zanotti-Cavazzoni, Latenser, Martinez, Rincon, and Zwank

Year Book of Dermatology and Dermatologic Surgery™: Dr Del Rosso

Year Book of Diagnostic Radiology®: Drs Elster, Abbara, Oestreich, Offiah, Rosado de Christenson, Stephens, and Strickland

Year Book of Emergency Medicine®: Drs Hamilton, Bruno, Handly, Minczak, Mullin, Quintana, and Ramoska

Year Book of Endocrinology®: Drs Schott, Apovian, Clarke, Eugster, Meikle, Oetgen, Ovalle, Schteingart, and Toth

Year Book of Hand and Upper Limb Surgery®: Drs Yao, Adams, Isaacs, Lee, and Rizzo

Year Book of Medicine®: Drs Barker, Garrick, Gersh, Khardori, LeRoith, Panush, Talley, and Thigpen

Year Book of Neonatal and Perinatal Medicine®: Drs Fanaroff, Benitz, Donn, Neu, Papile, Polin, and Van Marter

Year Book of Neurology and Neurosurgery®: Drs Klimo, Minagar, Gandhi, House, Kevill, Liu, Mazia, Panagariya, Ragel, Riesenburger, Robottom, Schwendimann, Shafazand, Uhm, and Yang

Year Book of Obstetrics, Gynecology, and Women's Health®: Drs Dungan and Shulman

Year Book of Oncology®: Drs Arceci, Bauer, Chiorean, Gordon, Lawton, Murphy, Thigpen, and Tsao

Year Book of Ophthalmology®: Drs Rapuano, Cohen, Flanders, Hammersmith, Milman, Myers, Nagra, Nelson, Penne, Pyfer, Sergott, Shields, Talekar, and Vander

Year Book of Orthopedics®: Drs Morrey, Huddleston, Rose, Swiontkowski, and Trigg

Year Book of Otolaryngology-Head and Neck Surgery®: Drs Sindwani, Balough, Franco, Gapany, and Mitchell

Year Book of Pathology and Laboratory Medicine®: Drs Raab and Bissell

Year Book of Pediatrics®: Dr Stockman

Year Book of Plastic and Aesthetic Surgery™: Drs Miller, Gosman, Gurtner, Gutowski, Ruberg, Salisbury, and Smith

Year Book of Psychiatry and Applied Mental Health®: Drs Talbott, Ballenger, Buckley, Frances, Krupnick, and Mack

Year Book of Pulmonary Disease®: Drs Barker, Jones, Maurer, Spradley, Tanoue, and Willsie

Year Book of Sports Medicine®: Drs Shephard, Cantu, Feldman, Galea, Jankowski, Janssen, Lebrun, and Nieman

Year Book of Surgery®: Drs Copeland, Behrns, Daly, Eberlein, Fahey, Huber, Klodell, Mozingo, and Pruett

Year Book of Urology®: Drs Andriole and Coplen

Year Book of Vascular Surgery®: Drs Moneta, Gillespie, Starnes, and Watkins

2012

The Year Book of ORTHOPEDICS®

Editor-in-Chief

Bernard F. Morrey, MD

Professor of Orthopedics, Mayo Graduate School of Medicine; Professor of Orthopedics, University of Texas, Health Science Center, San Antonio, Texas

ELSEVIER
MOSBY

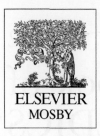

ELSEVIER
MOSBY

Vice President, Continuity: Kimberly Murphy
Developmental Editor: David Parsons
Production Supervisor, Electronic Year Books: Donna M. Skelton
Electronic Article Manager: Mike Sheets
Illustrations and Permissions Coordinator: Dawn Vohsen

2012 EDITION

Printed and bound by CPI Group (UK) Ltd, Croydon, CR0 4YY
Composition by TNQ Books and Journals Pvt Ltd, India
Transferred to Digital Print 2012

Editorial Office:
Elsevier, Inc.
Suite 1800
1600 John F. Kennedy Blvd
Philadelphia, PA 19103-2899

International Standard Serial Number: 0276-1092
International Standard Book Number: 978-0-323-08887-9

Editorial Board

Paul M. Huddleston III, MD

Assistant Professor of Orthopedic Surgery, Mayo Clinic College of Medicine, Rochester, Minnesota

Peter S. Rose, MD

Assistant Professor of Orthopedic Surgery, Mayo Clinic College of Medicine, Rochester, Minnesota

Marc F. Swiontkowski, MD

Professor, Department of Orthopaedic Surgery, University of Minnesota; Chief Executive Officer, TRIA Orthopaedic Center, Bloomington, Minnesota

Stephen D. Trigg, MD

Assistant Professor of Orthopedics, Mayo Graduate School of Medicine, Rochester, Minnesota; Consultant in Orthopedic Hand Surgery, Mayo Hospital, Jacksonville, Florida

Contributor

Christopher P. Beauchamp, MD

Associate Professor, Department of Orthopedics, Mayo Clinic, Scottsdale, Arizona

Table of Contents

Journals Represented

Journals represented in this YEAR BOOK are listed below.

Acta Anaesthesiologica Scandinavica
Acta Obstetricia et Gynecologica Scandinavica
AJR American Journal of Roentgenology
American Heart Journal
American Journal of Clinical Nutrition
American Journal of Clinical Pathology
American Journal of Epidemiology
American Journal of Medical Genetics (Part A)
American Journal of Obstetrics and Gynecology
Anesthesia & Analgesia
Archives of Internal Medicine
Australia & New Zealand Journal of Obstetrics & Gynaecology
Breast Journal
British Journal of Cancer
British Journal of Obstetrics and Gynaecology
British Medical Journal
Canadian Medical Association Journal
Cancer Epidemiology, Biomarkers & Prevention
Clinical Chemistry
Clinical Infectious Diseases
Contraception
European Journal of Obstetrics & Gynecology and Reproductive Biology
European Journal of Radiology
Fertility and Sterility
Genetics in Medicine
Gut
Gynecologic and Obstetric Investigation
Gynecologic Oncology
Headache
Human Pathology
Human Reproduction
Journal of Adolescent Health
Journal of Clinical Endocrinology & Metabolism
Journal of Clinical Microbiology
Journal of Clinical Oncology
Journal of Infectious Diseases
Journal of the American Medical Association
Journal of the National Cancer Institute
Journal of Ultrasound in Medicine
Journal of Urology
Lancet
Maturitas
Metabolism Clinical and Experimental
Modern Pathology
New England Journal of Medicine
Obstetrics & Gynecology
Pediatrics

Placenta
Proceedings of the National Academy of Sciences of the United States of America
Science Translational Medicine
Sleep
Ultrasound in Obstetrics & Gynecology

STANDARD ABBREVIATIONS

The following terms are abbreviated in this edition: acquired immunodeficiency syndrome (AIDS), anterior cruciate ligament (ACL), anteroposterior (AP), avascular necrosis (AVN), cardiopulmonary resuscitation (CPR), central nervous system (CNS), cerebrospinal fluid (CSF), computed tomography (CT), deoxyribonucleic acid (DNA), electrocardiography (ECG), health maintenance organization (HMO), human immunodeficiency virus (HIV), intensive care unit (ICU), intramuscular (IM), intravenous (IV), magnetic resonance (MR) imaging (MRI), range of motion (ROM), ribonucleic acid (RNA), total hip arthroplasty (THA), total knee arthroplasty (TKA), ultrasound (US), and ultraviolet (UV).

NOTE

The YEAR BOOK OF ORTHOPEDICS® is a literature survey service providing abstracts of articles published in the professional literature. Every effort is made to assure the accuracy of the information presented in these pages. Neither the editors nor the publisher of the YEAR BOOK OF ORTHOPEDICS® can be responsible for errors in the original materials. The editors' comments are their own opinions. Mention of specific products within this publication does not constitute endorsement.

To facilitate the use of the YEAR BOOK OF ORTHOPEDICS® as a reference tool, all illustrations and tables included in this publication are now identified as they appear in the original article. This change is meant to help the reader recognize that any illustration or table appearing in the YEAR BOOK OF ORTHOPEDICS® may be only one of many in the original article. For this reason, figure and table numbers will often appear to be out of sequence within the YEAR BOOK OF ORTHOPEDICS®.

Introduction

As we were reviewing articles for this year's volume, we considered the dramatic changes that have occurred in the manner in which physicians learn their specialty and become proficient at it. I was struck by the historical connection through the years between the YEAR BOOK and my home institution, the Mayo Clinic. The YEAR BOOK series started in 1901. Since 1959, the editor has been from the Mayo Clinic, except for a brief period during which Dr Clement Sledge, Boston, was the editor. The reason to mention this is that as we consider the periods during which these giants in orthopedics served as YEAR BOOK editor, it is most impressive to reflect on the dramatic changes in orthopedic content that has also occurred in our specialty. When the YEAR BOOK publication started, reconstruction of a diseased or dysfunctional joint was difficult, as joint replacement was not an option. Polio was rampant and management of sepsis dominated our specialty. Today everything has changed. We are investigating the genetic basis for orthopedic diseases and the ability to manipulate or at least screen patients and disease based on genetic profiles. Our interventions have become so sophisticated that we have come to expect a 95% satisfactory outcome for at least a decade. Our ability to treat orthopedic malignancies has dramatically improved both with regard to survival and function. Finally, our knowledge of and therefore ability to manage simple as well as complex trauma has been dramatically enhanced with the introduction of the AO influence both regarding implants, fixation philosophy and educational format. With this backdrop, this year's YEAR BOOK in my mind is truly a transitional volume. It is an attempt to bring the most up-to-date general orthopedic information to that surgeon who is faced with the daunting task of managing a broad spectrum of orthopedic conditions. I personally have intentionally avoided the more sophisticated subspecialty topics and made an attempt for the YEAR BOOK to continue to be a "general or mainstream resource."

This has been an invaluable opportunity for me to stay abreast of the broad spectrum of orthopedic activity. It is my hope that it will prove to be of significant benefit to those who read these pages in the ongoing management of their patients.

Bernard F. Morrey, MD

1 Basic Science

Introduction

Basic science of orthopedic surgery has dramatically changed since we began our careers. Our initial focus was that of biomechanics and joint kinematics. Since then the specialty, as well as medicine in general, has evolved to investigations at a cellular, molecular, genetic and proteogenomic level. We have tried to reflect this evolving level of sophistication and interest in the articles selected in this section. We have also attempted to characterize those articles we think highlight topics that may be more translatable to the bedside in the near future. Basic investigations going on in musculoskeletal diseases are truly exciting and offer significant opportunities for the future.

Bernard F. Morrey, MD

Chondrocytes or adult stem cells for cartilage repair: The indisputable role of growth factors

Freyria A-M, Mallein-Gerin F (Université Lyon, France)

Injury 43:259-265, 2012

Articular cartilage is easily injured but difficult to repair and cell therapies are proposed as tools to regenerate the defects in the tissue. Both differentiated chondrocytes and adult mesenchymal stem cells (MSCs) are regarded as cells potentially able to restore a functional cartilage. However, it is a complex process from the cell level to the tissue end product, during which growth factors play important roles from cell proliferation, extracellular matrix synthesis, maintenance of the phenotype to induction of MSCs towards chondrogenesis. Members of the TGF-β superfamily are especially important in fulfilling these roles. Depending on the cell type chosen to restore cartilage, the effect of growth factors will vary. In this review, the roles of these factors in the maintenance of the chondrocyte phenotype are discussed and compared with those of factors involved in the repair of cartilage defects, using chondrocytes or adult mesenchymal stem cells (Fig 1, Table 1).

▶ This review article is included to emphasize the known complexity of the issue of cartilage regeneration and the equally complex question of the value of

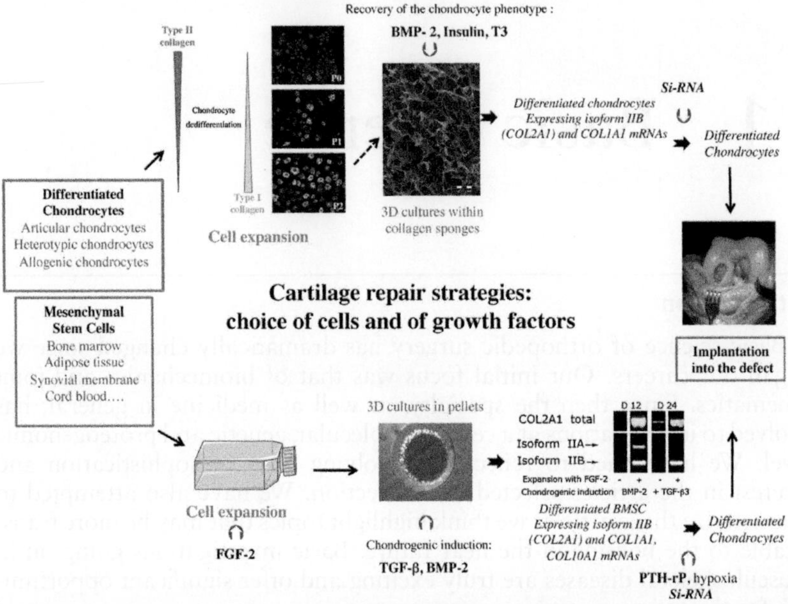

FIGURE 1.—Sequences of events leading to the production of cells to repair cartilage defects. The initial harvested cells (chondrocytes and mesenchymal stem cells) have to go through several culture conditions characterised by the addition of specific growth factors. At different stages the cell phenotype is analysed especially for the presence of the isoform IIB of type II collagen as a marker of differentiated chondrocytes. Whatever the type of cell used to construct a new cartilage, some drawbacks exist, such as the expression of type X and type I collagens that are not components of articular cartilage. Solutions to control these expressions could be the use of specific molecules as indicated. Si-RNA: small interfering RNA; T3: tri-iodothyronine; BMSC: bone marrow mesenchymal stem cell. (Reprinted from the Injury, International Journal of the Care of the Injured. Freyria A-M, Mallein-Gerin F. Chondrocytes or adult stem cells for cartilage repair: the indisputable role of growth factors. *Injury.* 2012;43:259-265, Copyright 2012, with permission from Elsevier.)

enhancement with growth factors. The review is short and easy to read. The important difference between differentiated condrocytes and mesenchymal stem cells is depicted (Fig 1) along with the implication of the introduction of growth factors. The complexity of the issues is highlighted by demonstrating differences in gender, age, variation of preparation, and timing (Table 1). Regardless, the enhancement of the process by the transforming growth factor-β super family is well documented. This nicely characterizes the current state of orthopedic research in this area.

B. F. Morrey, MD

TABLE 1.—Human Mesenchymal Stem Cells as a Source for Chondrogenesis: Relevant Literature Concerning the Different Growth Factors and a Variety of Experimental Models

Growth Factors: Cell Amplification	Growth Factors: Chondrogenic Induction	Method of Induction	Studies
BMSC	TGF-β1 (10 ng/ml)	Pellets (2.5 × 10^5 cells) ± TGF-β1 for 7, 14 and 21 days	Solchaga[79]
ADSC (p2)	TGF-β1 (10 ng/ml)	Pellets (5 × 10^5 cells) ± TGF-β1 in normoxia (20% oxygen) or hypoxia (5% oxygen) for 28 days	Merceron[50]
BMSC or ADSC (p2 + 10 ng/ml FGF-2)	TGF-β1 (10 ng/ml)	Alginate beads (4 × 10^6 cells/ml) + TGF-β1 for 14 and 21 days	Mehlhorn[47]
Fat pad or synovial membrane MSC (p2 ± 1 ng/ml TGF-β1 + 5 ng/ml FGF-2 + 10 ng/ml PDGF-bb)	TGF-β1 (10 ng/ml)	Pellets (5 × 10^5 cells) ± TGF-β1 on 3D orbital shaker (30 rpm) for 2 weeks	Marsano[45]
BMSC (p5-6 + 10 ng/ml FGF-2)	TGF-β1 (10 ng/ml)	Pellets (2 × 10^5 cells) ± TGF-β1 for 7, 14 and 28 days	Karlsson[34]
Muscle-derived cells (p2-3 + 10 ng/ml FGF-2 + 10^{-6} M Dexamethasone)	TGF-β1 (10 ng/ml)	Alginate βeads (5 × 10^6 cells/ml) ± TGF-β1 for 21 days	Andriamanalijaona[4]
BMSC	TGF-β1 (10 ng/ml) TGF-β2 (10 ng/ml) TGF-β3 (10 ng/ml)	Pellets (2 × 10^5 cells) ± TGF-β1, TGF-β2 or TGF-β3 for 35 days	Barry[7]
BMSC (+ 10 ng/ml FGF-2)	TGF-β1 (10 ng/ml) TGF-β3 (10 ng/ml)	Pellets (2 × 10^5 cells) ± TGF-β1 or TGF-β3 for 21 days	Varas[88]
BMSC (p3-4)	TGF-β3 (10 ng/ml)	Pellets (2.5 × 10^5 cells) ± TGF-β3 for 3, 7 and 14 days intermittent hydrostatic pressure (10MPa/1hz/4h per day)	Miyanishi[52]
BMSC (p2 + 1 ng/ml FGF-2)	TGF-β3 (10 ng/ml)	Pellets (5 × 10^6 cells) and aqueous-derived silk fibroin scaffolds ± TGF-β3 for 21 days	Wang[90]
BMSC (p2-3, + 10 ng/ml EGF and 10 ng/ml PDGF-bb)	TGF-β3 (10 ng/ml)	Pellets (4–5 × 10^5 cells) ± TGF-β3 for 14, 28 and 42 days	Peltari[61]
BMSC (p3 + 5 ng/ml FGF-2)	TGF-β3 (10 ng/ml)	Pellets (5 × 10^5 cells) ± TGF-β3 Transwell disks (5 × 10^5 cells) ± TGF-β3 for 28 days	Murdoch[54]
BMSC (p1)	BMP-2 (100 ng/ml) TGF-β1 (10 ng/ml)	Collagen hydrogel (2.5 × 10^5 cells/ml and 3 mg/ml Type I collagen) ± BMP-2 or TGF-β1 for 3 weeks	Noth[59]
ADSC (p2 + 1 or 10 ng/ml FGF-2)	BMP-2 (50 ng/ml) TGF-β1 (10 ng/ml)	Alginate beads (4 × 10^6 cells/ml) ± TGF-β1 and BMP-2 for 14 days	Mehlhorn[48]

(Continued)

TABLE 1.—(*Continued*)

Growth Factors: Cell Amplification	Growth Factors: Chondrogenic Induction	Method of Induction	Studies
BMSC or ADSC (p3)	BMP-7 (100 ng/ml) TGFβ-2 (5 ng/ml) PTH-rP (100 ng/ml)	Pellets (2.5×10^5 cells) ± TGFβ-2 (BM-MSC) and TGFβ-2 + BMP-7 (AT-MSC) for 4 weeks (Including 10 or 100 ng/ml PTH-rP after 14 days)	Kim[39]
BMSC or ADSC (p3)	BMP-2 (100 ng/ml) BMP-6 (100 ng/ml) BMP-7 (100 ng/ml) TGF-β2 (5 ng/ml)	Pellets (2.5×10^6 cells) + GF alone or in combinations (TGF-β2 ± BMP-2 or -6 or -7) for 4 weeks	Kim[38]
BMSC (p4)	IGF-1 (100 ng/ml) BMP-6 (500 ng/ml) TGF-β3 (10 ng/ml)	Pellets (2.5×10^5 cells) ± TGF-β3 and BMP-6 or IGF-1 in combination (TB or TI) or in cycling pattern for 21 days	Indrawattana[32]
BMSC (p3)	BMP-6 (500 ng/ml) TGF-β3 (10 ng/ml)	Pellets (2×10^5 cells) ± BMP-6 and TGF-β3 for 21 days	Sekiya[76]
BMSC (p2)	BMP-2 (500 ng/ml) BMP-4 (500 ng/ml) BMP-6 (500 ng/ml) TGF-β3 (10 ng/ml)	Pellets (2×10^5 cells) ± BMP-2 (or -4 or -6) and TGF-β3 for 21 days	Sekiya[75]
BMSC (p4)	BMP-2 (50 ng/ml) TGF-β3 (10 ng/ml)	Pellets (2.5×10^5 cells) ± TGF-β3 and BMP-2 for 2 weeks	Schmitt[74]
BMSC (p2-3)	BMP-2 (100 ng/ml) TGF-β3 (10 ng/ml)	Alginate beads (5×10^6 cells/ml) + TGF-β3 + BMP-2 for 21 days	Shen[77]
BMSC (p2 + 5 ng/ml FGF-2)	IGF-1 (100 ng/ml) TGF-β3 (10 ng/ml)	Pellets (5×10^5 cells) + TGF-β3 and IGF-1 in normoxia (20% oxygen) or hypoxia (5% oxygen) for 14 days	Khan[37]
BMSC (p1-2 + 1 ng/ml FGF-2)	IGF-1 (100 ng/ml) TGF-β1 (10 ng/ml) TGF-β3 (10 ng/ml)	Pellets (1×10^6 cells) + IGF-1 ± TGF-β3 or TGF-β1 ± dexamethasone for 16 days	Mwale[56]

BMSC or ADSC (p2-3 + 10 ng/ml EGF + 10 ng/ml PDGF-BB)	BMP-6 (10 ng/ml)	Pellets (4–5 × 10^5 cells) + 10 ng/ml TGF-β3 (BMSC) or + 10 ng/ml BMP-6 (ADSC)	Zimmermann[93]
	TGF-β3 (10 ng/ml)		
BMSC (p2-5 + 10 ng/ml EGF + 10 ng/ml PDGF-bb)	BMP-2, -4, -6, -7	Pellets (4–5 × 10^5 cells) + 10 ng/ml TGF-β3 or 10 ng/ml of various combinations of GF for 45 days	Weiss[91]
	IGF-1		
	FGF-1, -2		
	PTH-rP, TGF-β3		
ADSC (p1 no GF) BMSC (p2-4 + 1 ng/ml FGF-2)	BMP-2 (100 ng/ml)	Pellets (2.5 × 10^5 cells) + BMP-2 for 28 days	Noël[158]
BMSC (p1 + 1 ng/ml FGF-2) (cell infection at the end of p1 with 5 × 10^3 vp/cell Ad.BMP-2 or Ad.BMP-4)	BMP-2, -4 gene transfer	Pellets (2 × 10^5 cells) for 3, 7, 14, 21 days	Steinert[82]

Abbreviations: p, passage; ADSC, adipose tissue derived mesenchymal stem cell; BMSC, bone marrow mesenchymal stem cell; GF, growth factor; 3D, three-dimensional; vp, viral particles.
Editor's Note: Please refer to original journal article for full references.

Autologous Osteochondral Transplantation of the Talus Partially Restores Contact Mechanics of the Ankle Joint

Fansa AM, Murawski CD, Imhauser CW, et al (Hosp for Special Surgery, NY)
Am J Sports Med 39:2457-2465, 2011

Background.—Autologous osteochondral transplantation procedures provide hyaline cartilage to the site of cartilage repair. It remains unknown whether these procedures restore native contact mechanics of the ankle joint.

Purpose.—This study was undertaken to characterize the regional and local contact mechanics after autologous osteochondral transplantation of the talus.

Study Design.—Controlled laboratory study.

Methods.—Ten fresh-frozen cadaveric lower limb specimens were used for this study. Specimens were loaded using a 6 degrees of freedom robotic arm with 4.5 N·m of inversion and a 300-N axial compressive load in a neutral plantar/dorsiflexion. An osteochondral defect was created at the centromedial aspect of the talar dome and an autologous osteochondral graft from the ipsilateral knee was subsequently transplanted to the defect site. Regional contact mechanics were analyzed across the talar dome as a function of the defect and repair conditions and compared with those in the intact ankle. Local contact mechanics at the peripheral rim of the defect and at the graft site were also analyzed and compared with the intact condition. A 3-dimensional laser scanning system was used to determine the graft height differences relative to the native talus.

Results.—The creation of an osteochondral defect caused a significant decrease in force, mean pressure, and peak pressure on the medial region of the talus ($P = .037$). Implanting an osteochondral graft restored the force, mean pressure, and peak pressure on the medial region of the talus to intact levels ($P = .05$). The anterior portion of the graft carried less force, while mean and peak pressures were decreased relative to intact ($P = .05$). The mean difference in graft height relative to the surrounding host cartilage for the overall population was -0.2 ± 0.3 mm (range, -1.00 to 0.40 mm). Under these conditions, there was no correlation between height and pressure when the graft was sunken, flush, or proud.

Conclusion/Clinical Relevance.—Placement of the osteochondral graft in the most congruent position possible partially restored contact mechanics of the ankle joint. Persistent deficits in contact mechanics may be due to additional factors besides graft congruence, including structural differences in the donor cartilage when compared with the native tissue.

▶ Without question, biological reconstruction holds greater potential for long-term satisfactory function than does artificial replacement. This biomechanical study addresses a less common anatomic region, the talus. The concept is accepted as a transplant option at the knee and elbow. This study precisely creates Fig 2 in the original article and addresses a defect (Fig 4 in the original article) in the weight-bearing region of the talus. Despite the precision, although this restores some of the load distribution properties, the restoration is only partial

(Fig 8 in the original article). We have similar results at the elbow for radial head resection. The message is that these transplants imperfectly restore the load-bearing features of the joint. This does not even address issues related to healing or remodeling.

B. F. Morrey, MD

ACL Reconstruction Using Bone-Tendon-Bone Graft Engineered from the Semitendinosus Tendon by Injection of Recombinant BMP-2 in a Rabbit Model

Hashimoto Y, Naka Y, Fukunaga K, et al (Osaka City Univ Med School, Japan)
J Orthop Res 29:1923-1930, 2011

We attempted to generate a bone-tendon-bone structure by injecting human-type recombinant human bone morphogenetic protein-2 (rhBMP-2) into the semitendinosus tendon, and an anterior cruciate ligament (ACL) defect was reconstructed by grafting the engineered bone-tendon-bone graft. Two ossicles with a separation distance of 1 cm were generated within the left semitendinosus tendon of a rabbit 6 weeks after the injection of rhBMP-2 (15 μg at each site). The engineered bone-tendon-bone graft was transplanted in order to reconstruct the ACL by passing the graft through the bone tunnels. In the control group, the ACL was reconstructed with the semitendinosus tendon without BMP-2 using the same methods as those used in the experimental group. The animals were harvested at 4 or 8 weeks after surgery and examined by radiographic, histological, and

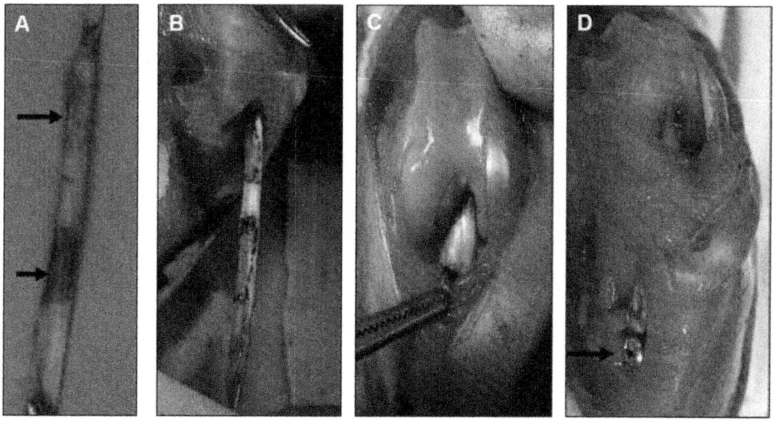

FIGURE 2.—Semitendinosus tendon harvested 6 weeks after BMP injection. Two calcified blocks (black arrows) appeared at the injection site, and they appeared red due to the blood (A). ACL reconstruction using a newly formed bone-tendon-bone graft passing through the bone tunnel (B,C). The graft was fixed with post-screws (black arrow) (D). For interpretation of the references to color in this figure legend, the reader is referred to web version of this article. (Reprinted from Hashimoto Y, Naka Y, Fukunaga K, et al. ACL reconstruction using bone-tendon-bone graft engineered from the semitendinosus tendon by injection of recombinant BMP-2 in a rabbit model. *J Orthop Res.* 2011;29:1923-1930, with permission from Orthopaedic Research Society.)

biomechanical methods. In the experimental group, ossicles in the bone-tendon-bone graft were successfully integrated into the host bone of the femur and tibia. Histological analysis revealed that characteristic features identical to the normal direct insertion morphology had been restored. Biomechanical pull-out testing showed that the ultimate failure load and stiffness of the reconstructed ACL in the experimental group were significantly higher than those in the control group at both 4 and 8 weeks ($p < 0.05$). These results indicate the potential of regenerative reconstruction of the ACL, and the reconstruction resulted in the restoration of morphology and function equivalent to those of the normal ACL (Fig 2).

▶ As in prior years, most of the sports literature focuses on the anterior cruciate ligament (ACL). This work is of interest because it offers a glimpse into what the future may hold. A bone morphogenetic protein enhanced engineered semitendinosus with osseous attachment to the femur and tibia is attractive (Fig 2). The functional and mechanical properties approach that of a normal ACL. Although like most basic investigations, the findings are not immediately transferable to the clinical setting, certainly the approach is worthy of aggressive investigation.

B. F. Morrey, MD

Collagen Production at the Edge of Ruptured Rotator Cuff Tendon is Correlated With Postoperative Cuff Integrity

Shirachi I, Gotoh M, Mitsui Y, et al (Kurume Univ, Japan; Kurume Univ Med Ctr, Japan)

Arthroscopy 27:1173-1179, 2011

Purpose.—The purpose was to evaluate the correlation between messenger RNA (mRNA) expression of collagen at the edge of the ruptured rotator cuff tendon and postoperative cuff integrity.

Methods.—The edge of the ruptured tendon was sampled during open rotator cuff surgery in 12 patients with full-thickness rotator cuff tears (mean age, 58.2 years). The mean period from symptom onset was 9.3 months (range, 1 to 36 months), and the mean tear size was 4.1 cm. As controls, rotator cuff tendons with no gross rupture were taken from 5 fresh cadavers. Production of type I and type III collagen was examined by real-time reverse transcription polymerase chain reaction. By use of magnetic resonance imaging, postoperative cuff integrity was evaluated based on the classification of Sugaya et al. and then scored, ranging from 5 points for type I to 1 point for type V.

Results.—Looking at the mRNA of type I and type III collagen in tendons, we found that the expression of mRNA for both collagen types in ruptured tendons was significantly greater than in control tendons ($P = .0462$ for type I collagen and $P = .0306$ for type III collagen). Correlating the mRNA of type I and type III collagen with repaired cuff integrity on postoperative magnetic

TABLE 3.—Correlation Between Collagen mRNA and Postoperative Cuff Integrity

	Type I Collagen mRNA Correlation Coefficient	*P* Value	Type III Collagen mRNA Correlation Coefficient	*P* Value
Postoperative cuff integrity	0.63	$P < .038$	−0.14	$P < .03$

NOTE. The relative ratios of the PCR products for the collagens in samples (ruptured tendons) compared with those in MG cells were calculated.

resonance imaging, we found a close relation between expression of mRNA for both collagen types and postoperative rotator cuff integrity ($r = 0.63$ [$P = .038$] for type I collagen and $r = 0.626$ [$P = .03$] for type III collagen). Furthermore, expression of type I collagen mRNA showed a significant inverse correlation with the period from symptom onset ($r = -0.845$, $P < .0005$).

Conclusions.—This study showed that expression of mRNA for type I and type III collagen at the edge of the ruptured rotator cuff tendon was significantly correlated with postoperative cuff integrity and that mRNA expression for type I collagen was significantly associated with the period from symptom onset. These results may suggest that conservative treatment should not be prolonged if patients do not respond within a certain period.

Level of Evidence.—Level III, prognostic case-control study (Table 3).

▶ This very interesting report uses a clever study design and addresses a subtle but relevant question. Using modern assay techniques, the authors were able to both demonstrate a correlation of the presence of type 1 and 3 collagen at the site of large rotator cuff tears and correlate the presence to healing of the repaired cuff (Table 3). The authors offer the most important comment, as they conclude expressions of increased levels of type 1 and 3 collagen might serve as a basis to offer earlier surgical intervention. Unfortunately, this is an extrapolation of the study data, and this conclusion is yet to be proven.

B. F. Morrey, MD

Cytokine Gene Expression After Total Hip Arthroplasty: Surgical Site Versus Circulating Neutrophil Response

Buvanendran A, Mitchell K, Kroin JS, et al (Rush Univ Med Ctr, Chicago, IL; Natl Inst of Dental and Craniofacial Res, Bethesda, MD)

Anesth Analg 109:959-964, 2009

Background.—After surgery, cytokines and chemokines are released at the surgical wound site, which can contribute to postoperative pain, local inflammation, and tissue repair. Multiple cell types are present that can release cytokines/chemokines at the wound site and, thus, the exact cellular source of these molecules is unclear. We sought to better understand the

TABLE 2.—Genes Upregulated or Downregulated in Hip Drain Neutrophils After Total Hip Arthroplasty Using Microarray Analysis

Symbol	Gene Name	Fold Change
IL8RB	Interleukin-8 receptor β/CXCR2	0.23
MIF	Macrophage migration inhibitory factor	2.7
IL18R1	Interleukin-18 receptor 1	3.1
IL1RN	Interleukin-1 receptor antagonist	3.2
CCL20	LARC/MIP-3α	5.3
CCR3	CC-CKR-3/CKR3	0.19
CX3CR1	CCRL1/CMKBRL1	0.35
CCR5	CC-CKR-5	0.43
LTB	Cytokine P33	0.26

Genes that show more than a twofold upregulation or downregulation in 24 h hip drain neutrophils versus presurgery blood neutrophils with $P < 0.05$.

contribution of neutrophils to cytokine/chemokine gene expression at the surgical wound site during the initial postsurgery phase of total hip arthroplasty (THA).

Methods.—Hip drain fluid was collected at 24 h postsurgery from six patients undergoing standardized THA. In addition, venous blood was collected presurgery and 24 h postsurgery. Neutrophils were isolated, total RNA extracted, and a biotinylated cRNA probe generated. The probes were hybridized with a cDNA microarray containing approximately 100 oligonucleotide sequences representing various human cytokines/chemokines or receptor genes. Changes in gene expression seen in the microarray were verified by reverse transcription polymerase chain reaction.

Results.—In the microarray analysis of hip drain neutrophils, interleukin-1 receptor antagonist (IL1RN), interleukin-18 receptor 1 (IL18R1), macrophage migration inhibitory factor (MIF), and macrophage inflammatory protein 3α (CCL20) were upregulated, whereas interleukin-8 receptor β (IL8RB/CXCR2) was consistently downregulated, compared with presurgery blood neutrophils. All of these changes were confirmed by reverse transcription polymerase chain reaction.

Conclusion.—There is a distinct cytokine gene expression profile in neutrophils at the THA surgical wound site at 24 h postsurgery when compared with that found in presurgery circulating neutrophils. Understanding these changes may allow us to knowledgeably manipulate neutrophil activity to reduce postoperative pain and inflammation without impairing wound healing (Table 2).

▶ This study was selected as much for the methodology and to emphasize the direction of much of the basic research in musculoskeletal medicine. Increased attention to gene expression in various pathologic or experimental states is a fundamental methodology being commonly adopted in orthopedic laboratories today. This study reveals a series of up- and down-regulated genes that control the behavior of white blood cells (Table 2). These changes are a function of the insult from the surgical intervention and, as the authors explain, may provide insights into more select means of managing postoperative pain without influencing motor function or recovery. The use of micro-arrays is very helpful as screening tools but in and of themselves do not offer targeted solutions. However, this is an effective first step when questioning the genetic control of various processes.

B. F. Morrey, MD

Effect of Graft Height Mismatch on Contact Pressures With Osteochondral Grafting of the Talus

Latt LD, Glisson RR, Montijo HE, et al (Univ of Arizona, Tucson; Duke Univ, Durham, NC; Carolinas Med Ctr, Charlotte, NC; et al)

Am J Sports Med 39:2662-2669, 2011

Background.—Osteochondral allograft transplantation is technically demanding. It is not always possible to place the surface of the graft perfectly flush with the surrounding cartilage. One must often choose between placing at least some portion of the surface of the graft slightly elevated or recessed. The effect of this choice on joint contact pressure is unknown.

Purpose.—This study was undertaken to determine the effect of graft height mismatch on joint contact pressure in the ankle.

Study Design.—Controlled laboratory study.

Methods.—Ten human cadaveric ankles underwent osteochondral grafting by removal then replacement of an osteochondral plug. Six conditions were tested: intact, graft flush, graft elevated 1.0 mm, graft elevated 0.5 mm, graft recessed 0.5 mm, and graft recessed 1.0 mm. Joint contact pressures were measured with a Tekscan sensor while loads of 200 N, 400 N, 600 N, and 800 N were sequentially applied.

Results.—The peak contact pressure at the graft site for the flush condition was not significantly different from the intact condition for either medial or lateral lesions. In contrast, peak pressure on the opposite facet of the talar dome was significantly increased during the flush condition for the medial but not the lateral grafts. Elevated grafts experienced significantly increased contact pressures, whereas recessed grafts experienced significantly decreased pressures. These changes were greater for lateral

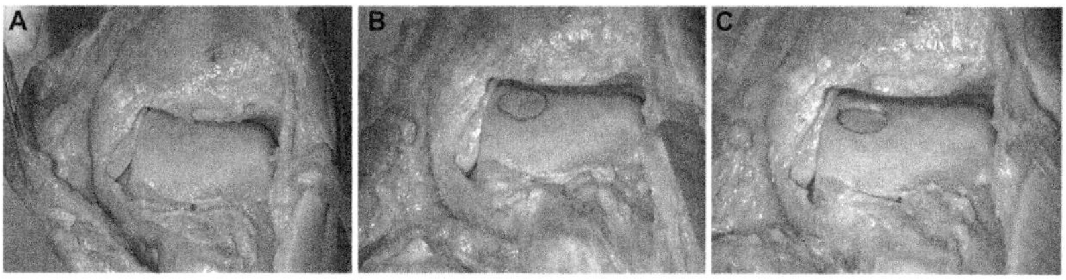

FIGURE 2.—Experimental conditions: (A) flush; (B) elevated 1.0 mm; and (C) recessed 1.0 mm. (Reprinted from Latt LD, Glisson RR, Montijo HE, et al. Effect of graft height mismatch on contact pressures with osteochondral grafting of the talus. *Am J Sports Med.* 2011;39:2662-2669, with permission from The Author(s).)

TABLE 2.—Normalized Peak Pressure Ratio (in Percentages; Normalized Peak Pressure/Normalized Peak Pressure During Intact Trial × 100) for All Loads (200, 400, 600, and 800 N) Averaged Together

Condition	Medial Lesion Graft Site	Medial Lesion Opposite Facet	Lateral Lesion Graft Site	Lateral Lesion Opposite Facet
Elevated 1.0 mm	255	126	675	66
Elevated 0.5 mm	151	119	396	72
Flush	68	149	121	98
Recessed 0.5 mm	25	162	69	108
Recessed 1.0 mm	23	155	56	110

than for medial lesions. Reciprocal changes in joint contact pressures were found on the opposite facet of the talus with elevated grafts on the lateral side and recessed grafts on the medial side.

Conclusion.—Flush graft placement can restore near-normal joint contact pressure. Elevated graft placement leads to significant increases in joint contact pressure at the graft site. Recessed graft placement leads to a transfer of pressure from the graft site to the opposite facet of the talus.

Clinical Relevance.—Osteochondral grafts in the talus should be placed flush if possible or else slightly recessed (Fig 2, Table 2).

▶ This is a nicely conceived and executed study with implications that go beyond the ankle joint. In surgery, we constantly wonder about this question—what happens if the graft is a little proud or recessed (Fig 2)? The answer is in. A prominent graft, even a fraction of a millimeter, is poorly tolerated, whereas if a recessed graft does transfer weight away from the graft, the impact is less adverse (Table 2). The findings are surely anatomically specific, but the basic concept and application would seem to be obvious: avoid a prominent osteochondral graft.

B. F. Morrey, MD

Does the source of hemarthrosis influence posttraumatic joint contracture and biomechanical properties of the joint?

Horisberger M, Kazemkhani S, Monument MJ, et al (Univ of Calgary, Alberta, Canada; Univ Hosp Basel, Switzerland)

Clin Biomech 26:790-795, 2011

Background.—Posttraumatic joint contracture is a common complication of intraarticular injuries and an associated traumatic hemarthrosis could be of importance for its development. The purpose of this investigation was to determine whether the source of the hemarthrosis (peripheral blood vs. bleeding from the bone marrow) affects the amount of contracture and its reversibility and biomechanical properties.

Methods.—46 New Zealand White rabbits were divided in 6 groups and 33 underwent 8 weeks immobilization with either hemarthrosis from bone marrow or peripheral blood. 16 rabbits underwent remobilization for another 8 weeks. 7 animals had only hemarthrosis (bone marrow) for 8 weeks, while 6 were used as controls. Analysis included mean contracture angle and biomechanical variables.

Findings.—The immobilized animals had an increased contracture angle, the knee angle vs. force curve had a greater hysteresis and showed higher initial stiffness. There was no difference in biomechanical properties of the knee between the different types of hemarthroses. After 8 weeks remobilization most biomechanical properties were not different from control.

Interpretation.—The origin of hemarthrosis, and therewith the presence of marrow-derived factors and pluripotential cells from bone marrow, does not seem to affect the severity of joint contractures nor their reversibility.

▶ Not only is joint contracture the most common complication of all joint injury, it is the most disabling consequence of elbow injury. This laboratory has been at the forefront to better understand the mechanisms of posttraumatic arthrofibrosis. This study is clean and asks a meaningful question as to a potential difference in the pathophysiology between circulatory and bone marrow blood elements as causative factors. The model and method failed to find a difference. Although this finding does not necessarily conclusively prove or disprove the hypothesis, it at least underscores the reality that the development of a contracted joint is a very complicated process.

B. F. Morrey, MD

Polyethylene Wear is Related to Patient-specific Contact Stress in THA

Košak R, Kralj-Iglič V, Iglič A, et al (Univ of Ljubljana, Med Centre, Slovenia; Univ of Ljubljana, Slovenia; et al)

Clin Orthop Relat Res 469:3415-3422, 2011

Background.—General numerical models of polyethylene wear and THA simulators suggest contact stresses influence wear. These models do not account for some patient-specific factors. Whether the relationship between patient-specific contact stress and wear apply in vivo is unclear.

Questions/Purposes.—We therefore determined whether (1) contact stress distribution at the prosthesis-cup interface and (2) hip geometry and cup inclination are related to wear in vivo.

Methods.—We retrospectively reviewed the radiographs of 80 patients who had aseptic loosening of their THAs as determined by radiographic criteria. We determined linear penetration and volumetric wear using postoperative and last followup radiographs. Contact stress distribution was determined by the HIPSTRESS method. The biomechanical model was scaled to fit the patient's musculoskeletal geometry of the pelvis, trochanteric position, and cup inclination using the standard postoperative radiograph.

Results.—Linear penetration and volumetric wear correlated with peak contact stress. Polyethylene wear was greater in THAs with a medial position of the greater trochanter and smaller inclination of the acetabular cup.

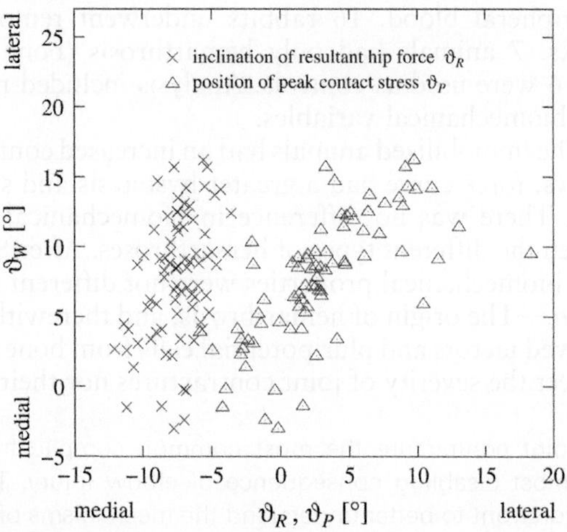

FIGURE 2.—The vector to the position of the peak contact hip stress p_{max} (ϑ_P) coincides with the direction of measured maximal linear wear ϑ_w, whereas the direction of the hip resultant force ϑ_R is located more medially compared with the direction of measured maximal linear wear ϑ_W. (Reprinted from Košak R, Kralj-Iglič V, Iglič A, et al. Polyethylene wear is related to patient-specific contact stress in THA. *Clin Orthop Relat Res*. 2011;469:3415-3422, with kind permission from Springer Science+Business Media.)

Conclusions.—Our observations suggest wear is specific to contact stresses in vivo.

Clinical Relevance.—Long-term wear in a THA can be estimated using contact stress analysis based on analysis of the postoperative AP radiograph (Fig 2).

► Useful information from biomechanical studies is not common today. This study helps us understand the rather dramatic host variation seen with some hip replacements. The important distinction between the resultant force vector and the location of maximum stress is not one that is usually considered (Fig 2). The important issue for the surgeon is recognition that the maximum stress is based on cup orientation, especially verticality. This may be more important to wear than to stability.

B. F. Morrey, MD

Interpretation of patient-reported outcomes for hip and knee replacement surgery: identification of thresholds associated with satisfaction with surgery

Judge A, Arden NK, Kiran A, et al (Univ of Oxford, UK)

J Bone Joint Surg Br 94-B:412-418, 2012

We obtained information from the Elective Orthopaedic Centre on 1523 patients with baseline and six-month Oxford hip scores (OHS) after undergoing primary hip replacement (THR) and 1784 patients with Oxford knee scores (OKS) for primary knee replacement (TKR) who completed a six-month satisfaction questionnaire.

Receiver operating characteristic curves identified an absolute change in OHS of 14 points or more as the point that discriminates best between patients' satisfaction levels and an 11-point change for the OKS. Satisfaction is highest (97.6%) in patients with an absolute change in OHS of 14 points or more, compared with lower levels of satisfaction (81.8%) below this threshold. Similarly, an 11-point absolute change in OKS was associated with 95.4% satisfaction compared with 76.5% below this threshold. For the six-month OHS a score of 35 points or more distinguished patients with the highest satisfaction level, and for the six-month OKS 30 points or more identified the highest level of satisfaction. The thresholds varied according to patients' pre-operative score, where those with severe pre-operative pain/function required a lower six-month score to achieve the highest levels of satisfaction.

Our data suggest that the choice of a six-month follow-up to assess patient-reported outcomes of THR/TKR is acceptable. The thresholds help to differentiate between patients with different levels of satisfaction, but external validation will be required prior to general implementation in clinical practice.

▶ With the ever increasing pressure to document outcomes, insight as to the most cost-effective means to accomplish this requirement is very important. Although not the stated reason for this study, it is the way I have interpreted the findings. Specifically, the investigators have employed a sophisticated methodology to demonstrate that a 6-month period of surveillance is adequate to reliably determine subjective patient satisfaction for both hip and knee replacement (Fig 2 in the original article). The implications are considerable, as this implies the traditional longer and hence more expensive, with greater dropout, surveillance period is not necessary, at least for patient satisfaction.

B. F. Morrey, MD

Cost-Effectiveness Analysis of the Most Common Orthopaedic Surgery Procedures: Knee Arthroscopy and Knee Anterior Cruciate Ligament Reconstruction

Lubowitz JH, Appleby D (Taos Orthopaedic Inst Res Foundation, Taos, NM; Smith & Nephew, Andover, MA)

Arthroscopy 27:1317-1322, 2011

Purpose.—The purpose of this study was to determine the cost-effectiveness of knee arthroscopy and anterior cruciate ligament (ACL) reconstruction.

Methods.—Retrospective analysis of prospectively collected data from a single-surgeon, institutional review board–approved outcomes registry included 2 cohorts: surgically treated knee arthroscopy and ACL reconstruction patients. Our outcome measure is cost-effectiveness (cost of a quality-adjusted life-year [QALY]). The QALY is calculated by multiplying difference in health-related quality of life, before and after treatment, by life expectancy. Health-related quality of life is measured by use of the Quality of Well-Being scale, which has been validated for cost-effectiveness analysis. Costs are facility charges per the facility cost-to-charges ratio plus surgeon fee. Sensitivity analyses are performed to determine the effect of variations in costs or outcomes.

Results.—There were 93 knee arthroscopy and 35 ACL reconstruction patients included at a mean follow-up of 2.1 years. Cost per QALY was $5,783 for arthroscopy and $10,326 for ACL reconstruction (2009 US dollars). Sensitivity analysis shows that our results are robust (relatively insensitive) to variations in costs or outcomes.

Conclusions.—Knee arthroscopy and knee ACL reconstruction are very cost-effective.

Level of Evidence.—Level I, economic analysis (sensible costs with multiway sensitivity analyses) (Table 3).

▶ This is really an important article. Not necessarily because of the exact findings, but to introduce the concept of cost effectiveness into the orthopedic

TABLE 3.—Ranking of Cost-Effectiveness per QALY of Different Medical Treatments Adjusted for Inflation[8] to Represent 2009 USD

Treatment	Cost/QALY
Phenylketonuria screening[16]	$1,100
Postpartum anti-D immunoglobulin[16]	$1,100
Antepartum anti-D immunoglobulin[16]	$2,630
Knee arthroscopy—reference case data	$5,783
Coronary artery bypass surgery for left main coronary artery disease[16]	$9,050
Total knee replacement arthroplasty[6]	$9,680
Neonatal intensive care, 1,000-1,499 g[16]	$9,690
ACL reconstruction—reference case data	$10,326
ACL reconstruction—previously published data[4,5]	$12,100
Thyroid (T4) screening[16]	$13,600
Total knee replacement arthroplasty[18]	$18,700
Treatment of severe hypertension (diastolic blood pressure ≥105 mm Hg) in men aged 40 yr[16]	$20,200
Treatment of mild hypertension (diastolic blood pressure ≥95-104 mm Hg) in men aged 40 yr[16]	$41,200
Estrogen therapy for postmenopausal symptoms in women without prior hysterectomy[16]	$58,200
Neonatal intensive care, 500-999 g[16]	$68,500
Coronary artery bypass surgery for single-vessel disease with mildly severe angina[16]	$78,200
School tuberculin testing program[16]	$94,100
Continuous ambulatory peritoneal dialysis[16]	$101,000
Hospital hemodialysis	$116,000

NOTE. Reference case data (representing our study results) are reported, along with additional data from previous references as indicated. ACL reconstruction is listed twice, indicating both reference data and previously published data.[4,5] Total knee replacement arthroplasty is listed twice, indicating different cost-effectiveness reported in two previously published studies.[6,18] Treatments with lower costs per QALY maximize the benefits to patients per unit of cost.[14] Treatments with a cost per QALY of less than $29,300 (2009 USD) are defined as very cost-effective.[7] Because studies use similar but not identical methods, reporting bias must be considered when one is comparing the relative cost-effectiveness.[5,16,17]

Editor's Note: Please refer to original journal article for full references.

community. I have placed this in the basic science category, since the methodology belongs here, health science research. While we all know the term *cost effectiveness* and probably have a personal sense of what it means, this article places it in context of methodology and relative value. Quality-adjusted life year is the currency of the realm for health science investigators dealing with cost effectiveness. While the orthopedic surgeon would and should have no clue as to the relevance of the absolute numbers for these 2 procedures, when placed in the context of other interventions (Table 3), we can get the point. I would argue that it is clearly in our profession's best interest to continue to portray our procedures in the context of cost effectiveness. If we do this, we win. Our patients win.

B. F. Morrey, MD

Achilles Tendon Healing in Rats is Improved by Intermittent Mechanical Loading during the Inflammatory Phase

Eliasson P, Andersson T, Aspenberg P (Linköping Univ, Sweden)
J Orthop Res 30:274-279, 2012

Tendons adapt to changes in mechanical loading, and numerous animal studies show that immobilization of a healing tendon is detrimental to the healing process. The present study addresses whether the effects of a few episodes of mechanical loading are different during different phases of healing. Fifty female rats underwent Achilles tendon transection, and their hind limbs were unloaded by tail suspension on the day after surgery. One group of 10 rats was taken down from suspension to run on a treadmill for 30 min/day, on days 2–5 after transection. They were euthanized on day 8. Another group underwent similar treadmill running on days 8–11 and was euthanized on day 14. Continuously unloaded groups were euthanized on days 8 and 14. Tendon specimens were then evaluated mechanically. The results showed that just four loading episodes increased the strength of the healing tendon. This was evident irrespective of the time point when loading was applied (early or late). The positive effect on early healing was unexpected, considering that the mechanical stimulation was applied during the inflammatory phase, when the calluses were small and fragile. A histological study of additional groups with early loading also showed some increased bleeding in the loaded calluses. Our results indicate that a short episodes of early loading may improve the outcome of tendon healing. This could be of interest to clinical practice.

▶ Optimal management of Achilles tendon rupture continues to be a source of debate. Although less invasive repair techniques have emerged, nonsurgical management continues to be preferred by many. This nicely done study offers some potentially beneficial insight into the healing process. The advantage of low-level stimulation is well documented, but the initiation of the stress on the tendon was performed early, in the inflammatory phase of the healing process.

This is a time most clinicians would continue to strictly protect the healing tendon. Based on this study, one may wish to revisit our treatment protocol and allow early, but well-controlled, stress to the healing tendon.

B. F. Morrey, MD

Augmented Tendon Achilles Repair Using a Tissue Reinforcement Scaffold: A Biomechanical Study

Giza E, Frizzell L, Farac R, et al (Dept of Orthopaedics, Sacramento, CA)
Foot Ankle Int 32:545-549, 2011

Background.—Missed or chronic Achilles tendon ruptures may have muscle atrophy and tendon retraction resulting in a defect that must be augmented with endogenous or exogenous materials. The Artelon® Tissue Reinforcement (ATR) scaffold is a readily available synthetic degradable poly(urethane urea) material used to augment tendon repair. The objective of this study was to compare human cadaveric Achilles tendon repairs with and without ATR.

Materials and Methods.—Eighteen fresh frozen human cadaver limbs were dissected and the tendon transected 2 cm proximal to the calcaneal insertion. The control group of nine specimens was repaired with sutures, while the experimental group was repaired with sutures and reinforced with a tubularized patch of ATR. Specimens were tested for ultimate load to failure in an Instron machine after preloading to 10 N followed by cyclic loading for 20 cycles from 2 to 30 N.

Results.—The ultimate load to failure in the control group was a mean of 248.1 N ± 19.6 (202 to 293 at 95% CI) versus 370.4 N ± 25.2 (312 to 428 at 95% CI) in the ATR group. The ultimate load to failure was 370.4 ± 25.2 N (312 to 428 at 95% CI) and 248.1 ± 19.6 N (202 to 293 at 95% CI) in the experimental and control groups, respectively

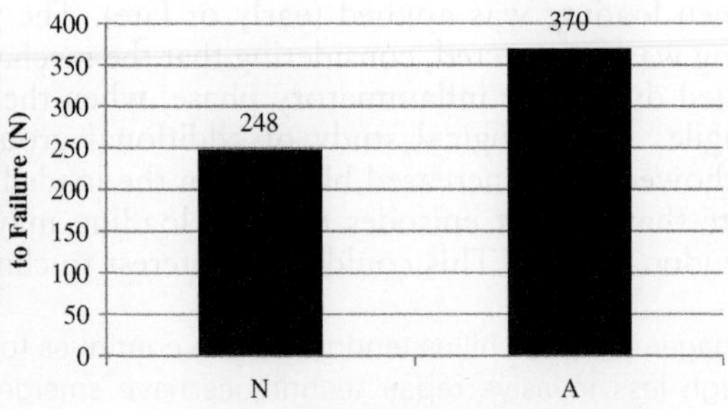

FIGURE 3.—Bar graph comparing the mean ultimate load to failure between the Non-Artelon Control Group (N) and Artelon Augment Group (A). (Reprinted from Giza E, Frizzell L, Farac R, et al. Augmented tendon Achilles repair using a tissue reinforcement scaffold: a biomechanical study. *Foot Ankle Int.* 2011;32:545-549, Copyright © 2011 by the American Orthopaedic Foot and Ankle Society, Inc., originally published in Foot & Ankle International 32:545-549 and reproduced here with permission.)

($p = 0.0015$). Creep of the ATR augmented group was 2.0 ± 0.5 mm, compared to 3.1 ± 1.1 mm for the control group ($p = 0.026$).

Conclusion.—ATR provided a statistically significant improvement in load to failure when compared to control specimens in a cadaver model.

Clinical Relevance.—This finding may allow for development of more aggressive rehabilitation techniques following chronic Achilles tendon repairs (Fig 3).

▶ Rupture of the Achilles tendon remains one of the most common and functionally disabling injuries to the foot and ankle. While the problem is usually well managed, rerupture remains one of the most common and difficult-to-manage complications. An effective synthetic augment is thus an attractive proposition. This biomechanical study demonstrates, as one might expect, the increased mechanical performance of the construct using this poly urethane urea scaffold (Fig 3). The key questions are how well tolerated is this substance just under the skin and what are its healing and gliding characteristics? If these are favorable, such an adjunct would be of value in both the acute and reoperative setting.

B. F. Morrey, MD

2 General Orthopedics

Introduction

This section is one of the most interesting to me, as it allows a review of a broad spectrum of topics. The issues and thus the content really don't change dramatically from year to year, but the emphasis might. In this section, we have tried to focus on diagnosis and effective treatments of common conditions. Over the course of this year, we have tried to review and introduce those articles we feel will be helpful to the broadest number of orthopedic surgeons caring for a broad spectrum of orthopedic pathology.

Bernard F. Morrey, MD

Level of Evidence of Presentations at American Academy of Orthopaedic Surgeons Annual Meetings

Voleti PB, Donegan DJ, Baldwin KD, et al (Hosp of the Univ of Pennsylvania, Philadelphia)

J Bone Joint Surg Am 94:e50.1-e50.5, 2012

Background.—The American Academy of Orthopaedic Surgeons (AAOS) Annual Meeting is a major international forum for scientific exchange and education. The purpose of this study was to evaluate the level of evidence of papers and posters presented at the 2001, 2004, 2007, and 2010 AAOS meetings to determine trends in the quality of study designs between the years 2001 and 2010.

Methods.—Abstracts for AAOS presentations from 2001 (288 papers and 468 posters), 2004 (290 papers and 466 posters), 2007 (525 papers and 541 posters), and 2010 (720 papers and 569 posters) were independently evaluated by three reviewers. The level of evidence of each presentation was determined based on the AAOS classification system. The results were subdivided according to orthopaedic subspecialty and type of presentation.

Results.—In subsequent years, there was a substantial increase in the percentage of Level I studies (2% in 2001, 3% in 2004, 5% in 2007, and 7% in 2010), Level II studies (15% in 2001, 18% in 2004, 23% in 2007, and 29% in 2010), and Level III studies (22% in 2001, 26% in 2004, 29% in 2007, and 33% in 2010), with a concomitant decrease in the percentage of Level IV studies (62% in 2001, 54% in 2004, 43% in 2007,

TABLE 3.—Number and Percentage of LOE of 2001, 2004, 2007, and 2010 AAOS Presentations

Year	2001	2004	2007	2010
Level I	13 (2%)	22 (3%)	54 (5%)	93 (7%)
Level II	113 (15%)	133 (18%)	245 (23%)	372 (29%)
Level III	165 (22%)	195 (26%)	309 (29%)	425 (33%)
Level IV	465 (62%)	406 (54%)	458 (43%)	399 (31%)
Level V	0 (0%)	0 (0%)	0 (0%)	0 (0%)
Total	756	756	1066	1289

and 31% in 2010). Overall, there was a significant nonrandom improvement in the level of evidence of presentations over the study period ($p < 0.001$). This trend was consistent across all orthopaedic subspecialties and in both the paper and the poster subgroups.

Conclusions.—The level of evidence of studies presented at the AAOS Annual Meeting is steadily increasing, which signifies a mark of continual improvement in the quality of the scientific program (Table 3).

▶ The levels of evidence hierarchy was introduced over 25 years ago to guide evaluation and interpretation of research papers. Although some practical aspects of orthopedic surgery interventions make level I evidence difficult to obtain, our field has justifiably been criticized for low-level scientific support of our treatments.

These authors essentially asked the question "Are things improving?" Thankfully, analyzing papers and posters at the American Academy of Orthopaedic Surgeons (AAOS) annual meeting at 4 time points between 2001 and 2010, the answer is yes. The decade saw a uniform drop in level IV evidence studies and a uniform rise in levels I through III evidence presentations, even as the number of presentations increased (Table III). This improvement held true across all subspecialties represented at the AAOS. Room for further progress remains, but these results assure us that our profession continues to improve our understanding of orthopedic care.

P. S. Rose, MD

Association of Smoking and Chronic Pain Syndromes in Kentucky Women

Mitchell MD, Mannino DM, Steinke DT, et al (Univ of Kentucky, Lexington)

J Pain 12:892-899, 2011

The objective of this project was to determine the relationship between cigarette smoking and the reporting of chronic pain syndromes among participants in the Kentucky Women's Health Registry. Data was analyzed on 6,092 women over 18 years of age who responded to survey questions on pain and smoking. The chronic pain syndromes included in the analysis were fibromyalgia, sciatica, chronic neck pain, chronic back pain, joint pain, chronic head pain, nerve problems, and pain all over the body. Analyses controlled

TABLE 2.—Reported Pain Frequencies

	Pain Reported
Any pain syndrome	2,662 (43.7%)
Fibromyalgia	318 (5.2%)
Sciatica	342 (5.6%)
Chronic neck	921 (15.1%)
Chronic back	1,469 (24.1%)
Joint	1,024 (16.8%)
Chronic head	306 (5.0%)
Nerve problems	619 (10.2%)
All over body	246 (4.0%)

NOTE. Frequencies in this table are not mutually exclusive. n = 6,092.

for age, body mass index, and Appalachian versus non-Appalachian county of residence. Results showed that women who were daily smokers reported more chronic pain (defined as the presence of any reported chronic pain syndromes) than women who were never smokers (adjusted odds ratio [aOR] = 2.04 and 95% confidence interval [CI] 1.67, 2.49). An increased risk was also seen for "some-day" smokers (aOR 1.68, 95% CI 1.24, 2.27), and former smokers (aOR 1.20, 95% CI 1.06, 1.37), though with less of an association in the latter group. This study provides evidence of an association between chronic pain and cigarette smoking that is reduced in former smokers.

Perspective.—This paper presents the association between smoking and musculoskeletal pain syndromes among Kentucky women. This finding may provide additional opportunities for intervention in patients with chronic pain (Table 2).

► I should admit a conflict: I am prone to review any article demonstrating the evils of smoking. Documentation of a statistical association between smoking and chronic musculoskeletal pain in women is yet another expression of the detrimental effects of smoking. What's more, the effect seems to influence a broad spectrum of pain patterns (Table 2). In addition to the simple awareness of the relationship, as the authors point out, it offers the surgeon an opportunity to advise our patients suffering from chronic pain.

B. F. Morrey, MD

An Economic Evaluation of a Systems-Based Strategy to Expedite Surgical Treatment of Hip Fractures

Dy CJ, McCollister KE, Lubarsky DA, et al (Hosp for Special Surgery, NY; Univ of Miami, FL)

J Bone Joint Surg Am 93:1326-1334, 2011

Background.—A recent systematic review has indicated that mortality within the first year after hip fracture repair increases significantly if the time from hospital admission to surgery exceeds forty-eight hours. Further investigation has shown that avoidable, systems-based factors contribute substantially to delay in surgery. In this study, an economic evaluation was conducted to determine the cost-effectiveness of a hypothetical scenario in which resources are allocated to expedite surgery so that it is performed within forty-eight hours after admission.

Methods.—We created a decision tree to tabulate incremental cost and quality-adjusted life years in order to evaluate the cost-effectiveness of two potential strategies. Several factors, including personnel cost, patient volume, percentage of patients receiving surgical treatment within forty-eight hours, and mortality associated with delayed surgery, were considered. One strategy focused solely on expediting preoperative evaluation by employing personnel to conduct the necessary diagnostic tests and a hospitalist physician to conduct the medical evaluation outside of regular hours. The second strategy added an on-call team (nurse, surgical technologist, and anesthesiologist) to staff an operating room outside of regular hours.

Results.—The evaluation-focused strategy was cost-effective, with an incremental cost-effectiveness ratio of $2318 per quality-adjusted life year, and became cost-saving (a dominant therapeutic approach) if ≥93% of patients underwent expedited surgery, the hourly cost of retaining a diagnostic technologist on call was <$20.80, or <15% of the hospitalist's salary was funded by the strategy. The second strategy, which added an on-call surgical team, was also cost-effective, with an incremental cost-effectiveness ratio of $43,153 per quality-adjusted life year. Sensitivity analysis revealed that this strategy remained cost-effective if the odds ratio of one-year mortality associated with delayed surgery was >1.28, ≥88% of patients underwent early surgery, or ≥339.9 patients with a hip fracture were treated annually.

Conclusions.—The results of our study suggest that systems-based solutions to minimize operative delay, such as a dedicated on-call support team, can be cost-effective. Additionally, an evaluation-focused intervention can be cost-saving, depending on its success rate and associated personnel cost.

▶ This contribution is included for review for a couple of reasons. The observations are important, and the finding would seem to be worth considering when managing the elderly patient with a hip fracture. Providing objective percentages that reflect the impact of the management decision being made is a powerful tool to influence thought (Fig 1 in the original article). But this also offers insight into the direction of practice management that is evidence based. There is no doubt we will be forced to follow such treatment algorithms in the future. Let's hope we will be the ones developing them.

B. F. Morrey, MD

Diabetes and Femoral Neck Strength: Findings from The Hip Strength Across the Menopausal Transition Study

Ishii S, Cauley JA, Crandall CJ, et al (Veterans Affairs Greater Los Angeles Healthcare System, CA; Univ of Pittsburgh, PA; David Geffen School of Medicine at Univ of California, Los Angeles; et al)

J Clin Endocrinol Metab 97:190-197, 2012

Context.—Diabetes mellitus is associated with increased hip fracture risk, despite being associated with higher bone mineral density in the femoral neck.

Objective.—The objective of the study was to test the hypothesis that composite indices of femoral neck strength, which integrate dual-energy x-ray absorptiometry derived femoral neck size, femoral neck areal bone mineral density, and body size and are inversely associated with hip fracture risk, would be lower in diabetics than in nondiabetics and be inversely related to insulin resistance, the primary pathology in type 2 diabetes.

Design.—This was a cross-sectional analysis.

Setting and Participants.—The study consisted of a multisite, multiethnic, community-dwelling sample of 1887 women in pre- or early perimenopause.

Outcome Measurements.—Composite indices for femoral neck strength in different failure modes (axial compression, bending, and impact) were measured.

Results.—Adjusted for age, race/ethnicity, menopausal stage, body mass index, smoking, physical activity, calcium and vitamin D supplementation, and study site, diabetic women had higher femoral neck areal bone mineral density [+0.25 SD, 95% confidence interval (CI) (+0.06, +0.44) SD] but lower composite strength indices [+0.20 SD, 95% CI (−0.38, −0.03) SD for compression, −0.19 SD, 95% CI (−0.38, −0.003) SD for bending, −0.19 SD, 95% CI (−0.37, −0.02) SD for impact] than nondiabetic women. There were graded inverse relationships between homeostasis model-assessed insulin resistance and all three strength indices, adjusted for the same covariates.

Conclusions.—Despite having higher bone density, diabetic women have lower indices of femoral neck strength relative to load, consistent with their documented higher fracture risk. Insulin resistance appears to play an important role in bone strength reduction in diabetes.

▶ This is a very well done study investigating the paradox between the known fact that the femoral neck in the diabetic patient is associated with greater bone density and a higher incidence of femoral neck fracture. After conclusively dismissing the usual suspects, age, race, body mass index, smoking, activity and the like, the authors offer a potential explanation. Development of insulin resistance is at least correlated to, if not the cause of, the increased fragility of the femoral neck in the diabetic patient. Interesting. One is left now to determine how to use this knowledge as a preventive measure.

B. F. Morrey, MD

Hip Arthroscopy for Femoroacetabular Impingement in Patients Aged 50 Years or Older

Philippon MJ, Schroder e Souza BG, Briggs KK (Steadman Philippon Res Inst, Vail, CO)
Arthroscopy 28:59-65, 2012

Purpose.—The purpose of this study was to investigate outcomes after hip arthroscopy in a consecutive series of patients aged 50 years or older and determine how long patients avoided total hip replacement.

Methods.—Between 2006 and 2008, prospectively collected data were retrieved from our database on 153 patients aged 50 years or older undergoing hip arthroscopy for femoroacetabular impingement. Data collected included range of motion, Modified Harris Hip Score (MHHS), Hip Outcome Score (HOS) for activities of daily living, HOS for sports, and Short Form 12 score. Survivors were defined as patients not requiring total hip replacement (THR). Survivorship was analyzed by use of the Kaplan-Meier method.

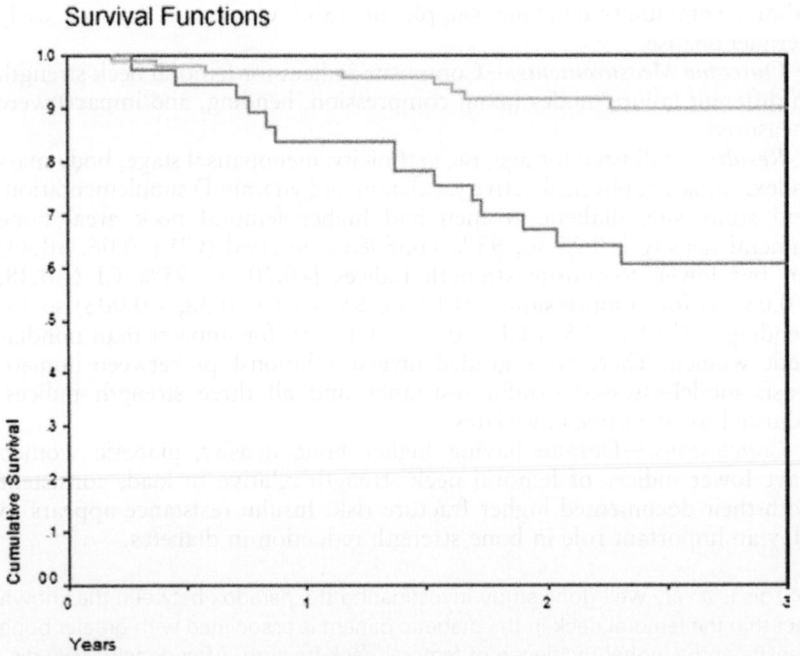

FIGURE 2.—Survivorship curve with patients divided by joint space. The green line represents the survivorship curve for patients with greater than 2 mm of joint space. The pink line is the survivorship curve for patients with 2 mm of joint space or less. Patients with greater than 2 mm of joint space show a gradual trend toward THR over the first 3 years. Patients with 2 mm of joint space or less show only 50% survivorship at 3 years. For interpretation of the references to color in this figure legend, the reader is referred to web version of this article. (Reprinted from Arthroscopy: The Journal of Arthroscopic and Related Surgery. Philippon MJ, Schroder e Souza BG, Briggs KK. Hip arthroscopy for femoroacetabular impingement in patients aged 50 years or older. *Arthroscopy.* 2012;28:59-65, Copyright 2012, with permission from the Arthroscopy Association of North America.)

Results.—THR was required after the arthroscopic treatment in 20% of patients (31 of 153). At 3 years (with data available in 64 patients), patients with greater than 2 mm of joint space had survivorship of 90% whereas those with 2 mm or less had survivorship of 57% (P =.001). In the patients who did not require THR, the MHHS improved from 58 to 84. The HOS for activities of daily living improved from 66 to 87 (P =.001), and the HOS for sports improved from 42 to 72 (P =.001). The physical component of the Short Form 12 improved from 38 to 49 (P =.001), whereas the mental component did not change (54 preoperatively *v* 53 postoperatively, P =.53). Median patient satisfaction was 9.

Conclusions.—On the basis of early results, patients with greater than 2 mm of joint space can expect improvement over preoperative status in pain and function after hip arthroscopy for femoroacetabular impingement. In patients aged 50 years or older with 2 mm of joint space or less and low preoperative MHHSs, early conversion to THR was seen.

Level of Evidence.—Level IV, therapeutic case series (Fig 2).

▶ Recognition of subtle dysplasia causing impingement and subsequent arthritis is one of the greatest insights into hip arthritis in the last 50 years. This knowledge must be translated into improved intervention if it is to reach its full potential value. This study from one of the leading experts in the field is of great benefit, as it offers a practical and well-documented treatment guideline. In the patient older than 50 years, arthroscopic debridement, at least in the hands of the experienced surgeon, is of statistical value—especially if there are 2 or more mm of joint space remaining (Fig 2). As is noted in mathematics after such a proof: Q.E.D.

B. F. Morrey, MD

Association Between Cam-Type Deformities and Magnetic Resonance Imaging–Detected Structural Hip Damage: A Cross-Sectional Study in Young Men

Reichenbach S, Leunig M, Werlen S, et al (Univ of Bern and Inselspital, Switzerland; Schulthess Clinic, Zurich, Switzerland; Hosp Sonnenhof, Bern, Switzerland; et al)

Arthritis Rheum 63:4023-4030, 2011

Objective.—Femoroacetabular impingement may be a risk factor for hip osteoarthritis in men. An underlying hip deformity of the cam type is common in asymptomatic men with nondysplastic hips. This study was undertaken to examine whether hip deformities of the cam type are associated with signs of hip abnormality, including labral lesions and articular cartilage damage, detectable on magnetic resonance imaging (MRI).

Methods.—In this cross-sectional, population-based study in asymptomatic young men, 1,080 subjects underwent clinical examination and completed a self-report questionnaire. Of these subjects, 244 asymptomatic men with a mean age of 19.9 years underwent MRI. All MRIs were read

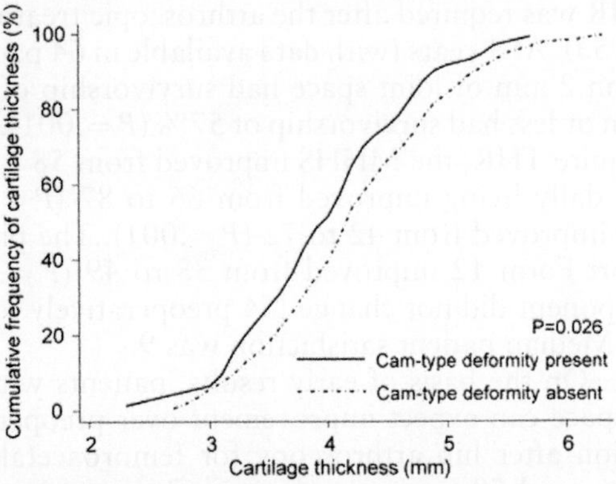

FIGURE 3.—Cumulative frequency curves for cartilage thickness in subjects with and subjects without a cam-type deformity. The cumulative frequency curve for cartilage thickness in those with a cam-type deformity was shifted to the left by ~0.20 mm. The *P* value was calculated using the 2-sided Wald test. (Reprinted from Reichenbach S, Leunig M, Werlen S, et al. Association between cam-type deformities and magnetic resonance imaging–detected structural hip damage: a cross-sectional study in young men. *Arthritis Rheum.* 2011;63:4023-4030, with permission from American College of Rheumatology.)

for cam-type deformities, labral lesions, cartilage thickness, and impingement pits. The relationship between cam-type deformities and signs of joint damage were examined using logistic regression models adjusted for age and body mass index. Odds ratios (ORs) and 95% confidence intervals (95% CIs) were determined.

Results.—Sixty-seven definite cam-type deformities were detected. These deformities were associated with labral lesions (adjusted OR 2.77 [95% CI 1.31, 5.87]), impingement pits (adjusted OR 2.9 [95% CI 1.43, 5.93]), and labral deformities (adjusted OR 2.45 [95% CI 1.06, 5.66]). The adjusted mean difference in combined anterosuperior femoral and acetabular cartilage thickness was −0.19 mm (95% CI −0.41, 0.02) lower in those with cam-type deformities compared to those without.

Conclusion.—Our findings indicate that the presence of a cam-type deformity is associated with MRI-detected hip damage in asymptomatic young men (Fig 3).

▶ Recognition of subtle impingement as an etiology of early osteoarthritis made by Ganz years ago has proven to be a real contribution to our understanding of the disease. This study furthers our knowledge by demonstrating a correlation of cartilage thickness and the presence of impingement by image analysis, even in the asymptomatic patient (Fig 3). The fact that almost 25% of asymptomatic individuals did have radiographic evidence of impingement is also worth noting. Such insight, coupled with knowledge of the outcome of early decompression, provides a basis for evidenced-based counseling of patients.

B. F. Morrey, MD

A Catastrophic Complication of Hip Arthroscopy

Bruno M, Longhino V, Sansone V (Universitá degli Studi di Milano, Milan, Italy)

Arthroscopy 27:1150-1152, 2011

We present the case of an unusual and serious complication of hip arthroscopy due to the severance of the inferior gluteal artery. The lesion induced a severe anemic condition and the formation of a large pseudoaneurysm, which compressed the sciatic nerve and left permanent neurologic sequelae. To our knowledge, this is the first reported case of its kind. We also describe how to establish a safe posterior hip joint arthroscopic portal to avoid such a complication (Fig 3).

► I rarely select case reports for the YEAR BOOK. I made an exception in this instance because as hip arthroscopy becomes more popular and legitimate, we will certainly see an increase in the complication rate, and, as demonstrated

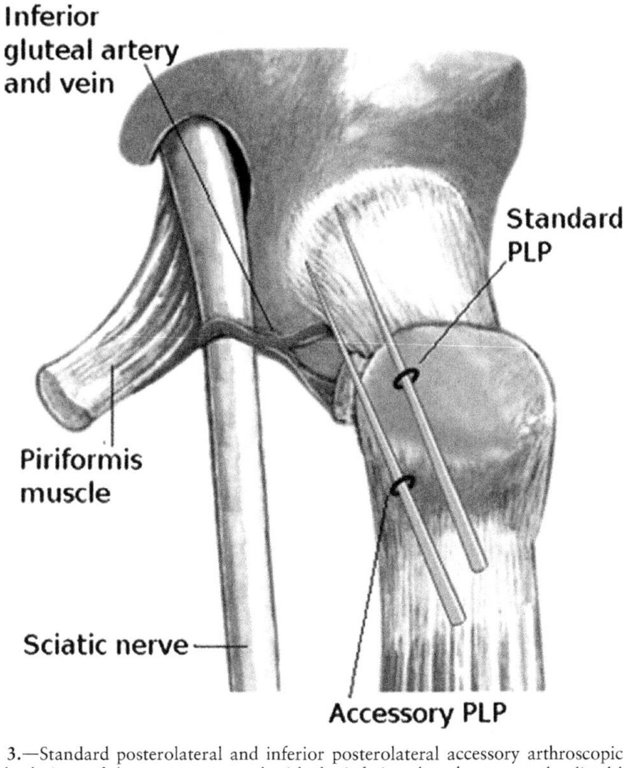

FIGURE 3.—Standard posterolateral and inferior posterolateral accessory arthroscopic hip portals. The potential relations of the accessory portal with the inferior gluteal artery at the distal border of the piriformis tendon should be noted. (Reprinted from Bruno M, Longhino V, Sansone V. A catastrophic complication of hip arthroscopy. *Arthroscopy.* 2011;27:1150-1152, Copyright 2011, with permission from the Arthroscopy Association of North America.)

here, some complications can be a disaster. In addition to pointing out the possibility of such an event as described here, the authors offer an explanation regarding the circumstances whereby this type of problem may occur. As is seen around all joints, prior surgery distorts the anatomy and tends to tether vulnerable structures. The authors offer a practical means of avoiding such a problem should a patient have prior surgery at the hip, especially if there is a prior posterior approach to the hip (Fig 3).

B. F. Morrey, MD

Association of Perioperative Use of Nonsteroidal Anti-Inflammatory Drugs With Postoperative Myocardial Infarction After Total Joint Replacement

Liu SS, Bae JJ, Bieltz M, et al (Weill College of Medicine of Cornell Univ, NY)

Reg Anesth Pain Med 37:45-50, 2012

Background and Objectives.—Use of nonsteroidal anti-inflammatory drug (NSAIDs) analgesics is controversial because of cardiovascular risk, but perioperative use may be advantageous for total joint replacement. Thus, we performed this single-center observational cohort study to determine any association between NSAID use and postoperative myocardial infarction (POMI).

Methods.—All patient admissions undergoing total hip or knee replacement between March 3, 2009, and September 1, 2010, were identified. Nonsteroidal anti-inflammatory drug use was identified. Postoperative myocardial infarction was defined as troponin I level greater than 0.1 ng/mL. Propensity scores were calculated to adjust for bias of receiving NSAIDs and troponin measurements. Propensity scores and other covariates were used in logistic regression to determine the independent association of NSAID use with POMI.

Results.—Of the 10,873 arthroplasty admissions, 1518 (14%) had serial troponins measured, and 97 had a POMI (0.9%). Incidence of POMI was 0.8% for the 9,831 who received NSAIDs and 1.8% for the 1,042 (10%) admitted patients who did not receive NSAIDs with a risk difference of −1% with 95% confidence interval (CI) of −0.2% to −1.9%. The adjusted odds ratio (0.95; 95% CI, 0.5−1.8) and relative risk (0.95; 95% CI, 0.5−1.8) indicated that NSAIDs were not significantly associated with the risk of POMI. Mean duration of NSAID use was 3 days. Length of stay (98 versus 115 hours) was significantly reduced in the NSAID group.

Conclusions.—Brief perioperative use of NSAIDs was not associated with increased risk for myocardial infarction after total hip and knee replacement; it may provide benefit in length of stay (Fig 2).

▶ The authors discuss an important but little studied issue regarding joint replacement. The ubiquitous nature of treating pain with nonsteroidal anti-inflammatory drugs poses a considerable concern if such treatment is associated with an increased risk of myocardial infarct as has been suggested. If this were so,

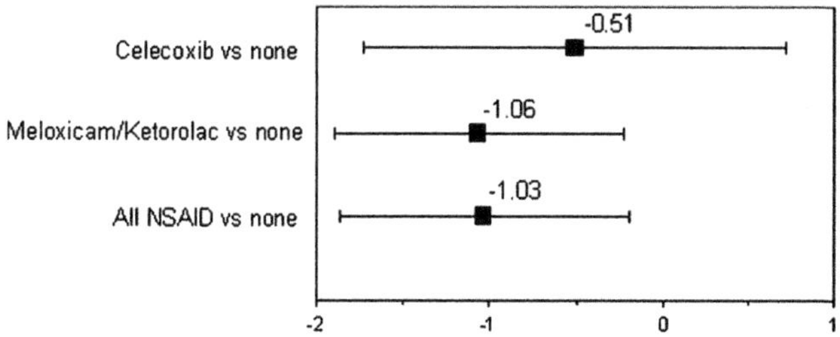

FIGURE 2.—Unadjusted risk difference for POMI. (Reprinted from Liu SS, Bae JJ, Bieltz M, et al. Association of perioperative use of nonsteroidal anti-inflammatory drugs with postoperative myocardial infarction after total joint replacement. *Reg Anesth Pain Med.* 2012;37:45-50, Copyright 2012, with permission from American Society of Regional Anesthesia and Pain Medicine.)

then we must reconsider our postoperative treatment of these patients. This large series seems to offer a rather definitive answer. They don't. Our response is thus obvious. We need not have a concern (Fig 2).

B. F. Morrey, MD

Delirium after fast-track hip and knee arthroplasty

Krenk L, Rasmussen LS, Hansen TB, et al (Univ of Copenhagen, Denmark; The Lundbeck Centre for Fast-Track Hip and Knee Arthroplasty, Denmark)
Br J Anaesth 108:607-611, 2012

Background.—Postoperative delirium (PD) is a serious complication after major surgery in elderly patients. PD is well defined and characterized by reduced attention and disorientation. Multimodal optimization of perioperative care (the fast-track methodology) enhances recovery, and reduces hospital stay and medical morbidity. No data on PD are available in fast-track surgery. The aim of this study was to evaluate the incidence of PD after fast-track hip (THA) and knee arthroplasty (TKA) with anticipated length of stay (LOS) of <3 days.

Methods.—In a prospective multicentre study to evaluate postoperative cognitive dysfunction, we included 225 non-demented patients with a mean age of 70 yr undergoing either THA or TKA in a fast-track set-up. Anaesthesia and postoperative pain management were standardized with limited opioid use. Nursing staff were trained to look for symptoms of PD which was assessed during interaction with healthcare professionals. Patients were invited for a clinical follow-up 1–2 weeks after surgery.

Results.—Clinical follow-up was performed in 220 patients at a mean of 12.0 days after surgery while five patients were followed up by telephone. The mean LOS was 2.6 days (range 1–8 days). Twenty-two patients received general anaesthesia, and the rest had spinal anaesthesia. No patients developed PD (95% confidence interval 0.0–1.6%).

TABLE 4.—Opioid Administered as Supplement to Standard Analgesic Regime According to Hospital (A, B, C, and D), in the PACU and During Hospitalization Where Median and Range are Reported

	A	B	C	D	Total
No. of patients	77	102	21	25	225
No. of patients receiving opioid in PACU	36	62	7	12	117
No. of patients receiving oxycodone in hospital	70	57	8	0	135
Oxycodone dose (mg kg^{-1} day^{-1})	0.14 (0.01–0.64)	0.14 (0.04–0.53)	0.16 (0.11–0.34)	NA	
No. of patients receiving morphine in hospital	0	56	8	13	77
Morphine dose (mg kg^{-1} day^{-1})	NA	0.14 (0.01–0.83)	0.10 (0.02–0.79)	0.13 (0.01–0.41)	
No. of patients receiving other opioid (ketobemidone)	0	4	0	1	5
Ketobemidone in equipotent morphine dose (mg kg^{-1} day^{-1})	NA	0.27 (0.11–0.65)	NA	0.18 (NA)	

Conclusions.—A fast-track set-up with multimodal opioid-sparing analgesia was associated with lack of PD after elective THA and TKA in elderly patients (Table 4).

► With the increased emphasis on reducing length of stay (LOS) now experienced worldwide, broader implications of the strategy are being investigated. Abbreviated LOS protocols were introduced about 15 years ago at Mayo, at which time the key roles of pain control and anesthesia protocols were recognized. This study form England reinforces the knowledge base by demonstrating the abbreviated LOS is associated with a decreased use of opiods and, hence, a decreased incidence in postoperative delirium. Once again, the key is the management of pain, as outlined in Table 4.

B. F. Morrey, MD

Leukocytosis is Common After Total Hip and Knee Arthroplasty

Deirmengian GK, Zmistowski B, Jacovides C, et al (The Rothman Inst of Orthopaedics at Thomas Jefferson Univ Hosp, Philadelphia, PA)

Clin Orthop Relat Res 469:3031-3036, 2011

Background.—Postoperative infection is a potentially devastating complication after THA and TKA. In the early postoperative period, clinicians often find nonspecific indicators of infection. Although leukocytosis may be a sign of a developing infection in the early postoperative period, it may also be part of a normal surgical response.

Questions and Purposes.—We determined (1) the natural history of white blood cell values after primary THA and TKA, (2) factors associated with early postoperative leukocytosis, and (3) the predictive value of white blood cell count for early postoperative periprosthetic joint infection.

Patients and Methods.—Using our institutional database, we identified all THA and TKA cases between January 2000 and December 2008. We determined the incidence of leukocytosis and characterized the natural history of postoperative white blood cell counts. We then investigated potential indicators of postoperative leukocytosis, including development of early periprosthetic infection.

Results.—The average postoperative white blood cell count increased to approximately 3×10^6 cells/μL over the first 2 postoperative days and then declined to a level slightly higher than the preoperative level by Postoperative Day 4. The incidence of postoperative leukocytosis for all patients was 38%. Factors associated with postoperative leukocytosis included TKA, bilateral procedures, older age, and higher modified Charlson Comorbidity Index. The sensitivity and specificity of white blood cell count for diagnosing early periprosthetic infection were 79% and 46%, respectively.

Conclusions.—Postoperative leukocytosis is common after THA and TKA and represents a normal physiologic response to surgery. In the absence of abnormal clinical signs and symptoms, postoperative leukocytosis may not warrant further workup for infection.

Level of Evidence.—Level III, diagnostic study. See Guidelines for Authors for a complete description of levels of evidence.

▶ I am including this study in the general section although it may be more specific for joint replacement surgery. Regardless, the surgeon is constantly faced with the interpretation of an elevated white blood cell (WBC) test in the postoperative period. My former resident, Dr Parvizi, and his colleagues provided us useful objective information about this phenomenon. Almost 40% have elevated WBC counts after joint replacement. The level peaks at day 3. While reasonably sensitive, it is not very specific. It is useful to know these specific data when interpreting a postoperative course.

B. F. Morrey, MD

Acute knee dislocation: An evidence based approach to the management of the multiligament injured knee

Howells NR, Brunton LR, Robinson J, et al (The Avon Orthopaedic Centre, Bristol, UK)

Injury 42:1198-1204, 2011

Traumatic knee dislocations are uncommon yet serious injuries that historically have had variable prognosis. The evaluation and management of traumatic knee dislocations remains controversial. Appropriate early management has been shown to have a significant impact on long term functional outcome. A comprehensive review of the recent literature is presented alongside our current approach to management.

The dislocated knee is an under diagnosed injury which relies on a high index of clinical suspicion on presentation of any knee injury. There is now a degree of consensus regarding need for surgery, timing of surgery, vascular investigations, surgical techniques and rehabilitation protocols.

Vigilant monitoring for neurovascular complications, appropriate investigations and early involvement of surgeons with a specialist interest in knee ligament surgeries is the key to successful management of these difficult injuries (Fig 2).

▶ Unfortunately, to get the full benefit of this worthwhile article, one must read the article because the abstract is rather generic. That said, a few points should be noted. About 40% of cases will be due to hyperextension injury and a third from a flexed knee "dashboard" type mechanism. The incidence of the well-recognized and dreaded vascular injury once reported as high as 65% today is more accurately in the 7% to 14% range. Diagnosis and management, although complex and somewhat debated, can be organized into several key perspectives (Fig 2). It is recognized today that surgical management is superior to closed treatment and should be done sooner rather than delayed several weeks. All torn structures should be addressed, and importantly, reconstruction in general is superior to repair, especially for the anterior and posterior cruciate ligaments

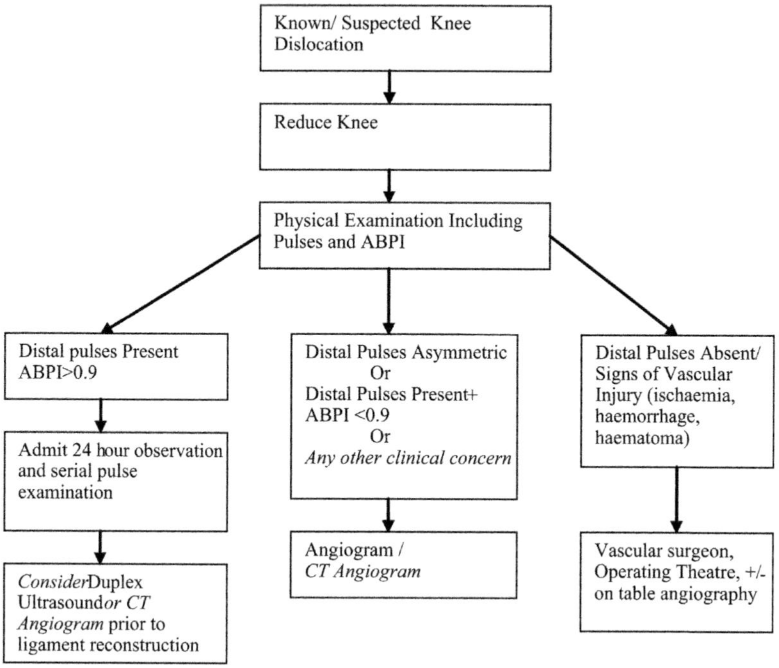

ABPI= ankle brachial pressure index, CT=computerised tomography

FIGURE 2.—Algorithm for diagnosis of vascular injury post-knee dislocation [46] (*italics* are authors modifications). *Editor's Note*: Please refer to original journal article for full references. (Reprinted from Howells NR, Brunton LR, Robinson J, et al. Acute knee dislocation: an evidence based approach to the management of the multiligament injured knee. *Injury.* 2011;42:1198-1204, Copyright 2011, with permission from Elsevier.)

and PCL. If arthroscopic techniques are to be used, a delay of at least a week is recommended to avoid excessive extravasation into the soft tissues. With the newer management philosophy, outcomes are improved, but objectively, they are still not functionally normal.

B. F. Morrey, MD

3 Trauma and Amputation

Introduction

This year we have a particularly large number of citations in this section of the YEAR BOOK. This is because we have held fairly steady with the number of controlled trials in various topics while adding cohort studies in subjects of relevance to those of us who treat injured patients and amputees. The one disappointment I have is that the number of selections for amputation topics of interest was way down. The articles available this year were for the most part related to esoteric aspects of prosthetic design and large database studies, which had minimal relevance to surgeons and practitioners treating amputees.

We have a large number of articles to bring to the readers' attention in regards to atypical femur fractures related to long term bisphosphonate use. This is a topic of increasing interest to our patients, and I tried to bring to your attention any article of potential relevance. There are the same large number of articles related to hip fracture management, which is a public health problem that will be with us for decades. In addition, there are important articles regarding how to manage patients who smoke or are on clopidogrel. A particularly large number of articles, including several controlled trials in reference to distal radius fracture management, are cited in the midst of a very comprehensive listing of upper extremity citations.

It is my sincere hope that you find these articles useful as you consider how to alter and improve your management of patients with these conditions.

Marc F. Swiontkowski, MD

General Topics

The effect of clopidogrel and aspirin on blood loss in hip fracture surgery

Chechik O, Thein R, Fichman G, et al (Tel Aviv Univ, Israel)
Injury 42:1277-1282, 2011

Introduction.—Anti-platelet drugs are commonly used for primary and secondary prevention of thrombo-embolic events and following invasive coronary interventions. Their effect on surgery-related blood loss and perioperative complications is unclear, and the management of trauma patients treated by anti-platelets is controversial. The anti-platelet effect is over in nearly 10 days. Notably, delay of surgical intervention for hip fracture repair for >48 h has been reported to increase perioperative complications and mortality.

Patients and Methods.—Intra-operative and perioperative blood loss, the amount of transfused blood and surgery-related complications of 44 patients on uninterrupted clopidogrel treatment were compared with 44 matched controls not on clopidogrel (either on aspirin alone or not on any anti-platelets).

Results.—The mean perioperative blood loss was 899 ± 496 ml for patients not on clopidogrel, 1091 ± 654 ml for patients on clopidogrel ($p = 0.005$) and 1312 ± 686 ml for those on combined clopidogrel and aspirin ($p = 0.0003$ vs. all others). Increased blood loss was also associated with a shorter time to operation ($p = 0.0012$) and prolonged surgical time ($p = 0.0002$). There were no cases of mortality in the early postoperative period.

Conclusions.—Patients receiving anti-platelet drugs can safely undergo hip fracture surgery without delay, regardless of greater perioperative blood loss and possible thrombo-embolic/postoperative bleeding events (Fig 1, Tables 2 and 3).

▶ With the increasing use of aspirin and clopidogrel for managing cardiac and peripheral vascular disease states, orthopedists are frequently faced with the

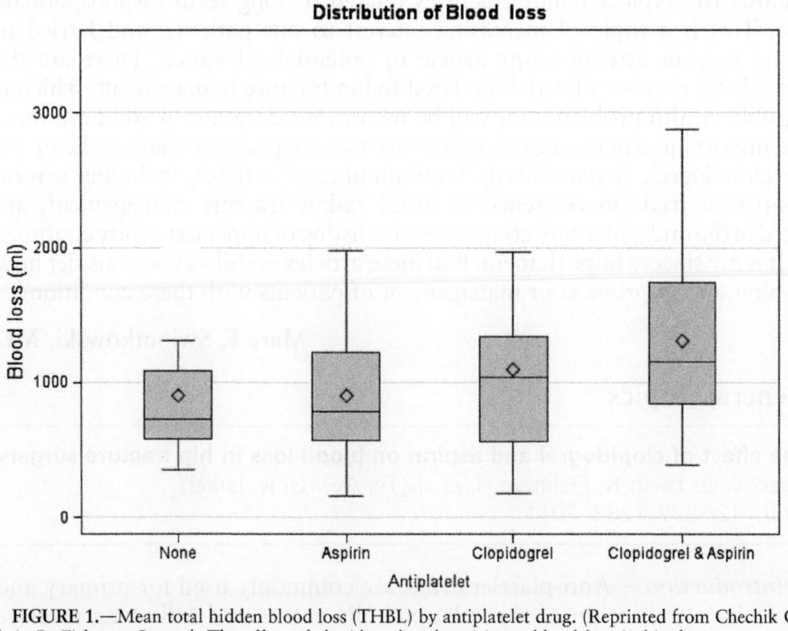

FIGURE 1.—Mean total hidden blood loss (THBL) by antiplatelet drug. (Reprinted from Chechik O, Thein R, Fichman G, et al. The effect of clopidogrel and aspirin on blood loss in hip fracture surgery. *Injury.* 2011;42:1277-1282, Copyright 2011, with permission from Elsevier.)

TABLE 2.—Mean Outcomes of Study Patients by Antiplatelet Treatment

	No Antiplatelets (N = 22)	Aspirin Alone (N = 22)	Clopidogrel Alone (N = 29)	Clopidogrel and Aspirin (N = 15)	Total (All Patients) (N = 88)
THBL[a] (ml)	898 ± 489	900 ± 513	1091 ± 654	1312 ± 686	1033 ± 599
MBL[b] (ml)	392 ± 277	430 ± 332	480 ± 491	309 ± 187	415 ± 363
Total transfusion (PC units)	1.09 ± 1.38	1.09 ± 1.27	1.38 ± 0.98	2.13 ± 1.6	1.36 ± 1.31
Hospitalisation time (days)	12.2 ± 3.4	12.3 ± 6.2	12.7 ± 6.3	13.1 ± 4	12.5 ± 5.2
Time to operation (h)	45 ± 27	35 ± 17	51 ± 25	77 ± 48	50 ± 32
Operation time (min)	66 ± 17	58 ± 15	65 ± 23	55 ± 16	61 ± 19

[a]Total hidden blood loss.
[b]Measured blood loss.

TABLE 3.—Complications in Hip Fracture Surgery and Antiplatelet Drugs

	No Antiplatelets (N = 22)	Aspirin Alone (N = 22)	Clopidogrel Alone (N = 29)	Clopidogrel and Aspirin (N = 15)	Total (All Patients) (N = 88)
Wound discharge	1	7	6	3	17 (19%)
Wound infection	0	1	2	0	3 (3%)
Reoperation (wound infection)	0	0	2	0	2 (2%)
Other systemic infection	1	1	2	3	7 (8%)
Acute renal failure	1	2	1	0	4 (5%)
Respiratory distress	0	1	2	2	5 (6%)
Cerebrovascular accident	1	0	1	0	2 (2%)
Acute coronary syndrome	0	0	2	3	5 (6%)
Gastrointestinal bleeding	0	0	3	0	3 (3%)
Surgical wound bleeding	0	1	0	1	2 (2%)
Total number of complications	4	13	21	12	50

situation of when it is safe to intervene for patients with fractures that need surgical intervention. This carefully conducted cohort study offers reassurance that proceeding directly to surgery without time for washout of the antiplatelet drugs or use of platelet transfusion is in the patient's best interest. This study should inform standardized treatment algorithms for patients in need of surgical stabilization of fractures.

M. F. Swiontkowski, MD

The Impact of Smoking on Complications After Operatively Treated Ankle Fractures—A Follow-Up Study of 906 Patients

Nåsell H, Ottosson C, Törnqvist H, et al (Karolinska Institutet, Stockholm, Sweden)
J Orthop Trauma 25:748-755, 2011

Objectives.—This study on patients with operatively treated ankle fractures aimed to investigate the impact of smoking on postoperative complications and especially deep wound infections.

Design.—Cohort study with prospective follow-up.

Setting.—University-associated teaching hospital with advanced trauma care.

Patients.—A consecutive series of patients (n = 906) operatively treated for an acute ankle fracture during a 3-year period was identified. For the analysis, the patients were categorized as nonsmokers (n = 721) and smokers (n = 185). Data were collected from the department database and completed with a review of the patients' medical charts.

Main Outcome Measures.—Postoperative complications.

Results.—Follow-up data at 6 weeks were available for 98.2% of the patients. Postoperative complications of any kind (30.1% versus 20.3%, $P = 0.005$) as well as deep wound infections (4.9% versus 0.8%, $P < 0.001$) were more common among smokers than nonsmokers. Multivariable analyses showed that smokers had six times higher odds of developing a deep infection compared with nonsmokers. A more complicated fracture, associated diabetes mellitus, and unsatisfactory operative fracture reduction also enhanced the risk of postoperative complications.

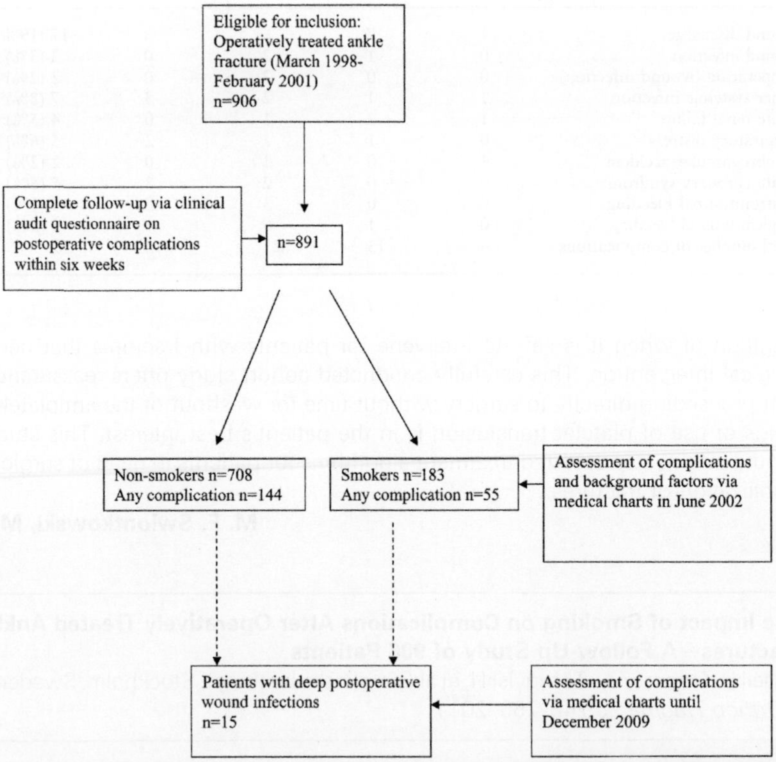

FIGURE 1.—Flowchart of patient inclusion and follow-up. (Reprinted from Nåsell H, Ottosson C, Törnqvist H, et al. The impact of smoking on complications after operatively treated ankle fractures—a follow-up study of 906 patients. *J Orthop Trauma.* 2011;25:748-755, with permission from Lippincott Williams & Wilkins.)

TABLE 2.—Registered Complications at 6 Weeks Among Patients With Complete Follow-Up Data (n = 891)

	Smokers (N = 183)		Nonsmokers (N = 708)		
	No.	Percent	No.	Percent	*P*
Any complication*	55	30.1	144	20.3	0.005
Deep wound infection (1)	9	4.9	6	0.8	<0.001
Superficial wound complication (2)	27	14.8	69	9.7	0.051
Deep vein thrombosis (3)	3	1.6	28	4.0	0.13
Pulmonary embolism (4)	3	1.6	3	0.4	0.07
Urinary tract infection (5)	4	2.2	7	1.0	0.19
Peripheral nerve injury (6)	1	0.5	1	0.1	0.30
Plaster-related complication (7)	3	1.6	9	1.3	0.70
Fracture malreduction/redislocation (8)	12	6.6	29	4.1	0.16
Compartment syndrome (9)	0	0	1	0.1	0.61
Perioperative vascular injury (10)	1	0.5	0	0	0.41

*Sum of complications 1–10: 1 = infection below the deep fascia, requiring surgical débridement; 2 = treated with antibiotics (93) or repeated dressings/control (3); 3 = diagnosed with ultrasound or phlebography; 4 = diagnosed with computed tomography scan; 5 = treated with antibiotics by the responsible doctor; 6 = clinical diagnosis; 7 = pressure wound or irritated skin from plaster; 8 = not ever reduced or losing congruency within 6–8 weeks; 9 = clinical diagnosis, fasciotomy performed in the foot; 10 = division of dorsalis pedis artery.

TABLE 4.—Factors Associated With Risk of Having a Deep Infection (15 of 891 Patients)

		Crude Measures		Univariable		Multivariable Adjusted for the Final Model†	
Predictor Variable	Level	No.	Deep Infection (%)	OR	95% CI	OR	95% CI
Smoking	Yes	183	4.9	6.1*	2.1–17.2	6.0	2.0–18.7
	No	708	0.8	Reference			
Primary postoperative x-ray	Yes	37	10.8	9.3*	2.8–30.7	8.1	2.2–30.3
unsatisfactory	No	854	1.3	Reference			
Secondary surgery resulting	Yes	23	8.7	6.3*	1.3–29.5		
from malreduction	No	868	1.5	Reference			
Trimalleolar fracture	Yes	250	4.4	7.3*	2.3–23.2	6.4	1.9–20.8
	No	641	0.6	Reference			
Insulin-dependent diabetes	Yes	27	7.4	5.2*	1.1–24.5	6.2	1.1–34.1
	No	864	1.5	Reference			
Open fracture	Yes	31	6.5	4.5	0.9–20.8		
	No	860	1.5	Reference			
Diabetes of any type	Yes	53	3.8	2.5	0.5–11.3		
	No	838	1.6	Reference			
Age 60 years or and older	Yes	258	1.9	1.2	0.4–3.6		
	No	633	1.6	Reference			
Sex	Male	415	1.2	Reference			
Female	Female	476	2.1	1.7	0.6–5.2		
Having any comorbidity	Yes	342	2.3	1.9	0.7–5.2		
except diabetes	No	549	1.3	Reference			
Drug and/or alcohol abuse	Yes	67	1.5	0.9	0.1–6.8		
	No	824	1.7	Reference			
High-energy injury (fall from	Yes	189	2.6	1.9	0.6–5.6		
height or more)	No	702	1.4	Reference			
Waiting more than 24 hours	Yes	199	1.0	0.5	0.1–2.4		
for surgery	No	692	1.9	Reference			
Surgery performed by	Yes	696	1.7	1.1	0.3–4.0		
a consultant	No	195	1.5	Reference			

Hosmer and Lemeshow: $P = 0.450$.
OR, odds ratio; CI, confidence interval.
*Statistically significant in univariable analysis.
†Associations adjusted for: smoking, primary postoperative x-ray unsatisfactory, secondary surgery resulting from malreduction, trimalleolar fracture, insulin-dependent diabetes, open fracture, diabetes of any type, age, having any comorbidity except diabetes, and sex.

Conclusions.—We conclude that cigarette smoking increases the risk of postoperative complications in patients operatively treated for an ankle fracture. Smoking is a considerable risk factor. Therefore, physicians, nurses, and other healthcare professionals should strive to support patients to stop smoking while still under acute treatment (Fig 1, Tables 2, 4, and 5).

▶ Orthopedic trauma surgeons have been aware of the negative impact of nicotine abuse on fracture healing complications for 2 decades. Robust clinical data sets to support these concerns have generally been lacking. This large single-center data sets focusing on ankle fractures presents us with an accurate picture of the association of smoking with complications. The biggest risk is with infectious complications with an incidence of nearly 5% in smokers versus less than 1% in nonsmokers. This relatively low rate in both groups attests to the surgical skill of the surgeons at this center. To a lesser degree, poor fracture reduction was also associated with increased risk of complications. These data will be useful

TABLE 5.—Factors Associated With Risk of Having a Superficial Wound Infection (96 of 891)

Predictor Variable	Level	No.	Crude Measures Percent With Superficial Wound Infection	Univariable OR	Univariable 95% CI	Multivariable Adjusted Model† OR	Multivariable Adjusted Model† 95% CI
Smoking	Yes	183	14.8	1.6	0.99–2.6	1.7	1.01–2.9
	No	708	9.7	Reference			
Primary postoperative x-ray unsatisfactory	Yes	37	16.2	1.6	0.7–4.0		
	No	854	10.5	Reference			
Secondary surgery resulting from malreduction	Yes	23	30.4	3.8*	1.5–9.6	3.5	1.4–9.2
	No	868	10.3	Reference			
Trimalleolar fracture	Yes	250	15.6	1.9*	1.2–2.9		
	No	641	8.9	Reference			
Insulin-dependent diabetes	Yes	27	25.9	3.0*	1.3–7.4		
	No	864	10.3	Reference			
Open fracture	Yes	31	51.6	10.4*	5.0–21.8	9.4	4.4–20.3
	No	860	9.3	Reference			
Diabetes of any type	Yes	53	20.8	2.3*	1.2–4.7		
	No	838	10.1	Reference			
Age 60 years and older	Yes	258	18.2	2.7*	1.7–4.1	2.8	1.8–4.4
	No	633	7.7	Reference			
Sex	Female	476	12.4	1.4	0.9–2.2		
	Male	415	8.9	Reference			
Having any comorbidity except diabetes	Yes	342	13.5	1.6*	1.01–2.4		
	No	549	9.1	Reference			
Drug and/or alcohol abuse	Yes	67	14.9	1.5	0.7–3.1		
	No	824	10.4	Reference			
High-energy injury (fall from height or more)	Yes	189	10.6	0.9	0.6–1.6		
	No	702	10.8	Reference			
Waiting longer than 24 hours for surgery	Yes	199	7.0	0.6	0.3–1.01		
	No	692	11.8	Reference			
Surgery performed by a consultant	Yes	696	9.9	0.7	0.4–1.1		
	No	195	13.8	Reference			

Hosmer and Lemeshow: $P = 0.563$.
*Statistically significant in univariable analysis.
†Associations adjusted: smoking, secondary surgery resulting from malreduction, trimalleolar fracture, insulin-dependent diabetes, age, and sex.

in counseling patients regarding the risks and benefits of operative management of ankle fractures, especially for those patients who smoke.

M. F. Swiontkowski, MD

Outcome in Patients With an Infected Nonunion of the Long Bones Treated With a Reinforced Antibiotic Bone Cement Rod

Selhi HS, Mahindra P, Yamin M, et al (Dayanand Med College & Hosp, Ludhiana, Punjab, India; et al)

J Orthop Trauma 26:184-188, 2012

Objectives.—This study looks at the treatment of 16 cases of infection in long bone fractures that had an adverse effect on healing. The goal was to find a method that may be effective in getting these most difficult injuries to heal. The use of reinforced antibiotic-impregnated bone cement rods was studied to see if this could be an effective form of treatment. The use of such devices makes sense because they provide stability that the fractures need for healing while also providing a high concentration of antibiotics locally. The concept was to reduce the amount of metal used for stability while still giving the fracture the correct milieu for healing.

Design.—This was a retrospective analysis of 16 patients with infected nonunions of long bones. A protocol for the use of intravenous and per oral antibiotics was developed based on the type of bacteria found from cultures of the infected sites. All cases included operative débridement and stabilization with a reinforced antibiotic-impregnated bone cement rod.

Patients.—The patient population was selected from all those who presented to the Department of Orthopaedic Surgery of Dayanand Medical College & Hospital, Ludhiana, India.

Main Outcome.—Success was considered when the nonunion healed and the limb became functional.

Results.—The infected nonunions were treated successfully in 14 of 16 cases. This represents an alternative to external fixation alone as a means of stabilizing nonunions while providing a high concentration of antibiotic locally for combating this most difficult problem.

Conclusions.—The use of reinforced antibiotic-impregnated bone cement rods with appropriate surgical débridement and antibiotics may be an effective way of treating infected nonunions of long bones.

Level of Evidence.—Therapeutic Level IV. See page 128 for a complete description of levels of evidence (Table 2).

▶ Deep infection following diaphyseal long bone fracture with nonunion is a serious complication that can jeopardize fracture healing and potentially lead to amputation. This retrospective cohort series utilizing antibiotic impregnated cement coating of intramedullary rods and systemic antibiotics based on culture profile shows that the majority of time this clinical situation can be

TABLE 2.—Sixteen Patients With Methods of Treatment and Outcome

Patient No.	Age and Sex	Bone Involved	Fracture Status	Smoker	Comorbidities	Fixation	Operating Room Culture	Core Metal	Union Time (Months)
1	32 years M	Femur	Closed	Yes		ILN	StaphA	Steel K nail	6
2	48 years M	Femur	Open	Yes	NIDD	ILN	NG	Steel ILN	6
3	47 years M	Tibia	Open	No	HTN	ExFix	StaphA	Steel K nail	6
4	40 years M	Tibia	Open	No		DCP	NG	Steel wire	6
5	18 years M	Femur	Closed	Yes		ILN	NG	Steel K nail	6
6	21 years M	Femur	Open	No		ExFix	StaphA	Steel K nail	8
7	28 years M	Femur	Open	No		ExFix	NG	Steel K nail	BG
8	42 years M	Femur	Open	No		ILN	NG	Steel K nail	NU
9	27 years M	Femur	Open	No		ILN	StaphA	Steel K nail	6
10	42 years F	Humerus	Open	No		Plate	Enterobacter	Steel K wire	8
11	54 years M	Femur	Open	No	NIDM/HTN	ExFix	StaphA	Steel K nail	NU
12	47 years M	Tibia	Open	Yes	NIDM	ExFix	Enterobacter	Steel wire	BG
13	43 years M	Tibia	Open	?		ILN	Enterobacter	Steel K nail	6
14	37 years F	Tibia	Closed	Yes	HTN	DCP	NG	Steel wire	BG
15	52 years M	Tibia	Closed	Yes	HTN	ILN	NG	Steel K nail	6
16	38 years M	Tibia	Open	?		ILN	NG	Steel K nail	6

M, male; F, female; NIDD, non insulin dependent diabetes mellitus; HTN, hypertension; NIDM, noninsulin-dependent diabetes mellitus; ILN, interlocking nail; ExFix, external fixation; StaphA, *Staphylococcus aureus*; NG, no growth; K, Kuntscher; NU, non union; BG, bone grafting.

salvaged. This is a useful technique that surgeons faced with this clinical situation should strongly consider.

M. F. Swiontkowski, MD

Oral Bisphosphonates and Risk of Subtrochanteric or Diaphyseal Femur Fractures in a Population-Based Cohort

Kim SY, Schneeweiss S, Katz JN, et al (Brigham and Women's Hosp, Boston, MA)

J Bone Miner Res 26:993-1001, 2011

Bisphosphonates are the primary therapy for postmenopausal and glucocorticoid-induced osteoporosis. Case series suggest a potential link between prolonged use of bisphosphonates and low-energy fracture of subtrochanteric or diaphyseal femur as a consequence of oversuppression of bone resorption. Using health care utilization data, we conducted a propensity score—matched cohort study to examine the incidence rates (IRs) and risk of subtrochanteric or diaphyseal femur fractures among oral bisphosphonate users compared with raloxifene or calcitonin users. A Cox proportional hazards model evaluated the risk of these fractures associated with duration of osteoporosis treatment. A total of 104 subtrochanteric or diaphyseal femur fractures were observed among 33,815 patients. The estimated IR of subtrochanteric or diaphyseal femur fractures per 1000 person-years was 1.46 [95% confidence interval (CI) 1.11—1.88] among the bisphosphonate users and 1.43 (95% CI 1.06—1.89) among raloxifene/calcitonin users. No significant association between bisphosphonate use and subtrochanteric or diaphyseal femur fractures was found [hazard ratio (HR) = 1.03, 95% CI 0.70—1.52] compared with raloxifene/calcitonin. Even with this large study size, we had little precision in estimating the risk of subtrochanteric or diaphyseal femur fractures in patients treated with bisphosphonates for longer than 5 years (HR = 2.02, 95% CI 0.41—10.00). The occurrence of subtrochanteric or diaphyseal femur fracture was rare. There was no evidence of an increased risk of subtrochanteric or diaphyseal femur fractures in bisphosphonate users compared with raloxifene/calcitonin users. However, this study cannot exclude the possibility that long-term bisphosphonate use may increase the risk of these fractures (Figs 3 and 4, Table 1).

► The orthopedic surgery community continues to follow the story of subtrochanteric/diaphyseal fractures in association with bisphosphonate long-term use. This investigation, utilizing a large administrative database, carefully examines this association with appropriate statistical tools. The comparison for the bisphosphonate group is raloxifene or calcitonin users, which is also appropriate. From this investigation, we can conclude that the risk/association is small and that there does not seem to be a differential risk between the groups that can be detected with any degree of precision. We will continue to follow up with this very important clinical association for the next several years, but in the meantime,

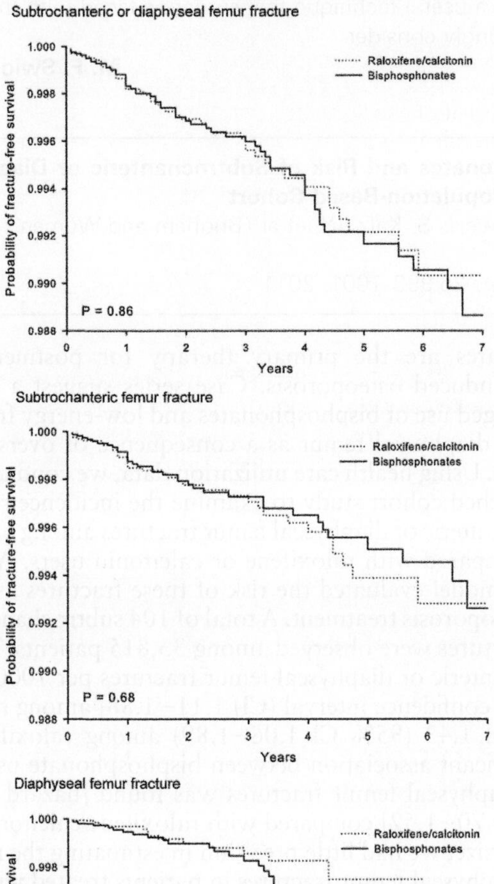

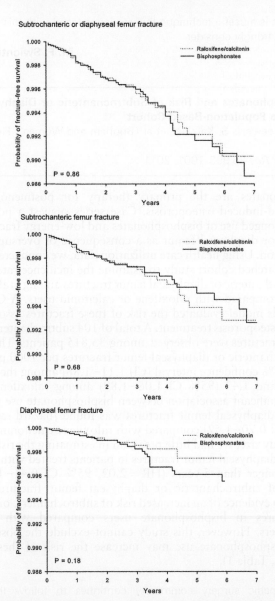

FIGURE 3.—Kaplan-Meier curves for fracture-free survival in oral bisphosphonates versus raloxifene/calcitonin nasal spray. (Reprinted from Kim SY, Schneeweiss S, Katz JN, et al. Oral bisphosphonates and risk of subtrochanteric or diaphyseal femur fractures in a population-based cohort. *J Bone Miner Res.* 2011 26:993-1001, with permission from American Society for Bone and Mineral Research.)

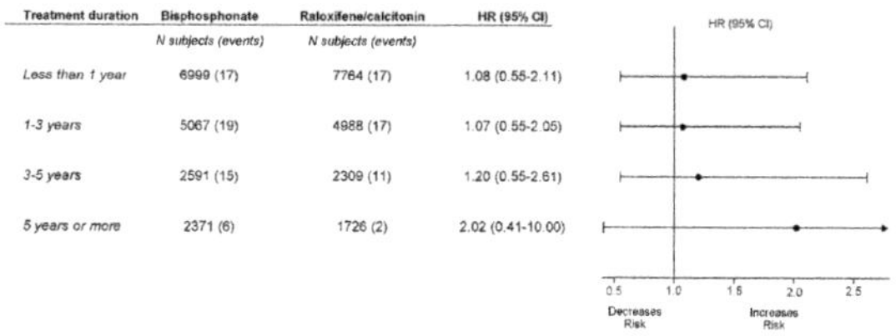

FIGURE 4.—Hazard ratios (HRs) for subtrochanteric or diaphyseal femur fractures according to osteoporosis treatment duration. (Reprinted from Kim SY, Schneeweiss S, Katz JN, et al. Oral bisphosphonates and risk of subtrochanteric or diaphyseal femur fractures in a population-based cohort. *J Bone Miner Res.* 2011 26:993-1001, with permission from American Society for Bone and Mineral Research.)

TABLE 1.—Characteristics of Propensity Score—Matched Study Population in 12 Months Prior to Filling Their First Osteoporosis Drug Prescription

	Bisphosphonates	Raloxifene/Calcitonin
n	17,028	16,787
Demographic factors		
Age, years, mean (SD)	79.9 (6.5)	80.0 (6.9)
Race, white	16,180 (95)	15,987 (95.2)
Sex, female	16,474 (96.8)	16,244 (96.8)
Health care utilization		
No. of visits, mean (SD)	10.6 (6)	10.5 (6.1)
ER visit	4,505 (26.5)	4,482 (26.7)
No. of all prescription drugs, mean (SD)	10.4 (6)	10.5 (6.1)
Hospitalization	6,089 (35.8)	6,146 (36.6)
Nursing home resident	1,882 (11.1)	1,991 (11.9)
Comorbidities		
Prior fall	2,094 (12.3)	2,119 (12.6)
Prior hip fracture	612 (3.6)	601 (3.6)
Prior vertebral fracture	1,858 (10.9)	1,890 (11.3)
BMD test	4,085 (24)	4,180 (24.9)
Hypertension	11,303 (66.4)	11,233 (66.9)
Chronic kidney disease	492 (2.9)	481 (2.9)
Chronic liver disease	207 (1.2)	191 (1.1)
Parkinson disease	586 (3.4)	598 (3.6)
Dementia	1,039 (6.1)	1,092 (6.5)
Diabetes mellitus	4,354 (25.6)	4,312 (25.7)
Congestive heart failure	3,664 (21.5)	3,728 (22.2)
Chronic obstructive pulmonary disease (COPD)	4,782 (28.1)	4,763 (28.4)
Inflammatory arthritis	1,267 (7.4)	1,258 (7.5)
Inflammatory bowel disease	241 (1.4)	226 (1.4)
Alcoholism	311 (1.8)	301 (1.8)
Comorbidity index, mean (SD)	1.9 (1.9)	2 (1.9)
Other medications		
Opioids	6,817 (40)	6,826 (40.7)
Antiepileptics	892 (5.2)	877 (5.2)
Proton pump inhibitors	4,361 (25.6)	4,441 (26.5)
Benzodiazepines	4,636 (27.2)	4,614 (27.5)
Selective serotonin reuptake inhibitors (SSRIs)	2,654 (15.6)	2,683 (16)
Warfarin	1,814 (10.7)	1,786 (10.6)
Inhaled steroid	1,389 (8.2)	1,391 (8.3)
Oral steroid	2,420 (14.2)	2,387 (14.2)

Note: New Jersey and Pennsylvania combined, second drug dispensing and a 90-day lag period are required. Data are presented in number (%), unless specified.

SD = standard deviation; ER = emergency room; BMD = bone mineral density.

we can be confident in reassuring patients that the risk of a hip or spine fracture from a low-energy fall is greater than this association and that bisphosphonate use is appropriate to continue. A year-long drug holiday after 5 to 7 continuous years of therapy is still advisable.

M. F. Swiontkowski, MD

Parathyroid Hormone 1-84 Accelerates Fracture-Healing in Pubic Bones of Elderly Osteoporotic Women

Peichl P, Holzer LA, Maier R, et al (Evangelisches Krankenhaus, Vienna, Austria; Thermenklinikum Baden, Austria; et al)

J Bone Joint Surg Am 93:1583-1587, 2011

Background.—Parathyroid hormone (PTH) has been shown to increase bone mineral density and to reduce the rate of fractures in patients with osteoporosis and also to improve fracture-healing. The purpose of the present prospective, randomized, controlled study was to evaluate the effect of PTH 1-84 on the course of pelvic fracture-healing and functional outcome in postmenopausal women.

Methods.—Sixty-five patients had a dual x-ray absorptiometry scan, radiographs, and a computed tomography scan to document pelvic fractures. Twenty-one patients received a once-daily injection of 100 μg of PTH 1-84 starting within two days after admission to the hospital, and forty-four patients served as the control group. All patients received 1000 mg of calcium and 800 IU of vitamin D. Computed tomography scans were repeated every fourth week until radiographic evidence of cortical bridging at the fracture site was confirmed. Functional outcome was assessed with use of a visual analog scale for pain and a Timed "Up and Go" test.

Results.—The mean time to fracture healing was 7.8 weeks for the treatment group, compared with 12.6 weeks for the control group ($p < 0.001$). At eight weeks, all fractures in the treatment group were healed and four fractures in the control group were healed (healing rate, 100% compared with 9.1%; $p < 0.001$). Both the visual analog scale score for pain and the result of the Timed "Up and Go" test improved in the study group as compared with the control group ($p < 0.001$).

Conclusions.—In elderly patients with osteoporosis, PTH 1-84 accelerates fracture-healing in pelvic fractures and improves functional outcome (Table 2).

▶ This is an important randomized trial that clarifies the role of PTH in fracture healing of osteoporotic individuals. This is a well-designed and conducted trial that confirms the utility of this pharmacologic approach in speeding fracture healing in the anterior pelvic ring. Radiographic and functional outcomes were improved with this intervention. Although there is a downside to the daily subcutaneous injection requirement, this issue would appear to be heavily outweighed by its favorable impact on pain and function. This is an important initial step in

TABLE 2.—Fracture-Healing, VAS Score, and Timed "Up and Go" Test

	PTH 1-84 Treatment Group (n = 21)	Control Group (n = 44)	P Value
Fracture-healing			
Week 4*	1 (4.8%)	0 (0%)	0.145†
Week 8*	21 (100%)	4 (9.1%)	<0.001†
Week 12*	21 (100%)	30 (68.2%)	0.004†
VAS score‡			
Week 0	7.6 ± 1.1	7.7 ± 1.1	0.743§
Week 8	3.2 ± 1.0	6.5 ± 0.9	<0.001§
Timed "Up and Go" at Week 12‡ (*s*)	22.9 ± 7.7	54.3 ± 19.9	<0.001§

*The values are given as the number of fractures, with the percentage in parentheses.
†Chi-square test.
‡The values are given as the mean and the standard deviation.
§Mann-Whitney U test.

evaluating the impact of this intervention on other fractures in patients with proven osteoporosis.

M. F. Swiontkowski, MD

The outcome of fractures in very elderly patients

Clement ND, Aitken SA, Duckworth AD, et al (The Royal Infirmary of Edinburgh, UK)

J Bone Joint Surg [Br] 93-B:806-810, 2011

We compared case-mix and outcome variables in 1310 patients who sustained an acute fracture at the age of 80 years or over. A group of 318 very elderly patients (≥ 90 years) was compared with a group of 992 elderly patients (80 to 89 years), all of whom presented to a single trauma unit between July 2007 and June 2008. The very elderly group represented only 0.6% of the overall population, but accounted for 4.1% of all fractures and 9.3% of all orthopaedic trauma admissions. Patients in this group were more likely to require hospital admission (odds ratio 1.4), less likely to return to independent living (odds ratio 3.1), and to have a significantly longer hospital stay (ten days, $p = 0.01$).

The 30- and 120-day unadjusted mortality was greater in the very elderly group. The 120-day mortality associated with non-hip fractures of the lower limb was equal to that of proximal femoral fractures, and was significantly increased with a delay to surgery > 48 hours for both age groups ($p = 0.04$). This suggests that the principle of early surgery and mobilisation of elderly patients with hip fractures should be extended to include all those in this vulnerable age group (Fig 1, Table 4).

▶ The authors report an analysis of a large cohort of fracture patients > 80 and > 90 years. This is the largest series of fracture patients in the later years of life

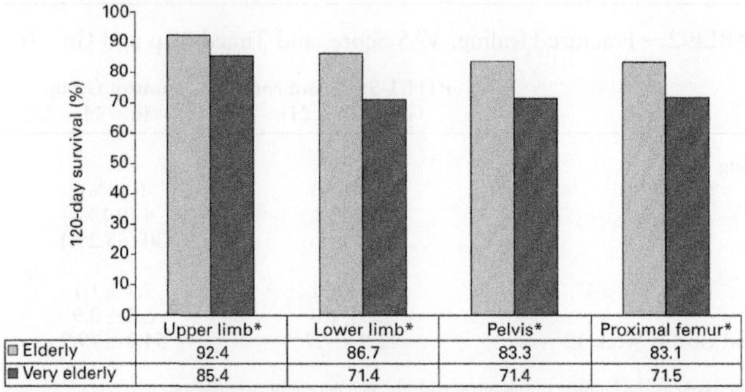

FIGURE 1.—Survival at 120 days according to age group and site of fracture. (*, univariate chi-squared test: upper limb $p = 0.02$, lower limb $p = 0.001$, pelvis $p = 0.007$, and proximal femur $p = 0.0006$). (Reprinted from Clement ND, Aitken SA, Duckworth AD, et al. The outcome of fractures in very elderly patients. *J Bone Joint Surg [Br]*. 2011;93-B:806-810, Copyright 2011 of the British Editorial Society of Bone and Joint Surgery.)

TABLE 4.—Outcome Measures According to Age Group

Outcome	Elderly	Very Elderly	p-Value*
30-day survival for all in-patients (%)			
Alive	*94.6*	*91.1*	
Dead	*5.4*	*8.9*	0.03 (OR† 1.7)
120-day survival for all in-patients (%)			
Alive	*85.5*	*74.0*	
Dead	*14.4*	*26.0*	0.0001 (OR 2.1)
Residence at 120 days if patient lived at home prior to fracture (%)			
Own home	*81.3*	*58.4*	0.004
Residential care	*9.3*	*15.7*	0.02
Nursing home	*6.6*	*18.9*	0.005
Rehabilitation ward	*3.0*	*6.5*	0.045
Hospital	*0*	*1.1*	0.08

*chi-squared test
†OR, odds ratio

ever reported. Individuals in these older decades primarily are injured with low-energy falls, and with loss of physiologic reserve, they have a high mortality risk. Because of the frail condition, hospital admission is more often required. This has important implications for all health systems regarding the aging of the postwar Baby Boomer population. The high mortality rate in both decades related to fracture is not surprising; it is well known in the hip fracture population and now is understood to be the same for all fractures.

M. F. Swiontkowski, MD

Femur Fractures

Nonoperative versus Prophylactic Treatment of Bisphosphonate-associated Femoral Stress Fractures

Banffy MB, Vrahas MS, Ready JE, et al (Brigham and Women's Hosp, Boston, MA)
Clin Orthop Relat Res 469:2028-2034, 2011

Background.—Several studies have identified a specific fracture in the proximal diaphysis of the femur in patients treated with bisphosphonates. The fractures typically are sustained after a low-energy mechanism with the presence of an existing characteristic stress fracture. However, it is unclear whether these patients are best treated nonoperatively or operatively.

Questions/Purposes.—What is the likelihood of nonoperatively treated bisphosphonate-associated femoral stress fractures progressing to completion and during what time period? If prophylactic fixation is performed, do patients have a shorter hospital length-of-stay compared with patients having surgical fixation after fracture completion?

Patients and Methods.—We retrospectively searched for patients older than 50 years receiving bisphosphonate therapy, with either incomplete, nondisplaced stress fractures or completed, displaced fractures in the proximal diaphysis of the femur between July 2002 and April 2009. After applying exclusion criteria, we identified 34 patients with a total of 40 bisphosphonate-associated fractures. The average duration of bisphosphonate use was 77 months. Twenty-eight of 40 (70%) fractures were completed, displaced fractures. Six of the 12 nondisplaced stress fractures initially were treated nonoperatively. The remaining six stress fractures were treated with prophylactic cephalomedullary nail fixation. The minimum followup was 12 months (mean, 36.5 months; range, 12–72 months).

Results.—Five of the six stress fractures treated nonoperatively progressed to fracture completion and displacement at an average of 10 months

TABLE 1.—Patient Demographics

Parameter	Value
Number of patients	34
Gender	
Male	0 (0%)
Female	34 (100%)
Age (years)*	68.5 (53–87)
Bisphosphonate	
Alendonate	29 (85.3%)
Zoledronic acid	3 (8.8%)
Pamidonate	2 (5.9%)
Duration of bisphosphonate use†	
<5 years	3 (15.8%)
>5 years	16 (84.2%)

*Values are expressed as mean, with range in parentheses.
†Only 19 of 34 patients had documentation of duration of bisphosphonate use.

(range, 3–18 months). The average hospital stay was 3.7 days for patients treated prophylactically and 6.0 days for patients treated after fracture completion.

Conclusions.—Our data suggest nonoperative treatment of bisphosphonate-related femoral stress fractures is not a reliable way to treat these fractures as the majority progress to fracture completion. Prophylactic fixation of femoral stress fractures also reduces total hospital admission time.

Level of Evidence.—Level IV, therapeutic study. See Guidelines for Authors for a complete description of levels of evidence (Table 1).

▶ This somewhat small retrospective cohort study of a fairly rare complication of bisphosphonate therapy again confirms that duration of therapy is a major risk factor; therapy for more than 5 years seems to be a clinically important concern. Additionally, with a very high rate of progression to complete fractures without prophylactic nailing, this intervention seems prudent in most cases.

M. F. Swiontkowski, MD

The Outcome of Surgically Treated Femur Fractures Associated With Long-Term Bisphosphonate Use

Weil YA, Rivkin G, Safran O, et al (Hadassah Hebrew Univ Hosp, Jerusalem, Israel; et al)

J Trauma 71:186-190, 2011

Introduction.—Bisphosphonates (BPs) evolved as the mainstay for the treatment of osteoporosis, reducing the incidence of fractures. Recently several publications described the occurrence of low-energy subtrochanteric and femoral shaft fractures associated with long-term BP use. The aim of this study was to describe the outcome of surgically treated femur fractures associated with prolonged BP use.

Patients.—Fifteen patients suffering from 17 atypical femoral fragility fractures associated with long-term (>3 years) BP use were located. Data included fracture type, time of BP use, last bone mineral density DEXA scores for the femoral neck and spine, type of surgery, and the need for revision.

Results.—Fourteen female patients and one male patient were identified. The median age was 73 years (range, 51–80 years). The mean BP use was 7.8 years (range, 4–13 years). Fourteen patients had low-energy traumatic femoral shaft (proximal and distal) or low subtrochanteric fractures. The mean lumbar spine (for 13 patients) bone mineral density T-score was −3.0, whereas mean femoral neck T-score was −1.8 with only three patients in the osteoporotic range.

Fracture healing after the first procedure for patients treated with nails was 54%, with 46% of patients requiring revision surgery. These included nail dynamization, exchange nailing, and one revision to a blade plate. All of these eventually healed.

Conclusions.—BP-related fractures are a recently described phenomenon. Despite initial osteoporosis, the DEXA scan may appear outside

TABLE 1.—Patient Demographics, Mechanism of Injury, and BMD Data

Patients SN	Age (Yr)	Gender	Fracture Mechanism	Duration of BP Treatment (yr)	DEXA Score Spine T-Score	DEXA Score Spine Z-Score	DEXA Score Femoral Neck T-Score	DEXA Score Femoral Neck Z-Score
1	80	Female	Fall	5	−2.7	0.0	−2.2	>0
2	73	Female	Fall	4	−3.5	−1.2	−2.8	−0.9
3	62	Female	Fall	8	−4.5	−2.9	−2.7	−1.3
4	72	Female	Fall	4	−4.4	−2.1	−2.6	−0.7
5	73	Female	Fall	12	−2.3	−0.3	−1.9	−0.1
6	85	Female	Fall	7	N/A	N/A	−1.4	1.1
7	62	Female	Fall	8	−1.3	−0.1	−0.2	1.0
8	72	Female	Fall	12	N/A	N/A	N/A	N/A
9	75	Female	Fall	7	N/A	N/A	N/A	N/A
9	75	Female	Fall	7	N/A	N/A	N/A	N/A
10	51	Female	Fall	5	N/A	N/A	−1.8	−1.1
10	51	Female	Fall	5	N/A	N/A	N/A	N/A
11	73	Female	Fall	11	−4.4	−2.0	N/A	N/A
12	52	Male	Fall	13	−2.5	−2.1	−2.3	−1.5
13	63	Female	Fall	5	−1.9	−0.6	0.5	1.7
14	73	Female	Atraumatic	12	−3.0	−0.7	−2.4	−0.4
15	76	Female	Fall	9	−2.9	−0.5	−1.4	0.7

TABLE 2.—Orthopedic Data Regarding Fracture Type, Index, and Revision Surgery

Patient SN	Fracture (AO/OTA)	Index Surgery	Open/Closed Reduction	First Revision	Second Revision
1	Shaft 32A3	IMN	Open + Bx	Dynamization	Exchange nail
2	Subtrochanteric 32A3.1	CMN	Open + Bx	Exchange nail	
3	Shaft 32A3	IMN	Open + Bx		
4	Shaft 32A3	IMN	Open + Bx		
5	Distal shaft 32A2	IMN	Closed		
6	Subtrochanteric 32A3.1	CMN	Closed	Blade plate	
7	Subtrochanteric 32A3.1	CMN	Open nailing	Dynamization	
8	Shaft 32A3	IMN	Open + Bx	Dynamization	
9	Distal shaft 32A2	IMN	Closed		
9	Distal shaft 32A2	IMN	Closed		
10	Shaft 32A3	IMN	Closed		
10	Shaft 32A3	IMN	Closed	Exchange nail	
11	Shaft 32A3	IMN	Open + Bx		
12	Shaft 32B1	IMN	Closed	Dynamization	
13	Distal shaft 32A3	IMN	Open nailing		
14	Distal shaft 32A3	LCP	Closed		
15	Subtrochanteric 32B1.1	CMN	Open + Bx		

IMN, intramedullary nail; CMN, cephalomedullary nail; LCP, locked compression plate; BX, biopsy.

the osteoporotic range for the femoral neck in these patients. In addition, a much higher failure rate with intramedullary nailing requiring revision surgery may occur with these patients (Tables 1 and 2).

▶ With the new focus on atypical femur fractures associated with long-term bisphosphonate use, data on the outcome of the surgical management of complete fractures is important. This retrospective review confirms the impression that these fractures are difficult to heal. With primary healing of just over 50%, we can expect that there will be high numbers of patients with this fracture association who need revision surgery. The use of teriparatide to aid in gaining fracture union is an important associated therapy that should be widely recommended until we have better data to evaluate its effectiveness in this setting. It is worth reemphasizing that bisphosphonate therapy effectively prevents hip and spine fractures, and this relatively rare complication does not outweigh the important impact of these drugs on patients with osteoporosis.

M. F. Swiontkowski, MD

Femoral Stress Fractures Associated With Long-Term Bisphosphonate Treatment

Ward WG Sr, Carter CJ, Wilson SC, et al (Wake Forest Univ School of Medicine, Winston Salem, NC)
Clin Orthop Relat Res 470:759-765, 2012

Background.—Recent studies have described unique clinical and radiographic characteristics of femoral stress fractures or low-energy fractures associated with long-term bisphosphonate therapy. However, it is unclear whether these fractures require subsequent surgery after the initial treatment.

Questions/Purposes.—We performed a cohort analysis of bisphosphonate-associated femoral stress fractures to (1) confirm the unique clinical and radiographic findings compared with existing literature, (2) determine whether any patients with completed fractures had no preexisting transverse stress fracture lines, (3) assess the need for additional surgical procedures, and (4) determine whether the hospital length of stay (LOS) differed for patients with prophylactic fixation of stress fractures versus fixation of completed fractures.

Methods.—We retrospectively reviewed 16 patients with 24 diaphyseal and subtrochanteric femoral stress fractures (14) or low-energy fractures (10) who had been on bisphosphonates for 3 to 10 years. Data included demographics, symptoms, medication history, radiographic characteristics, treatment parameters, LOS, and outcome. Minimum followup was 9 months (average, 44.0 months; median, 31 months; range, 9–112 months).

Results.—All patients had clinical and radiographic findings similar to those reported in the literature. Two of four patients sustained completed fractures after radiographs failed to reveal transverse lateral fracture lines. None of the 14 prophylactically treated impending fractures progressed or required additional surgery; however, in five of 10 femurs treated after fracture completion, six additional surgeries were performed. The average hospital LOS was shorter in patients who underwent prophylactic fixation (3.8 days) than in patients treated for completed fractures (5.6 days).

Conclusions.—Bisphosphonate-associated stress fractures and completed fractures are unique, possessing subtle characteristic radiographic features.

TABLE 1.—Literature Reports of Clinical and Radiographic Findings in Bisphosphonate-Associated Fractures

Study	Sex (F:M)	Age (Years)*	Number of Impending/ Completed Fractures	Patients with Prodromal Pain	Duration of Bisphosphonate Use (Years)*	Fractures with Transverse Line Before Fracture	Fractures with Lateral Cortical Thickening	Number of Prophylactic Reconstruction Nails that Failed/Total Number Treated with Nail	Patients with Bilateral Fractures
Banffy et al. [2]	34 F	All >50	12/28		6.4 (3–10)	100%	100%	0/6	0%
Capeci and Tejwani [4]	7 F	61 (53–75)	7 (impending)	57.10%	8.6 (5–13)		100%	0/3	100%
Koh et al. [9]	16 F	Median 68 (53–92)	12/4	100% (of completed fractures)	4.5 (2–7)	100%	100%		
Kwek et al. [10]	17 F	66 (53–82)	17 (completed)	76%	4.8 (2–8)	100%	100%		53%
Neviaser et al. [11]	25 F	69.4	25 (completed)		6.2 (1–10)	76%	76%		
Current study	15:1	69.1 (51–90)	14/10	100%	6.3 (3–10)	50% (2/4)	96% (22/23)	0/14	50%

Editor's Note: Please refer to original journal article for full references.
*Values are expressed as mean, with range in parentheses; F = female; M = male.

TABLE 2.—Clinical Data From Patients Treated with Bisphosphonates

Fracture Status	Patient	Age (Years)	Sex	Side	Alendronate	Duration (Years)	Other Bisphosphonates	Duration (Years)	Followup (Months)	Additional Surgery
Stress fracture treated prophylactically	1	76	Female	Left	Yes	3+	No		67	No
	2	76	Female	Right	Yes	3+	No		84	No
	3	74	Female	Right	Yes	3	No		72	No
	4	76	Female	Right	Yes	7	No		59	No
	4	76	Female	Left	Yes	7	No		59	No
	5	65	Female	Right	Yes	9+	No		42	No
	6	79	Male	Right	No		Zoledronic acid, pamidronate	10	25	No
	7	53	Female	Left	Yes	5+	Risedronate	1+	10	No
	8	90	Female	Right	Yes	9	Ibandronate	1+	20	No
	9	61	Female	Left	Yes	3+	Zoledronic acid	1.5	20	No
	9	61	Female	Right	Yes	3+	Zoledronic acid	1.5	19	No
	10	69	Female	Right	Yes	8.5	No		18	No
	11	64	Female	Right	Yes	4+	No		80	No
	12	84	Female	Left	No		Risedronate	6	10	No
Completed fracture after radiographic studies	3	74	Female	Left	Yes	3	No		74	No
	7	51	Female	Right	Yes	4	Risedronate	1+	28	Yes*
	10	69	Female	Left	Yes	8.5	No		18	No
	13	72	Female	Right	Yes	4+	Zoledronic acid	1	9	No
	14	66	Female	Left	Yes	10+	No		16	No
	14	66	Female	Right	Yes	9+	No		29	No
	16	66	Female	Right	Yes	7	No		73	Yes†
Completed fracture before any radiographic studies	5	60	Female	Left	Yes	4+	No		112	Yes‡
	15	65	Female	Left	Yes	10	No		11	Yes§
	16	65	Female	Left	Yes	6	No		89	Yes‖

*Dynamized at 6 months; revised at 10 months for broken intramedullary nail.
†Nonunion requiring revision reconstruction nail at 15 months.
‡Dynamized at 3 months.
§Dynamized at 7 months.
‖Nonunion requiring revision reconstruction nail at 18 months.

Completed fractures may occur through the thickened bone in the absence of an appreciable transverse stress fracture line. Our observations suggest prophylactic reconstruction nail fixation may avoid fracture completion and may be associated with a shorter hospital LOS and less morbidity than treatment of completed fractures.

Level of Evidence.—Level IV, diagnostic study. See the Guidelines for Authors for a complete description of levels of evidence (Tables 1-3).

▶ This cohort study adds further details regarding the radiographic criteria of bisphosphonate-related femoral fractures, also called *atypical femoral fractures*. These features have been described previously and are confirmed in this group of patients. Although the conclusions must be tempered by the fact that this is an uncontrolled observational cohort, it seems as if prohylactic nailing may well be the treatment of choice to prevent the difficulties associated with getting the

TABLE 3.—Radiographic Observations From Patients Treated with Bisphosphonates

Fracture Status	Patient	Black line on Plain Film	Black Line on CT	MRI	Bone Scan	Radiographic Thick Cortex	Transverse Lateral Cortical Fracture
Stress fracture treated prophylactically	1	NA	No	NA	NA	Yes	NA
	2	No	No	A, B, C	NA	Yes	NA
	3	Yes*	NA	A, B	E	Yes	NA
	4	Yes	NA	NA	E	Yes	NA
	4	Yes	NA	NA	E	Yes	NA
	5	No	No	NA	E	Yes	NA
	6	No	NA	NA	NA	Yes	NA
	7	No	NA	C	NA	No¶	NA
	8	NA	NA	A, B	NA	Yes	NA
	9	No	NA	NA	NA	Yes	NA
	9	Yes†	NA	NA	NA	Yes	NA
	10	No	No	A, B	NA	Yes	NA
	11	No‡	No	A, B	NA	Yes	NA
	12	No‡	NA	A, B	NA	Yes	NA
Completed fracture after radiographic studies	3	NA	NA	B, D	NA	Yes	Yes
	7	Yes*	Yes	B§	F§	Yes	Yes
	10	No	No	A, B	NA	Yes	Yes
	13	Yes*	NA	NA	E	Yes	Yes
	14	NA	NA	A, B	NA	Yes	Yes
	14	NA	NA	A, B‖	NA	Yes	Yes
	16	No	NA	NA	E	Yes	Yes
Completed fracture before any radiographic studies	5	NA	NA	NA	NA	Yes	Yes
	15	NA	NA	NA	NA	Yes	Yes
	16	NA	NA	NA	NA	NA#	Yes**

*Subtle.
†Partial-thickness black line.
‡Developed a thin black line in the zone of thickened cortical bone after intramedullary nail fixation.
§4 months before CT scan and fracture.
‖6 months before fracture (3 months before symptom onset).
¶Periosteal reactive bone present (she had minimal thickening on the opposite side before it fractured).
#Original fracture films not available.
**Original fracture films not available; transverse fracture exhibits rounding of edges on 16 months postoperative films; NA = not available; A = lateral cortical thickening; B = localized edema pattern; C = visible stress fracture line; D = lateral cortical irregularity, questionable thickening; E = focal lateral cortical increased activity; F = focal increased activity, medial greater than lateral.

displaced fractures to heal. Patients who present with proximal hip or thigh pain after a period of time on bisphosphonates deserve careful imaging and clinical evaluation to try and limit the number of patients who go on to displace these fractures.

M. F. Swiontkowski, MD

Bisphosphonate Use and Atypical Fractures of the Femoral Shaft

Schilcher J, Michaëlsson K, Aspenberg P (Linköping Univ, Sweden; Uppsala Univ, Sweden)

N Engl J Med 364:1728-1737, 2011

Background.—Studies show conflicting results regarding the possible excess risk of atypical fractures of the femoral shaft associated with bisphosphonate use.

Methods.—In Sweden, 12,777 women 55 years of age or older sustained a fracture of the femur in 2008. We reviewed radiographs of 1234 of the 1271 women who had a subtrochanteric or shaft fracture and identified 59 patients with atypical fractures. Data on medications and coexisting conditions were obtained from national registries. The relative and absolute risk of atypical fractures associated with bisphosphonate use was estimated by means of a nationwide cohort analysis. The 59 case patients were also compared with 263 control patients who had ordinary subtrochanteric or shaft fractures.

Results.—The age-adjusted relative risk of atypical fracture was 47.3 (95% confidence interval [CI], 25.6 to 87.3) in the cohort analysis. The increase in absolute risk was 5 cases per 10,000 patient-years (95% CI, 4 to 7). A total of 78% of the case patients and 10% of the controls had received bisphosphonates, corresponding to a multivariable-adjusted odds ratio of 33.3 (95% CI, 14.3 to 77.8). The risk was independent of co-existing conditions and of concurrent use of other drugs with known effects on bone. The duration of use influenced the risk (odds ratio per 100 daily doses, 1.3; 95% CI, 1.1 to 1.6). After drug withdrawal, the risk diminished by 70% per year since the last use (odds ratio, 0.28; 95% CI, 0.21 to 0.38).

Conclusions.—These population-based nationwide analyses may be reassuring for patients who receive bisphosphonates. Although there was a high prevalence of current bisphosphonate use among patients with atypical fractures, the absolute risk was small. (Funded by the Swedish Research Council.) (Tables 1 and 4).

▶ Orthopaedic surgeons are regularly questioned about the risk of continued bisphosphonate use by women who are taking these drugs or are contemplating it and have heard of the issue of atypical femur fractures in the lay press. This large database study provides important information for our patients who are asking these questions. The patients who had femur subtrochanteric or diaphyseal fractures and were on bisphosphonates were compared with a cohort of age-matched patients with fractures in the same area. The duration

TABLE 1.—Risk of Atypical Femoral Fracture Associated with Bisphosphonate Use During the 3 Years (2005–2008) Preceding the Fracture*

Variable	No. of Women	Cases of Atypical Fracture: No. of Atypical Fracture Cases	Cases of Atypical Fracture: Crude Incidence *No./10,000 Patient-yr*	Age-Adjusted Relative Risk (95% CI)	Age-Adjusted Absolute Risk (95% CI)
Bisphosphonate use					
Never	1, 437,820	13	0.09	1.0 (reference)	
Ever	83,311	46	5.5	47.3 (25.6–87.3)	0.0005 (0.0004–0.0007)
Duration of use					
<1.0 yr	15,672	3	1.9	18.4 (5.3–64.3)	0.0002 (0.0000–0.0004)
1.0–1.9 yr	21,406	4	1.9	17.0 (5.7–50.7)	0.0002 (0.0000–0.0004)
≥2.0 yr	46,233	39	8.4	67.0 (35.8–125.8)	0.0008 (0.0006–0.0011)
Time since last use					
<1.0 yr	83,311	42	5.0	42.9 (22.9–80.4)	0.0005 (0.0004–0.0007)
1.0–1.9 yr	70,036	1	0.1	3.5 (1.0–11.9)	<0.0001 (0.0000–0.0000)
≥2.0 yr	75,583	3	0.4	3.2 (1.0–10.1)	<0.0001 (0.0000–0.0001)

*CI denotes confidence interval.

TABLE 4.—Odds Ratios for Atypical Femoral Fractures Associated with Bisphosphonate Use*

Variable	Case Patients (N = 59)	Controls (N = 263)	Odds Ratio (95% CI): Age-Adjusted	Odds Ratio (95% CI): Multivariable-Adjusted†
Bisphosphonate use				
Never	13	237	1.0 (reference)	1.0 (reference)
Ever	46	26	27.2 (12.8–58.1)	33.3 (14.3–77.8)
Type of bisphosphonate				
Alendronate	38	18	34.1 (15.2–76.6)	38.8 (15.9–94.6)
Risedronate	6	4	19.7 (4.7–83.0)	41.2 (6.9–247.7)
Etidronate	0	5	NA	NA
Ibandronate	2	0	NA	NA
Risk of fracture per 100 defined daily doses	NA	NA	1.4 (1.2–1.6)	1.3 (1.1–1.6)
Duration of use				
<1.0 yr	3	7	6.8 (1.5–31.4)	9.8 (1.9–49.9)
1.0–1.9 yr	4	6	7.1 (1.6–30.7)	9.5 (2.1–43.3)
≥2.0 yr	39	13	49.3 (20.6–118.0)	51.1 (20.3–128.2)
Time since last use				
<1.0 yr	42	16	44.0 (19.0–102.0)	47.5 (19.2–117.6)
1.0–1.9 yr	1	4	2.4 (0.2–24.7)	3.7 (0.3–41.6)
≥2.0 yr	3	6	6.4 (1.3–31.9)	9.0 (1.8–45.8)
Risk of fracture per yr since last use	NA	NA	0.29 (0.22–0.38)	0.28 (0.21–0.38)

*NA not applicable.
†Variables were adjusted for age (as a continuous variable), use or nonuse of a glucocorticoid, and Charlson index score (as a continuous variable).

of therapy is an important risk factor. The increasingly recommended "drug holiday" after 5 years on bisphosphoate therapy is supported by this analysis. An important take-home to be shared with patients is the rapid decrease in risk after stopping the therapy. This study adds important information to the developing story of atypical femur fractures with bisphosphonate use. The most important message for the public is that the benefit of these drugs far outweighs the risk of this rather rare complication.

M. F. Swiontkowski, MD

Functional Outcome Following Intramedullary Nailing of the Femur: A Prospective Randomized Comparison of Piriformis Fossa and Greater Trochanteric Entry Portals

Stannard JP, Bankston L, Futch LA, et al (Univ of Missouri, Columbia; Baton Rouge Orthopedic Clinic, LA; Univ of Alabama at Birmingham Sports Medicine; et al)

J Bone Joint Surg Am 93:1385-1391, 2011

Background.—The purpose of the study was to prospectively compare the functional outcome of intramedullary nailing of the femur performed with use of a trochanteric and a piriformis fossa entry portal.

Methods.—One hundred and ten patients with a femoral shaft fracture were enrolled in a prospective, randomized study. Fifty-four patients were randomized to Group A (piriformis fossa portal) and fifty-six to Group B (trochanteric portal). Outcome measures included the Western Ontario and McMaster Universities (WOMAC) Osteoarthritis Index hip function score, pain, and blinded functional evaluation by a physical therapist.

Results.—Most measures of hip function did not differ between the two groups. The WOMAC score at three, six, and twelve months did not differ significantly between the piriformis fossa and trochanteric nailing groups. Functional tests included the chair stand test and the timed up and go test. Patients in Group B had significantly better scores on the chair stand test (13.3 compared with 11.1 in Group A, $p = 0.04$) at six months postoperatively, but there was no difference at twelve months (14.0 compared with 13.6). The two groups did not differ significantly on the timed up and go test at either six or twelve months. The two groups also did not differ on the muscle strength testing. Intraoperative parameters differed significantly between the groups with respect to operative time, fluoroscopy time, and incision length, with the difference favoring Group B for each parameter. Analog pain scale values were similar in Group A (2.49) and Group B (2.15) at twelve months postoperatively.

Conclusions.—Patients in our prospective randomized study who were treated with trochanteric nailing did not differ in hip function at one year postoperatively compared with patients treated with intramedullary nailing through the piriformis fossa. The values of several intraoperative parameters were significantly better in the trochanteric nailing group. Our data indicate that the functional hip outcome of femoral intramedullary nailing performed through the greater trochanter is equal to that of intramedullary nailing performed through the piriformis fossa (Tables 3, 4, and 6).

▶ This well-conducted randomized, controlled trial compared trochanteric starting point nailing with piriformis starting point nailing with patients in the

TABLE 3.—Functional Outcome

Test	Group A*	Group B*	*P* Value
At 6 months			
Chair stand test† (*no. of repetitions*)	11.07	13.27	0.0424
Timed up and go test‡ (*sec*)	12.52	9.55	0.2524
Tensor fasciae latae strength (*lb*)			
Injured side	12.95	14.67	0.3816
Contralateral side	16.34	17.25	0.4143
Gluteus medius strength (*lb*)			
Injured side	13.47	16.28	0.0894
Contralateral side	16.86	18.05	0.1921
At 12 months			
Chair stand test† (*no. of repetitions*)	13.63	14.03	0.4929
Timed up and go test‡ (*sec*)	9.72	8.72	0.7126
Tensor fasciae latae strength (*lb*)			
Injured side	15.61	17.38	0.2981
Contralateral side	18.01	16.99	0.9781
Gluteus medius strength (*lb*)			
Injured side	16.45	18.38	0.1361
Contralateral side	18.39	18.12	0.6313

*The values are given as the mean.
†In 30 seconds. A higher value indicates better performance.
‡3-m (108-cm) distance; unsupported. A lower value indicates better performance.

TABLE 4.—Heterotopic Ossification*

Brooker Grade	Total	Group A	Group B	*P* Value
I	12 (11)	6 (11)	6 (10)	>0.05
II	21 (18)	10 (18)	11 (19)	>0.05
III	10 (9)	9 (16)	1 (2)	0.0033
IV	1 (1)	1 (2)	0 (0)	0.0033
Total	44 (39)	26 (47)	18 (31)	0.1

*The values are given as the number of fractures that developed heterotopic ossification, with the percentage in parentheses.

TABLE 6.—Secondary Outcomes Involving Intraoperative Parameters

	Group A	Group B	*P* Value
Operative time* (*min*)	104 (41 to 233)	75 (35 to 187)	<0.0001
Incision length* (*mm*)	72 (25 to 190)	38 (20 to 85)	<0.0001
Fluoroscopy time* (*sec*)	149 (48 to 311)	118 (29 to 320)	0.0005

*The values are given as the mean, with the range in parentheses.

supine position. The investigators noted smaller incisions and shorter operating and fluoroscopy times. These outcome measures may well have been impacted by surgeon bias although they do make intuitive sense. Although functional testing at 6 months favored the trochanteric nails, there was no difference at

12 months, nor was there a difference in validated functional outcome questionnaire measures at that timeframe. It must be emphasized that these patients were treated in the supine position. Many surgeons favor the lateral position as originally recommended by Kuntscher for better exposure, shorter incisions even in obese patients, and greater ease at identifying either starting point with fluoroscopy. The choice of patient position and nail starting point is one that will still be impacted by surgeon experience and training.

M. F. Swiontkowski, MD

Femur

Intramedullary nailing versus submuscular plating in adolescent femoral fracture

Park K-C, Oh C-W, Byun Y-S, et al (Hanyang Univ Guri Hosp, Republic of Korea; Kyungpook Natl Univ Hosp, Daegu, Republic of Korea; Fatima Hosp, Daegu, Republic of Korea; et al)
Injury 43:870-875, 2012

Background.—Femoral fractures in adolescents usually need operative treatment, but the optimal method is unclear. The purpose of this study is to compare intramedullary nailing (IN) and submuscular plating (SP) in adolescent femoral fractures.

Materials and Methods.—We performed the prospective, comparison study of IN and SP in adolescent femoral shaft fractures at a mean age of 13.9 years (11–17.4). Twenty-two cases of IN and 23 cases of SP were followed for a minimum of 1 year. We compared radiological and clinical results, surgical parameters, and complications of two techniques.

Results.—Bony union was achieved in all cases except one case of IN. Time to union was similar in both groups. None showed mal-union over 10° or limb length discrepancy over 1 cm. None of SP group and 2 in IN group experienced re-operation; one patient had deep infection with nonunion. The other patient sustained mal-rotation. Both patients healed after revision procedure. All patients showed excellent or satisfactory results of Flynn's criteria. The time to full-weight bearing was shorter in IN (IN: 57.3 days, SP: 89.2 days, $p < 0.05$). In surgical parameters, operative time seemed shorter in IN (IN: 94.7 min, SP: 104 min, $p = 0.095$), and fluoroscopy time was shorter in IN (IN: 58 s, SP: 109 s, $p < 0.05$) than SP group.

Conclusion.—Although both IN and SP yield good results and minimal complication in adolescent femoral fractures, IN may be advantageous in less need of fluoroscopy, technical easiness in reduction and early weight bearing (Tables 3 and 4).

▶ Adolescent femoral shaft fractures can be treated with multiple surgical methods. This comparative study focuses on the 2 most commonly used methods. Fractures in adolescents heal quite reliably, which is demonstrated here by the high union rates. As with adult femoral shaft fractures, intramedullary nailing seems to have low complication rates and is technically more straightforward.

TABLE 3.—Results After Operation

	Intramedullary Nailing	Submuscular Plating
Radiological results		
Union rate	95.5% (21/22)	100% (23/23)
Time to union (weeks)	16.3	16.7
Nonunion	1	None
Delayed union	1	1
LLD over 1 cm	None	None
Mal-rotation	1	None
Clinical results		
Deep infection	1	None
Patients needed re-operation	2	None
Time to weight bearing (days)	57.3	89.2
Functional outcome (Flynn)		
Excellent	13	12
Satisfactory	9	11
Poor	None	None

TABLE 4.—Optional Demographics

	Intramedullary Nailing	Submuscular Plating
Surgical demographics		
Operation time (min)	94.7	104
Bleeding amount (cc)	185	220
Radiation exposure (s)	58	109
Difficulty in hardware removal	None	3

Difficulty in hardware removal – It means the removal procedure needed other additive procedures or implants except the original equipments.

The advantages in fluoroscopy time are significant and should encourage us to continue to use intramedullary nails with the exception of metaphyseal fractures, especially distal fractures.

M. F. Swiontkowski, MD

A Comparison of Locked Versus Nonlocked Enders Rods for Length Unstable Pediatric Femoral Shaft Fractures

Ellis HB, Ho CA, Podeszwa DA, et al (Steadman Philippon Sports Medicine Fellowship, Vail, CO; Univ of Texas Southwestern, Dallas)
J Pediatr Orthop 31:825-833, 2011

Background.—Stainless steel flexible Enders rods have been used for intramedullary fixation of pediatric femur fractures with good success. Despite intraoperative anatomic alignment, length unstable femur fractures can present postoperatively with fracture shortening. The purpose of this study was to review all length unstable pediatric femoral shaft fractures in which Enders rods were used and compare those that were locked to those that were not locked.

Methods.—A retrospective clinical and radiographic review of all patients at a single institution undergoing flexible intramedullary fixation for length unstable femoral shaft fractures from 2001 to 2008. A length unstable fracture was defined as either a comminuted fracture or a spiral fracture longer than twice the diameter of the femoral shaft. A total of 107 length unstable femoral shaft fractures fixed with Enders rods were identified, of which 37 cases (35%) had both Enders rods "locked" through the eyelet in the distal femur with a 2.7 mm fully threaded cortical screw. Patient demographics, clinical course, complications, fracture characteristics, and radiographic outcomes were compared for the locked and nonlocked groups.

Results.—There were no statistical differences between the groups in demographic data, operative variables, fracture pattern, fracture location, time to union, femoral alignment, or major complications. Shortening of the femur and nail migration measured at 1 to 6 weeks postoperatively was significantly greater for the nonlocked cases. The medial and lateral locked Enders rods moved 1.3 and 1.9 mm, respectively, and the unlocked Enders each moved 12.1 mm ($P < 0.05$). At final follow-up there were significantly more ($P < 0.05$) clinical complaints in nonlocked group, including limp, clinical shortening, and painful palpable rods.

Conclusions.—Locking Enders rods for length unstable pediatric fractures is an excellent option to prevent shortening and resulted in no additional complications, added surgical time, or increased blood loss.

Level of Evidence.—Level III (Tables 2 and 4).

▶ Flexible nails have generally been used for pediatric femoral shaft fractures that are length stable. This is a large retrospective cohort study that compares 2 cohorts of children with length-unstable femoral shaft fractures, 1 in which screws were placed through the eyelet of the Enders nails to prevent back out and 1 in which this was not done. The cohorts are relatively comparable, but the outcomes are not (Tables 2 and 4). It must be noted that Enders nails are one of the only flexible implants in which screws can be used to control implant backout and prevent fracture shortening. Other types of flexible implants should be restricted to use with length-stable (transverse and short oblique patterns) femoral fracture patterns. It seems safe to conclude from this study that Enders

TABLE 2.—Results After First Follow-up and Fracture Union

	Unlocked Enders	Locked Enders Group	P
Fracture shortening (mm)	12	4.75	$P < 0.0001$
Union alignment (degrees)			
Coronal plane (valgus)	3.2	1.7	$P = 0.17$
Sagittal plane (anterior)	4	3.3	$P = 0.53$
Change of position of enders nail (mm)			
Medial	12.08	1.32	$P \leq 0.0001$
Lateral	12.07	1.89	$P \leq 0.0001$

TABLE 4.—Clinical Observations (Minor Complications)

	Unlocked Enders	Locked Enders Group	P
Palpable/prominent hardware	8	2	
Limp	5	0	
Leg length discrepancy	5	0	
Rotational alignment	2	0	
Knee stiffness	3	0	
Knee effusion	0	1	
Total	23	3	0.03

nails can be used for length-unstable femoral shaft fracture patterns in children as long as screws are placed through the eyelets of the nails.

M. F. Swiontkowski, MD

Calcaneus Fractures

Comparison of Percutaneous Screw Fixation and Calcium Sulfate Cement Grafting Versus Open Treatment of Displaced Intra-Articular Calcaneal Fractures

Chen L, Zhang G, Hong J, et al (The Second Affiliated Hosp of Wenzhou Med College, Wenzhou Zhejiang Province, China; et al)
Foot Ankle Int 32:979-985, 2011

Background.—The conventional treatment for displaced intra-articular fractures of the calcaneus (DIACF), with open reduction and internal plate fixation (ORIF), carries the risk of wound infection and delayed recovery. Alternatively percutaneous fixation techniques offer the possibility of equivalent outcomes with a reduction in soft tissue complications. The goal of the present study was to evaluate the outcome of percutaneous reduction (PR), screw fixation, and calcium sulphate cement (CSC) grafting in the treatment of DIACF.

Methods.—Ninety patients were randomly assigned to PR and CSC grafting or ORIF between January 2006 and August 2008. The blood loss, Böhler's angle, calcaneal width, length, height and articular congruity of the posterior facet, wound complication, range of joint motion were compared, function scores such as American Orthopaedic Foot and Ankle Society score (AOFAS) and Maryland foot score (MFS) were measured.

Results.—The quality of reduction was not significantly different between the two groups. There were significant differences favoring PR in blood loss ($p < 0.01$), range of joint motion ($p < 0.01$), AOFAS ($p < 0.01$) and MFS ($p < 0.01$) between the two groups. Postop infection was 12% ORIF and 3% PC ($p = 0.23$). Earlier weightbearing in the PR group did not result in a greater frequency of redisplacement than in the OR group.

Conclusion.—Our results indicate that compared with ORIF, the percutaneous reduction, fixation and CSC grafting for treatment of DIACF

TABLE 2.—Clinical Outcomes

	ORIF (Average)	PR+CSC (Average)	P
Blood loss (ml) (mean ± SD)	75 ± 21	9 ± 3	<0.01
Bohler's injury (°)	1.4	1.5	0.98
Bohler's postoperatively (°)	30.6	32.1	0.04
Δ Bohler's (°)	29.1	30.1	0.34
Bohler's–healed (°)	28.9	30.4	0.04
Δ Bohler's at healing (°)	1.7	1.7	0.84
Reduction of calcaneus width (mm)	−2.7	−2.8	0.61
Change in calcaneal length (mm)	6.7	7.0	0.28
Infection	5/40	1/38	0.23
AOFAS (max. 100)	85.8	91.7	<0.01
MFS (max. 100)	86.0	91.5	<0.01
Subtalar joint range of motion (°)	25.5	31.7	<0.01
Ankle joint range of motion (°)	50.5	52.2	<0.01

AOFAS, American Orthopaedic Foot and Ankle Society score. MFS, Maryland foot score. Radiological followup data at the time of trauma, immediate postoperatively, and 2 years after the surgery.

might allow accelerated weightbearing activity, reduce joint stiffness and improve the patients' satisfaction (Table 2).

▶ This is a well-done randomized, controlled trial comparing percutaneous reduction and screw fixation techniques with open reduction and internal plate fixation (ORIF) for displaced intra-articular joint depression–type fractures. The radiographic outcomes were clearly better with ORIF, but that was the only measure with better outcomes. Percutaneous reduction and screw fixation with calcium phosphate cementation of the defect had clinically important lower rates of infection and better functional outcomes. Surgeon skill and experience is an important variable for both techniques, and some would argue that the high level of wound complication is indicative of lower levels of surgeon experience. It may also indicate detection bias, as there are no details about how this determination was made. Either way this is an important study that should push us to continued evaluation of percutaneous reduction and fixation techniques to lower patient morbidity and improve functional outcomes.

M. F. Swiontkowski, MD

Pelvic and Acetabular Fracture

Survivorship of the native hip joint after percutaneous repair of acetabular fractures in the elderly

Gary JL, Lefaivre KA, Gerold F, et al (Univ of Texas Southwestern Med School, Dallas; Univ of British Columbia, Vancouver, Canada)
Injury 42:1144-1151, 2011

Our purpose was to examine survivorship of the native hip joint in patients ages 60 and over who underwent percutaneous reduction and fixation of acetabular fractures. A retrospective review at a University Level I

Trauma Center was performed. Our institutional trauma database was reviewed. Patients aged 60 or older treated with percutaneous reduction and fixation of acetabular fractures between 1994 and 2007 were selected. 79 consecutive patients with 80 fractures were identified. Rate of conversion to total hip arthroplasty were used to construct a Kaplan—Meier curve showing survivorship of the native hip joint after treatment. 75 fractures had adequate clinical follow-up with a mean of 3.9 years (range 0.5—11.9 years). Average blood loss was 69 cc and there were no postoperative infections. 19/75 (25%) were converted to total hip arthroplasty at a mean time of 1.4 years after the index procedure. Survivorship analysis demonstrated a cumulative survival of 65% at 11.9 years of follow-up. There were no conversions to arthroplasty beyond 4.7 years postoperatively. There were no statistically significant associations between conversion to arthroplasty and age, sex, closed vs. limited open reduction, and simple vs. complex fracture pattern. Percutaneous fixation is a viable treatment option for patients age 60 or greater with acetabular fractures. Rates of conversion to total hip arthroplasty are comparable to open treatment methods and if conversion is required, soft tissues are preserved for future surgery (Figs 5 and 6, Table 2).

▶ This is a well-done survivorship study evaluating closed and limited open reduction and percutaneous fixation in patients older than 60. The longevity of this surgical approach was better in men than women but without statistical significance, likely related to the issue of osteoporosis. It appears that if posttraumatic arthritis has not progressed significantly in the first 16 to 18 months postoperatively, the patient's native hip will likely be retained with rare exception.

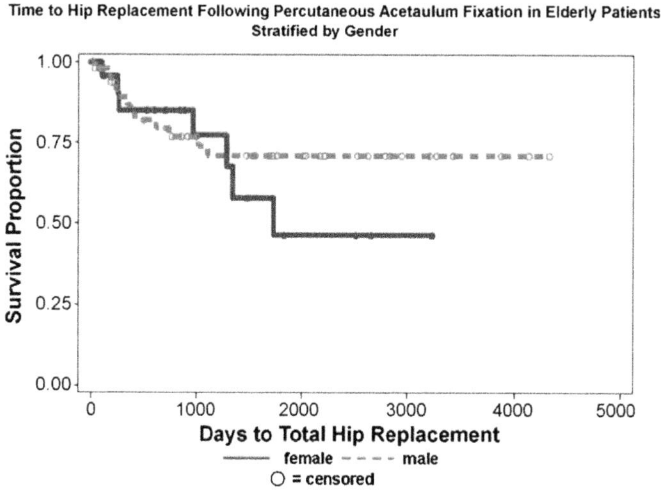

FIGURE 5.—Survivorship of native hip joint after percutaneous acetabular fixation: stratified by gender. (Reprinted from Gary JL, Lefaivre KA, Gerold F, et al. Survivorship of the native hip joint after percutaneous repair of acetabular fractures in the elderly. *Injury*. 2011;42:1144-1151, with permission from Elsevier.)

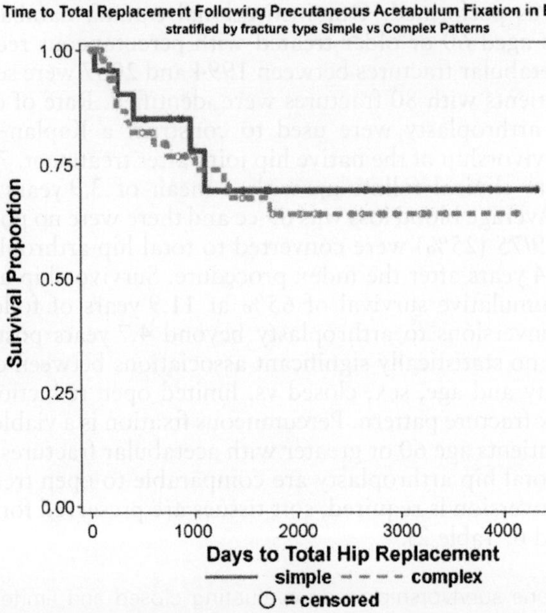

FIGURE 6.—Survivorship of native hip joint after percutaneous acetabular fixation: stratified by complex vs. simple fracture pattern. (Reprinted from Gary JL, Lefaivre KA, Gerold F, et al. Survivorship of the native hip joint after percutaneous repair of acetabular fractures in the elderly. *Injury.* 2011;42:1144-1151, with permission from Elsevier.)

TABLE 2.—Conversion to Total Hip Arthroplasty by Fracture Pattern

Fracture Patterns	Number	# Total Hip	% Total Hip
Anterior column	13	1	7.7
Posterior column	1	0	0
Posterior wall	3	2	66.7
Anterior wall	1	0	0
Transverse	5	2	40.0
Anterior column with posterior hemitransverse	17	4	23.5
Both column	28	6	21.4
T-type	7	2	28.6
Transverse posterior walls	5	2	40.0

There is a trend toward complex patterns having a higher risk of earlier conversion to total hip resurfacing arthroplasty than simple patterns, as expected. This is a highly experienced center with high volumes—these results should be applicable to other centers/surgeons.

M. F. Swiontkowski, MD

Immediate Full Weightbearing After Percutaneous Fixation of Anterior Column Acetabulum Fractures

Kazemi N, Archdeacon MT (Univ of Cincinnati, OH)

J Orthop Trauma 26:73-79, 2012

Objective.—To present clinical, radiographic, and functional outcomes of patients allowed immediate full weightbearing after closed reduction and percutaneous fixation of anterior column component acetabulum fractures.

Design.—Retrospective review.

Setting.—Academic Level I trauma center.

Patients.—Between September 2001 and December 2008, 28 patients with anterior column or anterior column posterior hemitransverse acetabulum fractures that were determined to be amenable to percutaneous fixation (at the discretion of the senior author [M.T.A.]) were selected.

Intervention.—All patients underwent closed reduction and anterior to posterior supra-acetabular percutaneous screw fixation followed by immediate postoperative full weightbearing.

Main Outcome Measurements.—Primary outcome measures included clinical, radiographic, and functional outcomes assessed with the modified Merle d'Aubigne Score and the Short Musculoskeletal Function Assessment questionnaire.

Results.—Six patients were lost to follow-up (less than 1 year), and the remaining 22 (79%) had a mean follow-up of 39 months (range, 12–74 months). There were no intraoperative complications. Radiographic grades were excellent in 19 patients, good in two patients, and fair in one patient. The mean modified Merle d'Aubigné Score was 17.4 (range, 11–18). The mean Short Musculoskeletal Function Assessment function and bothersome index were 20.2 (range, 0–72.8) and 20.1 (range, 0–72.9), respectively.

Conclusion.—Clinical, radiographic, and functional outcomes of patients in this study are comparable to other reported studies. Despite an immediate full weightbearing protocol, complications, particularly poor final radiographic grade, do not appear common. The advantage of this protocol lies in the ability to immediately ambulate postoperatively with early return to work and recreation. We believe this technique is safe and offers a reasonable alternative for anterior column acetabulum fractures.

▶ The subject of postoperative weight-bearing limitation has been understudied in the orthopedic trauma clinical research environment. Here is a cohort study in which patient weight bearing was allowed to progress as tolerated in a series of patients with anterior column acetabular fractures. The majority of the fractures were nondisplaced or minimally displaced, and the percutaneous screw fixation probably provided the assurance to the authors that progressive weight bearing was of minimal risk to the patients. One wonders in how many situations in which we limit patient postoperative weight bearing for 6 to 8 weeks would the findings be similar!

M. F. Swiontkowski, MD

Percutaneous screw fixation for the acetabular fracture with quadrilateral plate involved by three-dimensional fluoroscopy navigation: Surgical technique

Ruan Z, Luo C-F, Zeng B-F, et al (Shanghai Jiao Tong Univ, China)
Injury 43:517-521, 2012

Background.—The percutaneous three-dimensional (3D)-fluoroscopic-navigated screw directing to the quadrilateral plate was attempted.

Materials and Methods.—Five patients with acetabular fractures were treated by 3D navigated percutaneous screw. The quadrilateral plate was involved in all the patients. The Arcadis 3D (ARCADIS Orbic 3D®; Siemens AG Healthcare Sector, Erlangen, Germany) and computer navigation system (stryker navigation system) were employed, screwing trajectory was attempted to anchor the quadrilateral plate perpendicularly to the

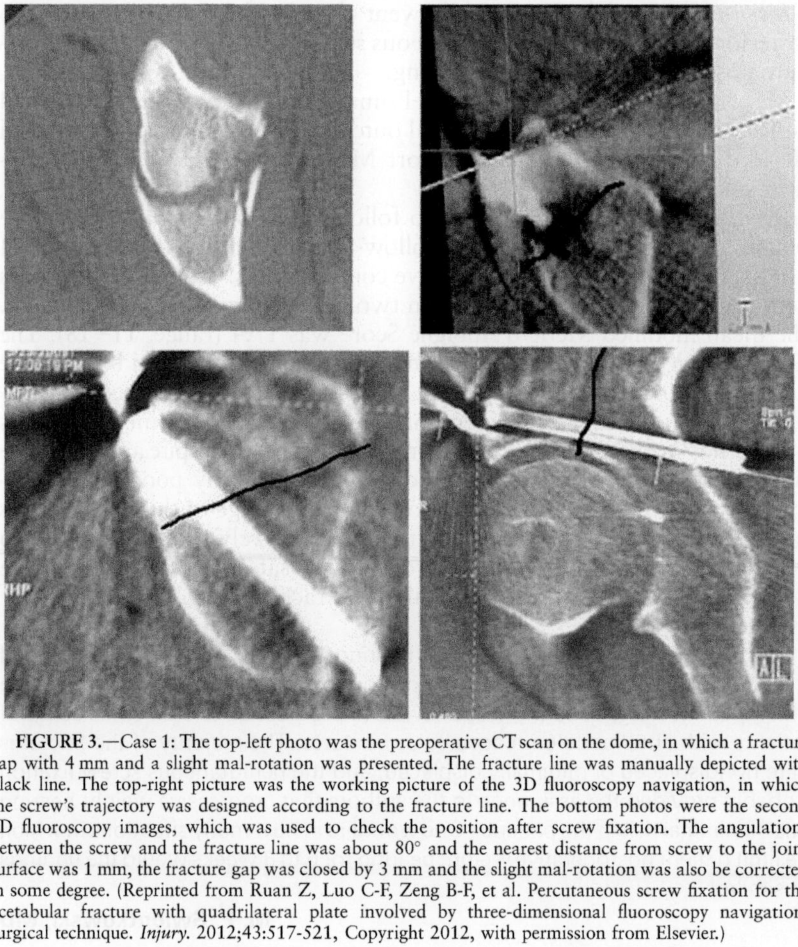

FIGURE 3.—Case 1: The top-left photo was the preoperative CT scan on the dome, in which a fracture gap with 4 mm and a slight mal-rotation was presented. The fracture line was manually depicted with black line. The top-right picture was the working picture of the 3D fluoroscopy navigation, in which the screw's trajectory was designed according to the fracture line. The bottom photos were the second 3D fluoroscopy images, which was used to check the position after screw fixation. The angulations between the screw and the fracture line was about 80° and the nearest distance from screw to the joint surface was 1 mm, the fracture gap was closed by 3 mm and the slight mal-rotation was also be corrected in some degree. (Reprinted from Ruan Z, Luo C-F, Zeng B-F, et al. Percutaneous screw fixation for the acetabular fracture with quadrilateral plate involved by three-dimensional fluoroscopy navigation: surgical technique. *Injury.* 2012;43:517-521, Copyright 2012, with permission from Elsevier.)

fracture line and close to the joint cartilage as much as possible. Parameters including fracture gap closure (P1), distance to the joint cartilage (P2), angulations between the screw and the fracture line (P3), were measured with the software installed on the machine of Arcadis 3D.

Result.—Seven screws were inserted with the use of 3D fluoroscopic navigation. The quadrilateral plate was hold by percutaneous screws. The closure of fracture gap was achieved in 3 patients by 2–3 mm. The nearest distance from the screw to the joint cartilage was ranged from <1 mm to 6 mm. The angulations between the screw and the fracture line was 80–90° in three patients, it was 60° and 65° respectively on the rest two patients. All patients felt pain free 1 week after the operation. No complication was noted postoperatively.

Conclusion.—The surgical technique of percutaneous screwing for the acetabular fracture with three-dimensional fluoroscopy-based navigation was demonstrated (Fig 3).

▶ There is much interest in intraoperative surgical navigation systems used with limited exposure surgery to improve patient functional outcomes. Acetabular surgery is no exception. This small cohort series shows what is possible. Whether these patients needed surgery to improve outcome is not answered by this study. Longer-term and better designed trials are needed to appropriately clarify the role of this technology in acetabular fracture surgery.

M. F. Swiontkowski, MD

Functional Outcomes in Elderly Patients With Acetabular Fractures Treated With Minimally Invasive Reduction and Percutaneous Fixation

Gary JL, Vanhal M, Gibbons SD, et al (Univ of Texas Southwestern Med School, Houston)

J Orthop Trauma 26:278-283, 2012

Objectives.—To present the functional outcomes of elderly patients treated with percutaneous acetabular surgery and compare them with those treated with traditional open reduction and internal fixation in previously published series.

Design.—Retrospective.

Setting.—University level I trauma center.

Patients.—All patients aged 60 and older treated with percutaneous screw fixation for acetabular fractures from 1994 to 2007 were included. Seventy-nine consecutive patients were identified. Thirty-six patients died before functional outcomes were obtained, leaving 43 patients and fractures in our study group. Functional outcomes were obtained in 35 of 43 (81.3%) patients at an average of 6.8 years after the index surgery.

Intervention.—Minimally invasive reduction and percutaneous fixation of acetabular fractures.

Main Outcome Measurement.—Short musculoskeletal functional assessment and Harris Hip Score.

Results.—One-year mortality was 13.9% (11 of 79). Average short musculoskeletal functional assessment dysfunction and bother indices were 23.3 and 21.3, respectively, in 24 patients who maintained their native hip. When compared with Short Musculoskeletal Functional Assessment data from 2 other series of patients treated with formal open reduction and internal fixation, no differences existed in the dysfunction ($P = 0.49$) or bother ($P = 0.55$) indices. Conversion to total hip arthroplasty occurred in 11 of 36 patients (30.6%). Average Harris Hip Scores in patients with their native hip was 77 (range, 33–100). In the 11 patients converted to total hip arthroplasty, average Short Musculoskeletal Functional Assessment dysfunction and bother indices were 24.3 and 23.9, respectively. No differences were found in the dysfunction ($P = 0.93$) or bother ($P = 0.16$) indices when compared with patients converted from open reduction and internal fixation to total hip arthroplasty. Average Harris Hip Score in patients converted to total hip arthroplasty was 83 (range, 68–92), and this was not significantly different from the best scores reported with acute total hip arthroplasty.

Conclusions.—Functional outcomes and rates of conversion to total hip arthroplasty of acetabular fractures in elderly patients treated with percutaneous reduction and fixation show no significant differences when compared with published series of patients treated with formal open reduction and internal fixation.

Level of Evidence.—Therapeutic Level IV. See Instructions for Authors for a complete description of levels of evidence (Table 3).

▶ Percutaneous acetabular fracture surgery, particularly for the older patients, has been an area of interest for the orthopedic trauma community for a decade. Concerns have centered around the lack of accuracy of reduction, leading to inferior long-term outcomes. This carefully done retrospective analysis assures us that these outcomes are at least equivalent to open approaches and that conversion to total hip arthroplasty leads to an acceptable long-term result (Table 3). For centers where there is surgical commitment to focus on percutaneous reduction and fixation techniques for acetabular fractures in the older

TABLE 3.—Analysis of Variance Comparing SMFA Outcomes Between 2 Subgroups and Population Norms for Patients >60 Years Old

	Native Hip (n = 24)		Delayed THA (n = 11)		Population Norms (Age >60 Years)		
	Average	SD	Average	SD	Average	SD	*P*
Function index	23.3	19.6	24.3	15.4	18.9	17.4	0.31
Bother index	21.3	21.5	23.9	19.4	18.5	19.3	0.54
Daily activities	29.9	29.3	22.7	18.5	20.2	22.5	0.12
Emotional status	24.3	19.0	32.5	19.1	23.3	17.7	0.23
Arm and hand function	8.7	13.8	13.6	15.5	10.7	15.3	0.67
Mobility	28.2	23.7	29.0	14.7	21.7	20.6	0.17

THA, total hip arthroplasty.

patient, this article adds reassurance that the efforts are not harming patients in the long term.

M. F. Swiontkowski, MD

Functional Outcomes in Women After High-Energy Pelvic Ring Injury

Vallier HA, Cureton BA, Schubeck D, et al (Metro Health Med Ctr, Cleveland, OH)
J Orthop Trauma 26:296-301, 2012

Objectives.—Residual dysfunction after pelvic trauma has been previously described, but limited functional outcome data are available in the female population after high-energy pelvic ring injury. The purposes of this study were to determine functional outcomes and to characterize factors predictive of outcome.

Design.—Prospective collection of functional outcomes data.

Setting.—Level I trauma center.

Patients/Participants.—Eighty-seven women with mean age of 33.5 years and mean Injury Severity Score of 23.1 were included. The Orthopaedic Trauma Association classification included 32 B-type and 55 C-type fractures. Four were open fractures and six had bladder ruptures.

Intervention.—Forty-nine patients were treated operatively and 38 nonoperatively.

Main Outcome Measurements.—Musculoskeletal Functional Assessment (MFA) questionnaires were completed after a minimum of 16 months and a mean of 41 months of follow-up.

Results.—The mean MFA score was 33. Only 15 women (17.2%) had MFA scores comparable with an uninjured reference value (9.3), and 34 (39.1%) had better than the reference value for prior hip injury (25.5). Anteroposterior compression injuries had worse scores versus other patterns (48.3 vs 31.0, $P = 0.01$), and trends toward worse outcomes were noted after symphyseal disruption ($P = 0.11$) and transsymphyseal plating ($P = 0.09$). Sacral fracture or sacroiliac injury, amount of initial or final displacement, and type of posterior ring treatment were not associated with MFA scores. Mean scores were 32.3 after surgery and 34.0 after nonoperative management ($P = 0.67$). Functional outcomes were not related to age or Injury Severity Score, but isolated pelvis fractures had better MFA scores (21.1 vs 35.5, $P = 0.008$) and worse MFA scores (41.7 vs 29.1, $P = 0.004$) were seen with other lower extremity fractures. Those with bladder ruptures ($n = 6$) also had poor outcomes, mean MFA 50.0 ($P = 0.078$).

Conclusions.—Wide variation is seen in functional outcome of women after high-energy pelvic ring fracture as measured by the MFA with mean scores demonstrating substantial residual dysfunction. Better outcomes were noted after isolated fractures and in women who had not sustained other fractures in their lower extremities. History of bladder rupture or anteroposterior compression injury was associated with poor MFA scores.

TABLE 3.—Functional Outcomes After Pelvic Ring Injury*

	MFA Score	*P*
Fracture classification		
B-type fractures (n = 32)	34.3	0.68 versus C-type
C-type fractures (n = 55)	32.2	
APC (n = 12)	48.3	0.01 versus non-APC
LC (n = 57)	32.9	
VS (n = 9)	23.3	
CMI (n = 9)	26.4	
Open fracture (n = 4)	40.3	0.48 versus closed fracture
Closed fracture (n = 83)	31.8	
Bladder rupture (n = 6)	50.0	0.078 versus intact bladder
Symphysis disruption (n = 28)	38.2	0.11 versus intact symphysis
Sacral fracture (n = 58)	32.3	0.89 versus intact sacrum
Sacroiliac joint dislocation (n = 34)	36.7	0.27 versus intact SI joint
Nonoperative (n = 38)	34.0	0.67 versus operative
Operative (n = 49)	32.3	
Age		0.40 over all groups
Younger than 26 years (n = 42)	30.3	
26–35 years (n = 15)	28.1	
36–45 years (n = 19)	40.8	
Older than 45 years (n = 9)	40.1	
Injury Severity Score		0.21 over all groups
Less than 18 (n = 22)	32.1	
Less than 20 (n = 37)	33.0	
Less than 25 (n = 51)	33.3	
25 or greater (n = 36)	32.2	
Isolated pelvic ring injury (n = 15)	21.1	0.008 versus multiple injury
Associated lower extremity fracture (n = 27)	41.7	0.004 versus no lower extremity fracture

APC, anteroposterior compression; LC, lateral compression; VS, vertical shear; CMI, combined mechanism of injury; SI, sacroiliac.

Editor's Note: Please refer to original journal article for full references.

*Eighty-seven patients completed questionnaires with a mean Musculoskeletal Functional Assessment (MFA) score of 33 for all patients. Fractures were classified according to the Orthopaedic Trauma Association (OTA) classification and by the method of Young and Burgess.[29–31]

Level of Evidence.—Prognostic Level IV. See Instructions for Authors for a complete description of levels of evidence (Table 3).

▶ Multiple cohort studies have indicated that pelvic fracture functional outcomes are highly variable and generally result in moderate to severe long-term functional deficits. This well-done outcome study focused on multiple outcomes in women who sustained pelvic fracture. The results as assessed by the Musculoskeletal Functional Assessment are in line with prior publications. Associated other injuries have the biggest impact toward worse functional outcomes. There are wide variations in outcome that probably relate to issues such as education, social support, income, health habits, and level of preinjury fitness. These factors have been identified in other studies, such as the Letrozole, Exemestane, and Anastrozole Pharmacodynamics trial, as heavily impacting the outcomes from severe musculoskeletal injury.

Our efforts should continue to be on prevention and on rehabilitation strategies and approaches after these types of injuries.

M. F. Swiontkowski, MD

Anterior Pelvic External Fixator Versus Subcutaneous Internal Fixator in the Treatment of Anterior Ring Pelvic Fractures

Cole PA, Gauger EM, Anavian J, et al (Univ of Minnesota–Regions Hosp, St Paul; Brown Univ, Providence, RI; et al)

J Orthop Trauma 26:269-277, 2012

Objectives.—To compare the short-term results of anterior pelvic external fixation (APEF) versus anterior pelvic internal fixation (APIF) applied subcutaneously in the context of surgical treatment of pelvic ring injuries.

Design.—A single center retrospective chart review.

Setting.—A level 1 trauma center.

Methods.—A consecutive series of 48 patients who underwent surgical stabilization of their anterior pelvic ring (24 utilizing APIF and 24 utilizing APEF) by 2 surgeons at a single hospital were studied. The choice to use either APEF or APIF was left up to each surgeon, the indications for use are the same. Data collected included surgical or postoperative complications including infection, implant failure, reoperation, documented surgical

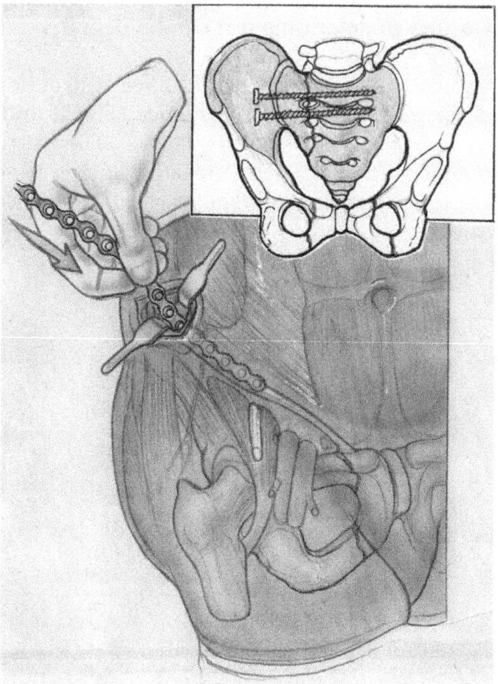

FIGURE 2.—Insertion of the reconstruction plates can be done by hand after creating a tunnel carefully above the external oblique muscle with a cob or periosteal surfer. The plate slides over the area of the conjoint tendon, well anterior to the neurovasculature below. The posterior pelvic ring must be either stable or stabilized as the primary consideration of treatment for pelvic ring injuries. (Reprinted from Cole PA, Gauger EM, Anavian J, et al. Anterior pelvic external fixator versus subcutaneous internal fixator in the treatment of anterior ring pelvic fractures. *J Orthop Trauma.* 2012;26:269-277, with permission from Lippincott Williams & Wilkins.)

site pain persisting to clinical follow-up visits, and radiographic union. Measurements on inlet and outlet pelvic radiographs were made immediately postoperation and at all follow-up clinic visits to determine whether there were differences in maintaining pelvic fracture reduction. Statistical analysis was performed to evaluate significant differences between the 2 groups with regard to each of these variables.

Results.—The APIF group was found to have a significantly lower incidence of wound complication ($P < 0.05$) and a lower occurrence of associated morbidity events as compared with the APEF group. In addition, the APIF group was found to have a significantly lower rate of surgical site pain persisting through all clinical follow-up intervals ($P = 0.05$). There was no difference between the 2 groups in terms of maintenance of pelvic reduction in the early postoperative phase or at final follow-up. No other significant differences were observed between the 2 groups.

Conclusions.—The present study, which was based on our initial experience with the subcutaneous anterior pelvic fixator, demonstrated encouraging clinical outcomes in terms of a lower wound complication rate and associated morbidity, and surgical site symptoms, although maintaining equivalent reduction. These findings suggest that further analysis of this technique is warranted to determine if it can be definitively recommended for general use.

Level of Evidence.—Therapeutic Level III. See Instructions for Authors for a complete description of levels of evidence (Figs 2 and 3, Table 3).

▶ This relatively new concept of "internal/external" pelvic fixation for anterior pelvic ring disruption is appealing on multiple levels, the most important of

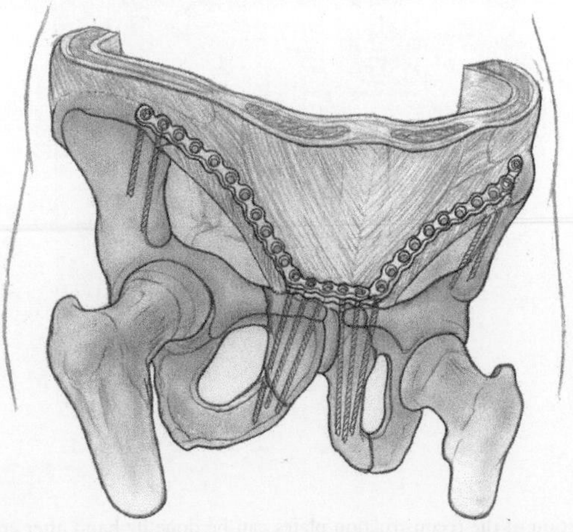

FIGURE 3.—The final construct for bilateral APIF with the plates overlapping in the midline. Screws are placed through both plates into the pubic rami for increased stability. This slightly oblique view demonstrates the curvature of the plates, leaving at least a few millimeters between the plate and the inguinal ligament so that there is no compression through this region. (Reprinted from Cole PA, Gauger EM, Anavian J, et al. Anterior pelvic external fixator versus subcutaneous internal fixator in the treatment of anterior ring pelvic fractures. *J Orthop Trauma*. 2012;26:269-277, with permission from Lippincott Williams & Wilkins.)

TABLE 3.—Incidence of Complication and Increased Morbidity

	APIF, n (%)	APEF, n (%)
Complications		
Surgical wound/pin site infection	1 (4)	6 (25)
Loss of fixation	0 (0)	3 (12)
Loosening of implants	0 (0)	1 (4)
Any of the above*	1 (4)	9 (38)
Morbidity		
Admission to hospital	0 (0)	2 (8)
Nonroutine clinic visit	1 (4)	1 (4)
Emergency department visit	1 (4)	1 (4)
Premature removal of hardware	0 (0)	1 (4)
Any of the above	1 (4)	5 (21)

*$P < 0.05$, Fisher exact test.

which are patient acceptance and lack of pin track problems. Although it is clearly a technique that requires more invasive dissection and surgical experience, the advantages clearly outweigh these disadvantages in experienced hands. This is obviously not a technique for an inexperienced pelvic fracture surgeon, and perhaps the reason why the complication rate for pelvic ex fix is so high is that it has been thought of as a technique for first-line trauma surgeons. This technique is one that should be studied with greater levels of scrutiny in multicenter randomized controlled trial studies.

M. F. Swiontkowski, MD

Quality of Radiographic Reduction and Perioperative Complications for Transverse Acetabular Fractures Treated by the Kocher-Langenbeck Approach: Prone Versus Lateral Position

Collinge C, Archdeacon M, Sagi HC (Harris Methodist Fort Worth Hosp/John Peter Smith Orthopedic Surgery Residency, Fort Worth, TX; Univ of Cincinnati, OH; Tampa General Hosp/Florida Orthopedic Inst)

J Orthop Trauma 25:538-542, 2011

Objective.—To compare radiographic reduction, intraoperative factors, and perioperative complications for transversely oriented acetabular fractures treated by the Kocher-Langenbeck approach with the patient in either the prone or lateral position.

Design.—Retrospective study.

Setting.—Two regional referral trauma centers.

Participants.—Sixty-six skeletally mature individuals with transversely oriented acetabular fractures treated operatively through the Kocher-Langenbeck approach in either the prone or lateral position.

Intervention.—Operative fixation of an acute transverse acetabular fracture through the Kocher-Langenbeck approach.

Main Outcome Measures.—This study primarily assessed the radiographic reduction of two similar consecutive cohorts of patients surgically treated for transversely oriented acetabular fractures using the Kocher-Langenbeck approach with the patient positioned in either the lateral or prone position. Secondary outcome measures included operative time, estimated blood loss, and perioperative complications.

Results.—Thirty-three transversely oriented acetabular fractures were reduced and stabilized with the patient in the lateral position, whereas 33 fractures were treated with the patient in the prone position. Demographic and injury variables as well as surgical time and estimated blood loss were similar between the two groups. Two postoperative infections occurred in each group, and one incomplete iatrogenic sciatic nerve palsy was recognized in the lateral group. The mean maximum fracture residual displacement measured on postoperative radiographs was 2.1 mm (range, 0–7 mm) in the lateral group compared with 1.3 mm (range, 0–7 mm) in the prone group ($P = 0.08$). The quality of reduction according to Matta's criteria was graded in prone positioned patients as anatomic in 20 patients (61%), imperfect in 11 patients (33%), and poor in two patients (6%), whereas lateral-positioned patients were graded as anatomic in 14 patients (42%), imperfect in 13 patients (40%), and poor in six (18%) patients ($P = 0.21$).

Discussion and Conclusion.—This study demonstrated a trend toward higher radiographic residual fracture displacement in patients with transversely oriented acetabular fractures reduced and stabilized through the Kocher-Langenbeck approach in the lateral position compared with those positioned prone. However, no significant differences were observed in operative time, estimated blood loss, or perioperative complications between the two groups (Tables 1 and 2).

► This is an interesting comparative cohort study evaluating the clinical outcomes of transverse acetabular fractures treated with open reduction internal fixation in the prone versus lateral positions. This research design has issues with selection and detection bias that accompany its structure. It makes inherent sense that

TABLE 1.—Summary of Patient and Injury Characteristics

Operative Position	Lateral (n = 33)	Prone (n = 33)	*P*
Mean age (years)	36.7 (range, 19–57)	38.1 (range, 20–59)	0.48
Gender (% male)	67	73	1.00
Body mass index[13]	30.9 (range, 22.1–47.9)	27.5 (range, 17–39.5)	0.30
Fracture pattern[1]			
Pure transverse	5	3	1.00
Transverse-PW	18	22	
T-type	10	8	
ASA Class			
I	1	0	1.00
II	12	14	
III	117	16	
IV	3	3	
Multiple system injuries (%)	64%	70%	0.18

PW, posterior wall; ASA, American Society of Anesthesiologists
Editor's Note: Please refer to original journal article for full references.

TABLE 2.—Summary of Clinical and Radiographic Results

	Lateral Position (n = 33)	Prone Position (n = 33)	*P*
Operative time (minutes)	263 (range, 160–472)	258 (range, 156–450)	0.82
Estimated blood loss (mL)	532 (range, 300–1500)	644 (range, 200–3000)	0.25
Complications (total)	3 (2 infections, 1 sciatic nerve palsy that recovered completely)	2 (2 infections)	N/A
Additional approaches	2	1	N/A
Mean postoperative residual radiographic displacement (mm)	2.1 (range, 0–7)	1.3 (range, 0–7)	0.08
Matta's radiographic grading[15] based on postoperative radiographs			
Anatomic (%)	41	60	0.24
Imperfect (%)	41	35	
Poor (%)	18	5	

Editor's Note: Please refer to original journal article for full references.

the lateral position would have higher residual displacement because the compression forces related to gravity have to be neutralized. The fact that there is no difference in blood loss, operative time, or complications confirms that the individual surgeon is a major factor in these outcomes, and these are expert acetabular surgeons. Given equivalent surgeon experience, the prone position is probably the best choice to address these fractures.

M. F. Swiontkowski, MD

Hip Fracture

Postoperative Opioid Consumption and Its Relationship to Cognitive Function in Older Adults with Hip Fracture

Sieber FE, Mears S, Lee H, et al (Johns Hopkins Bayview Med Ctr, Baltimore, MD)
J Am Geriatr Soc 59:2256-2262, 2011

Objectives.—To determine the relationship between opioid consumption and cognitive impairment after hip fracture repair.

Design.—Prospective study of consecutive patients.

Setting.—Johns Hopkins Bayview Medical Center, Baltimore, Maryland.

Participants.—Two hundred thirty-six participants aged 65 and older undergoing hip fracture repair.

Measurements.—Older adults without preoperative delirium who underwent hip fracture repair between April 2005 and July 2009 were followed for pain, opioid consumption, and postoperative delirium. Participants were tested for delirium using the Confusion Assessment Method preoperatively and midmorning on Postoperative Day 2. The nursing staff assessed pain on a numeric oral scale (range 0–10). Opioid analgesia was provided in response to pain at rest to achieve scores of 3 or less. Opioid consumption was analyzed with respect to the occurrence of incident postoperative delirium, presence of dementia, and other demographic variables.

Results.—Of the 236 participants, 66 (28%) had dementia, and 213 (90%) received opioids postoperatively, including 55 (83%) with dementia and 158 (93%) without. There was no association between the use of any postoperative opioid and incident delirium ($P = .61$) in participants with ($P = .33$) and without ($P = .40$) dementia. Dementia, but not postoperative delirium, was associated with less opioid use ($P < .001$ for dementia; $P = .12$ for delirium; $P = .04$, for their interaction; Wald chi-square = 142.8, $df = 7$). Opioid dose ($P \geq .59$) on Postoperative Days 1 and 2 was not predictive of incident delirium. Dementia ($P < .001$) and intensive care unit admission ($P = .006$), not opioid consumption, were the most important predictors of incident postoperative delirium.

Conclusion.—Concern for postoperative delirium should not prevent the use of opioid analgesic therapy sufficient to achieve a generally accepted

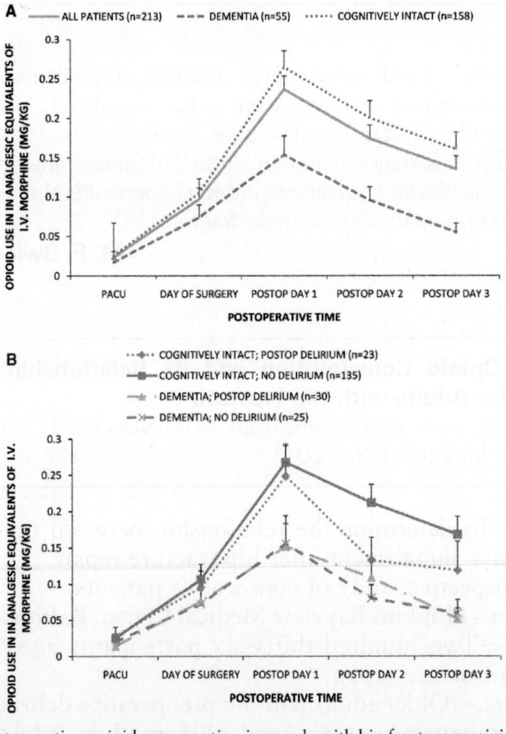

FIGURE 1.—Postoperative opioid consumption in people with hip fracture receiving any postoperative opioid: (A) with and without probable dementia (mean ± SE of the mean (SEM)). (B) as a function of probable dementia, postoperative delirium, neither, or both (mean ± SEM). In the total participant population, postoperative delirium was not associated with alterations in opioid consumption. As longitudinal analysis revealed, probable dementia, but not postoperative delirium, was associated with significantly less opioid use ($P < .001$ for dementia; $P = .12$ for delirium; $P = .04$, for their interaction; Wald chi-square = 142.8, $df = 7$). Furthermore, opioid dose ($P = .59$) on Postoperative Days 1 and 2 was not predictive of incident delirium. All opioids were converted to their analgesic equivalent of intravenous (i.v.) morphine sulfate, as described in the text. (Reprinted from Sieber FE, Mears S, Lee H, et al. Postoperative opioid consumption and its relationship to cognitive function in older adults with hip fracture. *J Am Geriatr Soc.* 2011;59:2256-2262, with permission from The American Geriatrics Society.)

TABLE 3.—Postoperative Factors

Factor	Overall (N = 236)	Probable Dementia No (n = 170)	Probable Dementia Yes (n = 66)	*P*-Value¶	Delirium No (n = 176)	Delirium Yes (n = 60)	*P*-Value¶
Receiving any opioids, n (%)	213 (90)	158 (93)	55 (83)	**.047**	160 (91)	53 (88)	.61
Using patient-controlled analgesia, n (%)	60 (25.4)	50 (29.4)	10 (15.2)	**.03**	54 (30.7)	6 (10.0)	**.001**
Opioid dose, cumulative for PACU through POD-3 (morphine equivalents, mg/kg), mean ± SD*	0.62 ± 0.77	0.71 ± 0.82	0.36 ± 0.55	**.005**	0.66 ± 0.82	0.49 ± 0.59	.18
Pain averaged over POD0 to POD3 (range 0–10), mean ±SD	2.4 ± 1.9	2.7 ± 1.9	1.5 ± 1.8	**<.001**	2.6 ± 1.9	1.7 ± 1.8	**.007**
Severe pain (>6/10), n (%)	29 (12.3)	24 (14.1)	5 (7.6)	.19	24 (13.6)	5 (8.3)	.36
Admitted to ICU, n (%)	53 (22.5)	35 (20.6)	18 (27.3)	.30	31 (17.6)	22 (36.7)	**.004**
Stay in ICU, days, mean ± SD†	4.3 ± 4.8	4.3 ± 5.5	4.1 ± 3.2	.87	3.3 ± 2.5	5.7 ± 6.7	.07
Receiving erythrocyte transfusion, n (%)	136 (57.6)	94 (55.3)	42 (63.6)	.30	96 (54.5)	40 (66.7)	.13
Erythrocytes transfusion (units of packed erythrocytes), mean ± SD†	1.9 ± 1.1	1.9 ± 1.1	1.8 ± 1.2	.77	1.8 ± 1.0	2.1 ± 1.4	.10
Experiencing infectious complications, n (%)‡	73 (30.9)	51 (30.0)	22 (33.3)	.64	49 (27.8)	24 (40.0)	.10
Experiencing cardiovascular complications, n (%) §	49 (20.8)	31 (18.2)	18 (27.3)	.15	27 (15.3)	22 (36.7)	**.001**

PACU = postanesthesia care unit; POD = postoperative day; SD = standard deviation.

*All opioids were converted to their equivalent dose of intravenous morphine sulfate using 100 µg of intravenous fentanyl, 2 mg of intravenous hydromorphone, and 30 mg of oral oxycodone as equivalent to 10 mg of intravenous morphine sulfate.[14,15]

†Averaged only over the subset of the population admitted to the intensive care unit (ICU) or receiving erythrocyte transfusion.

‡Infectious complications include urinary tract infection and pneumonia.

§Cardiovascular complications include congestive heart failure, myocardial infection, and new arrhythmia.

¶Mean ± SD for continuous data, median (lower quartile, upper quartile) for ordinal data, and number (percent of total) for frequency data. Values in bold indicate $P < 0.05$.

level of comfort in individuals with or without preexisting cognitive impairment (Fig 1, Table 3).

▶ This is a carefully done cohort study focused on the impact of narcotic use in hip fracture patients with and without cognitive impairment and its impact on delirium. The study does confirm that we are not as aggressive with narcotic use in patients with cognitive impairment compared with patients who are cognitively intact—this is an area deserving of further research, as it is conceivable that the lack of pain control in patients who are incapable of expressing themselves may lead to worse outcomes. The study reassures us that the use of narcotics does not prompt a higher incidence of delirium, which is the main take home point. This is not a subject that can be addressed in a controlled trial; therefore, this evidence should prompt us to be a little more liberal in the use of narcotics for pain control in patients with hip fracture.

M. F. Swiontkowski, MD

Less Invasive Stabilization System (LISS) Versus Proximal Femoral Nail Anti-Rotation (PFNA) in Treating Proximal Femoral Fractures: A Prospective Randomized study

Zhou F, Zhang ZS, Yang H, et al (Peking Univ Third Hosp, Beijing, China)
J Orthop Trauma 26:155-162, 2012

Objective.—To evaluate the outcome and efficacy of LISS (Less Invasive Stabilization System; Synthes USA, Paoli, PA) for the treatment of proximal femoral fractures to find another appropriate minimally invasive surgery for these fractures in which intramedullary nailing may be difficult.

Design.—A consecutive prospective randomized clinical study.

Setting.—University teaching hospital.

Patients.—Between May 2006 and March 2008, 64 consecutive patients who had a proximal femoral fracture were randomized to be treated with fixation with either LISS or PFNA (Proximal Femoral Nail Anti-rotation; Synthes USA).

Intervention.—LISS or PFNA fixation of proximal femoral fractures.

Main Outcome Measurements.—Intraoperative time, intraoperative blood loss, length of hospitalization, hip function (Harris score), general complications, fracture complications.

Results.—Fifty-nine patients were evaluated with a mean follow-up time of 26.8 months (range, 21–36 months). No statistical differences in general complications, intraoperative blood loss, length of hospitalization, or hip function could be found between the two groups. The average operative time was longer in the LISS group (98.25 minutes) compared with the PFNA group (65.36 minutes) ($P < 0.05$). One PFNA case had intrapelvic penetration of the helical blade; two LISS cases had breakage of the screws.

Conclusion.—There were no major differences in outcome or complications between the treatment groups. LISS can be used effectively in treating

TABLE 3.—Postoperative Data

	LISS	PFNA	P
Hospital stay (days)			
Average	7.61	10.33	0.457
Range	5–13	5–14	
General complications	5	5	
Fracture complications	2	1	
Hip function (Harris score)			
Average	86.04	84.09	0.247
Range	34–100	61–100	
Death	4	4	
In 1 month	1	2	
In 6 months	3	2	

LISS, Less Invasive Stabilization System; PFNA, Proximal Femoral Nail Anti-rotation.

proximal femoral fractures, especially for complex fractures patterns in which intramedullary nailing may be difficult.

Level of Evidence.—Therapeutic Level II. See page 128 for a complete description of levels of evidence (Table 3).

► This randomized, clinical study that compares intramedullary nailing fixation with locked plate fixation for proximal tibial fractures is likely underpowered to show significant differences in patient functional outcome and complication rates. However, it does show that the estimated blood loss and operative treatment are so similar that any significant differences would likely be clinically unimportant. The length of stay data reveal a significant difference in the way postoperative hip fracture patients are treated outside of North America. The take-home message from this study is that the surgeon is the major critical variable in terms of patient outcome and complications—the device may account for a small part of these results, but patient (fracture pattern and related bone quality) and surgeon factors account for at least 90% to 95% of the critical elements.

M. F. Swiontkowski, MD

Delayed Surgery for Patients With Femur and Hip Fractures—Risk of Deep Venous Thrombosis

Smith EB, Parvizi J, Purtill JJ (Rothman Inst of Orthopaedics at Thomas Jefferson Univ Hosp, Philadelphia, PA)
J Trauma 70:E113-E116, 2011

Background.—This prospective study explores the incidence of preoperative deep venous thrombosis (DVT) in a group of patients with hip and femur fracture who for various reasons experienced a delay of >24 hours from the time of injury until time of surgery. We also evaluated the results of preoperative treatment with inferior vena cava (IVC) filter.

Methods.—There were 101 consecutive patients with a mean age of 75.8 years. The mean time to surgery from injury was 3.5 days. All patients were evaluated for signs and symptoms of DVT and underwent Doppler ultrasound before surgery. All patients received preoperative prophylactic anticoagulation. Those patients with DVT underwent IVC filter insertion before surgical intervention.

Results.—No patient exhibited signs or symptoms of DVT; however, preoperative ultrasound detected DVT in 10 patients. Despite negative ultrasound, two additional patients developed pulmonary embolus preoperatively for an overall incidence of thromboembolic disease of 11.9%. The average delay in surgery was 5.7 days for patients with DVT versus 3.2 days for those without ($p = 0.021$). The incidence increased each day from 14.5% if surgery was delayed >1 day to 33.3% if surgery was delayed >7 days. Relative risk increased from 2.32 to 3.71 over the same period. There were no postoperative thromboembolic complications or complications related to IVC filter placement in these patients.

Discussion.—In this prospective study, we observed that patients experiencing a delay in surgical care for an acute hip or femur fracture are at a relatively high risk for development of thromboembolic disease despite prophylactic anticoagulation. There was a direct correlation between the period of delay and the incidence of thromboembolism. Clinical examination in this setting is unreliable as none of these patients had signs or symptoms suggestive of DVT. We suggest that all patients with delayed (>24 hours) surgical intervention undergo preoperative Doppler ultrasound to rule out DVT. Appropriate measures such as placement of an IVC filter and aggressive postoperative anticoagulation should then be implemented for those with DVT and/or pulmonary embolus (Table 1).

▶ Delay in operative stabilization for elderly patients with hip fracture has been shown in numerous retrospective cohort studies to increase morbidity and mortality. This prospective study focuses on the increased risk of deep venous thrombosis (DVT) with this delay. Routine Doppler ultrasound scan is a sound recommendation, based on this report, for patients delayed to the operating room more than 24 hours. The early complications with inferior vena cava filter were not apparent in this series; longer-term issues with these filters can occur

TABLE 1.—The Incidence and Relative Risk for Thromboembolic Disease Following an Acute Injury

Delay to Surgery (> No. of Days)	Incidence (%)	Relative Risk
1	14.5	2.32
2	17.0	2.72
3	17.1	2.72
4	23.8	1.89
5	27.8	3.30
6	26.7	2.87
7	33.3	3.71

and were not reported here. The report should serve to increase our vigilance for DVT in patients who are delayed to the operating room for stabilization of a hip fracture. In addition to vigilance, aggressive therapy should be considered in this circumstance.

M. F. Swiontkowski, MD

Gotfried Percutaneous Compression Plating Compared with Sliding Hip Screw Fixation of Intertrochanteric Hip Fractures: A Prospective Randomized Study

Yang E, Qureshi S, Trokhan S, et al (Elmhurst Hosp Ctr, NY; Mount Sinai School of Medicine, NY)

J Bone Joint Surg Am 93:942-947, 2011

Background.—The use of a Gotfried percutaneous compression plate provides a minimally invasive technique for the fixation of intertrochanteric proximal femoral fractures. The purpose of this study was to determine if the percutaneous compression plate provided advantages compared with the sliding hip screw for treatment of A1 and A2 AO/OTA intertrochanteric proximal femoral fractures.

Methods.—An institutional review board-approved, prospective, randomized, single-blinded study was conducted at a level-I trauma center between July 2004 and September 2007. All patients who met the study criteria and provided informed consent were randomized to treatment with a sliding hip screw or percutaneous compression plate. Of the sixty-six patients who consented to participate, thirty-three were randomized to be treated with a sliding hip screw and thirty-three, with a percutaneous compression plate. Data evaluated included surgical time, incision length, blood loss, need for blood transfusion, and postoperative functional status. Follow-up included clinical findings, radiographs until healing was confirmed, functional and pain assessment scores, and the Short Form-36. The median follow-up period for surviving patients was thirty-six months.

Results.—Sixty-six patients, forty-seven women and nineteen men, with a mean age of seventy-seven years were entered into the study. The treatment groups were similar with respect to study variables ($p > 0.05$). Operative times (forty-eight vs. seventy-eight minutes), incision length (56 vs. 82 mm), and blood loss (41 vs. 101 mL) significantly favored the percutaneous compression plate group ($p < 0.001$). The groups were similar immediately postoperatively; however, by discharge, fewer patients with a percutaneous compression plate required walking aids (40% vs. 59%). This trend continued throughout the study but was not significant. Pain with activity was lower throughout the study for the percutaneous compression plate group, but the difference was significant only at the three-month interval.

Conclusions.—Previously published reports showing shorter operative times and less blood loss with the percutaneous compression plate were reaffirmed. Compared with the sliding hip screw, the percutaneous compression plate resulted in a larger percentage of patients who were able to walk independently, consistently lower levels of pain with activity, and improved quality of life according to multiple scales of the Short Form-36, but the differences were not significant. Significant differences favoring the percutaneous compression plate were found with regard to operating times, incision length, and blood loss.

▶ This fairly well-done randomized clinical trial documents the clinical advantages of the Gottfried percutaneous plate in the management of patients with intertrochanteric fractures amenable to treatment with a sliding screw implant. The device has certain biomechanical differences compared with the standard sliding hip screw, which may explain the advantage demonstrated in early functional independence. The other parameters of blood loss, shorter operative times, and so on can be explained in part by detection bias and increased technical familiarity with the Gottfried implant. The lack of health-related quality-of-life differences between the 2 implants makes clinical sense. Patient factors likely outweigh the mechanical and perioperative value of the percutaneous application of the Gottfried device. Percutaneous application of the standard hip screw has been documented in other studies, and it is likely that in expert hands, those patient advantages would be negligible.

M. F. Swiontkowski, MD

Treatment of post-operative infections following proximal femoral fractures: Our institutional experience

Theodorides AA, Pollard TCB, Fishlock A, et al (Univ of Leeds, UK; Univ of Oxford, UK)

Injury 42:S28-S34, 2011

Proximal femoral fractures (PFFs) are a major health concern in the elderly population. Improvements made in implants and surgical techniques resulted in faster rehabilitation and shorter length of hospital stay. Despite this, the reduced physiological reserve, associated co-morbidities and polypharmacy intake of the elderly population put them at high risk of postoperative complications particularly of infectious origin.

Out of 10 061 patients with proximal femoral fractures 105 (1.05%) developed surgical site infection; 76 (72%) infections occurred in patients who had sustained intracapsular (IC) fractures with the remaining 29 (28%) infections occurring in patients with extracapsular (EC) neck of femur fractures. The median number of additional surgical debridements was 2 (range 1–7). MRSA was isolated in 49 (47%) of the cases; 38 patients (36%) ultimately underwent a Girdlestone's excisional arthroplasty.

Mortality at 30 days and 3 months was 10% and 31%, respectively. It was noted that post-operative hip infection predisposed to a prolonged

TABLE 4.—Mortality at 30 Days, 3 Months and 1 Year, From the Oxford Matched cohorts of 87 Infected and 162 Control Cases

Time Post Initial Fracture Surgery	Infected Case Mortality (%)	Control Case Mortality (%)	Odds Ratio	p-Value
30 days	9 (10)	18 (11)	0.92	1.0
3 months	26 (30)	34 (21)	1.61	0.12
1 year	37 (43)	57 (35)	1.36	0.28

TABLE 5.—Recently Published Studies Reporting on Infection and Mortality Rates Following Proximal Femoral Fractures

Authors	Year	Patients	Deep Wound Infection Rate N	(%)	Mortality Rate
Edwards et al.[19]	2008	3563	41	1.15	30% (12 mo)
Cumming and Parker[20]	2007	3180	26	0.82	33% (12 mo)
Partanen et al.[21]	2006	2276	25	1.10	34.5% (12 mo)
Johnston et al.[22]	2006	3571	25	0.70	28.2% (12 mo)
Roche et al.[23]	2005	2448	27	1.10	33% (12 mo)
Dorotka et al.[24]	2003	182	2	1.10	13.7% (6 mo)[a]
Varley and Milner[25]	1995	177	6	3.39	n/a

Editor's Note: Please refer to original journal article for full references.
[a]In patients operated within less than 18 h from the fracture.

length of stay in the acute unit and subsequently to a more dependent destination after discharge (Tables 4 and 5).

▶ This is a carefully analyzed hip fracture cohort study focused on the differential outcomes in patients who develop infections after hip fracture surgery and the differential outcomes compared with patients who do not develop infections. Although the percentages of mortality at 30 days and 1 year are higher in patients who develop infections than in those who do not, there is no statistical difference. The risk for infection after prosthetic replacement is greater than the risk after internal fixation, which is consistent with recent meta-analyses. The impact in terms of return to the operation room, use of resources, length of stay, and patient morbidity is substantial. Every effort should always be made to prevent these serious complications.

M. F. Swiontkowski, MD

Factors affecting the incidence of deep wound infection after hip fracture surgery

Harrison T, Robinson P, Cook A, et al (Peterborough City Hosp, UK)
J Bone Joint Surg Br 94-B:237-240, 2012

Prospective data on 6905 consecutive hip fracture patients at a district general hospital were analysed to identify the risk factors for the development of deep infection post-operatively. The main outcome measure was infection beneath the fascia lata.

A total of 50 patients (0.7%) had deep infection. Operations by consultants or a specialist hip fracture surgeon had half the rate of deep infection compared with junior grades ($p = 0.01$). Increased duration of anaesthesia was significantly associated with deep infection ($p = 0.01$). The method of fracture fixation was also significant. Intracapsular fractures treated with a hemiarthroplasty had seven times the rate of deep infection compared with those treated by internal fixation ($p = 0.001$). Extracapsular fractures treated with an extramedullary device had a deep infection rate of 0.78% compared with 0% for those treated with intramedullary devices ($p = 0.02$).

The management of hip fracture patients by a specialist hip fracture surgeon using appropriate fixation could significantly reduce the rate of

TABLE 1.—Influence of Factors on the Rate of Deep Sepsis After Hip Fracture Surgery (the Proforma on Which Data was Collected Evolved Over Time and Some Pieces of Information were Not Collected in Earlier Patients)

Factor	Deep Sepsis	No Deep Sepsis	Rate of Sepsis	p-Value
Mean age	81.3 (57 to 102)	79.9 (16 to 106)		0.36*
Mean pre-operative mobility†	3.8 (0 to 8)	3.6 (0 to 9)		0.64*
Mean pre-operative mental test score‡	5.2 (0 to 10)	5.5 (0 to 10)		0.64*
Mean pre-operative haemoglobin (g/dl)	12.7 (10.1 to 15.6)	12.4 (5.0 to 19.4)		0.25*
Gender (n)				
Male	11	1499	0.73%	1.00§
Female	39	5356	0.72%	
Residential status (n)				
Independent	37	5016	0.73%	0.87§
Institution	13	1839	0.70%	
Pathological (n)				
No	45	6233	0.72%	1.00§
Yes	1	191	0.52%	
ASA¶ grade (n)				
1 to 2	10	2277	0.44%	0.06§
3 to 4	36	4089	0.87%	
Fracture type (n)				
Intracapsular	25	3224	0.77%	0.25§
Extracapsular	13	2442	0.53%	
Mean duration of anaesthesia (min)	76.0 (30 to 380)	65.1 (45 to 150)		0.01*
Mean duration of surgery (min)	64.7 (15 to 300)	60.8 (35 to 135)		0.39*
Intracapsular fixation method (n)				
Hemi-arthroplasty	28	2202	1.26%	0.0001§
Internal fixation	3	1638	0.18%	
Extracapsular fixation method (n)				
Extramedullary	19	2411	0.78%	0.02§
Intramedullary	0	602	0.00%	

Editor's Note: Please refer to original journal article for full references.
*Student's *t*-test.
†Graded on a scale from 9 to 0, with 9 representing unimpaired mobility and 0 representing confined to bed[9].
‡Scored from 10 (highest) to 0 (lowest)[10].
§Fisher's exact test.
¶ASA, American Society of Anesthesiologists[8].

TABLE 2.—Comparison of the Grade of Operating Surgeon in Relation to Deep Infection

Grade of Operating Surgeon	Number of Deep Infection *Versus* no Deep Infection (% rate)	p-Value*
Consultant and specialist hip surgeon *vs* Junior surgeon	27/4862 (0.55%) *vs* 23/1979 (1.15%)	0.012
Consultant *vs* Specialist hip surgeon	1/394 (0.25%) *vs* 26/4468 (0.58%)	0.72
Specialist hip surgeon *vs* Junior surgeon	26/4468 (0.58%) *vs* 23/1979 (1.15%)	0.019
Consultant *vs* Junior surgeon	1/394 (0.25%) *vs* 23/1979 (1.15%)	0.17

*Fisher's exact test.

deep infection and associated morbidity, along with extended hospitalisation and associated costs (Tables 1 and 2).

▶ Deep infection after hip fracture surgery is a serious complication with increased risk for mortality. This database analysis of a large number of hip fracture patients with a variety of fracture patterns and surgical treatments informs us regarding the factors that play a role in increasing risk. Surgeon experience plays an important role, which is an issue to be dealt with in our orthopedic residency. This also speaks to the issues of limiting surgical exposure, prevention of devitalizing muscle, and preserving tissue planes—a greater focus on how well we perform these procedures contrasted with how fast we perform these procedures. The higher risk for deep infection following hemiarthroplasty contrasted with internal fixation is again confirmed in this analysis with a 7-fold greater risk. Intramedullary devices with percutaneous application appear to greatly limit the risk of deep infection following management of extracapsular fracture as well.

M. F. Swiontkowski, MD

Sliding hip screw *versus* the Targon PF nail in the treatment of trochanteric fractures of the hip: A randomised trial of 600 fractures

Parker MJ, Bowers TR, Pryor GA (Peterborough and Stamford Hosp NHS Foundation Trust, UK)

J Bone Joint Surg Br 94-B:391-397, 2012

In a randomised trial involving 598 patients with 600 trochanteric fractures of the hip, the fractures were treated with either a sliding hip screw (n = 300) or a Targon PF intramedullary nail (n = 300). The mean age of the patients was 82 years (26 to 104). All surviving patients were reviewed at one year with functional outcome assessed by a research nurse blinded to the treatment used. The intramedullary nail was found to have a slightly increased mean operative time (46 minutes (SD 12.3) *versus* 49 minutes (SD 12.7), $p < 0.001$) and an increased mean radiological screening time (0.3 minutes (SD 0.2) *versus* 0.5 minutes (SD 0.3), $p < 0.001$). Operative difficulties were more common with the intramedullary nail. There was no statistically significant difference between implants for wound healing

TABLE 2.—Operative Details

	Sliding Hip Screw	Targon PF Nail	p-Value
Mean (SD) length of anaesthesia (mins)	57 (12.3)	61 (13.7)	0.0008
Mean (SD) length of surgery (mins)	46 (12.3)	49 (12.7)	<0.0001
Mean (SD) x-ray screening time (mins)	0.3 (0.2)	0.5 (0.3)	<0.0001
Open reduction of fracture (n, %)	13 (*4*)	0	0.0002
Difficult proximal screw insertion (n, %)	3 (*1*)	17 (*6*)	0.002
Difficult distal locking (n, %)	0 (*0*)	39 (*13*)	<0.0001
Reaming of the femur (n, %)	0 (*0*)	4 (*1*)	0.12
Required blood transfusion (n, %)	99 (*33*)	100 (*33*)	1.0
Mean (SD) units blood transfused	0.64 (0.95)	0.70 (1.1)	0.46

complications ($p = 1$), or need for post-operative blood transfusion ($p = 1$), and medical complications were similarly distributed in both groups. There was a tendency to fewer revisions of fixation or conversion to an arthroplasty in the nail group, although the difference was not statistically significant (nine *versus* three cases, $p = 0.14$). The extent of shortening, loss of hip flexion, mortality and degree of residual pain were similar in both groups. The recovery of mobility was superior for those treated with the intramedullary nails ($p = 0.01$ at one year from injury).

In summary, both implants produced comparable results but there was a tendency to better return of mobility for those treated with the intramedullary nail (Table 2).

▶ This well-done randomized clinical trial (RCT) compares the use of the sliding hip screw with an intramedullary (IM) device in patients with trochanteric fracture. This trial confirms the results of other trials in that the technical difficulties with the IM implant are greater than the sliding hip screw. This is accompanied by greater imaging time and operating room time. However, these downsides may be offset by the better functional recovery in patients treated with the IM device. Surprisingly, the radiographic outcomes were similar; I would have expected somewhat less shortening and malunion in the IM group. The choice of which device approach to use will remain up to the surgeon. This trial, perhaps more than any RCT I have seen, gives impetus to consider the IM device because of the functional outcome differences. Cost differences are not considered in this study, and a follow up cost-effectiveness analysis will be welcome.

M. F. Swiontkowski, MD

Foot and Ankle

Reliability and Necessity of Computerized Tomography in Distal Tibial Physeal Injuries

Thawrani D, Kuester V, Gabos PG, et al (Nemours Children's Clinic, Wilmington, DE)
J Pediatr Orthop 31:745-750, 2011

Objective.—Complex distal tibial physeal fractures can be difficult to characterize on plain radiographs. The role of computed tomography

(CT) scans in the evaluation and treatment decision of these injuries is unclear. We aimed to determine whether or not the addition of CT would improve the reliability of fracture classification and treatment decision.

Methods.—Five independent observers evaluated 50 distal tibial physeal fractures on 2 separate occasions for Salter Harris (SH) classification and treatment decision (surgical/nonsurgical) using plain radiographs (round 1) and combination of radiographs and CT (round 2). During round 1, observers were asked if they would order a CT, and during round 2, they were asked if the CT was useful. These rounds were repeated at 2 to 4 weeks to assess intraobserver reliability. Statistical analyses were performed to assess inter and intraobserver reliability using Kappa coefficient (κ).

Results.—Intraobserver reliability for SH classification showed substantial agreement, $\kappa = 0.76$ and $\kappa = 0.80$, respectively, during round 1 and 2. Interobserver agreement on the SH class was lower during round 1 and 2 ($\kappa = 0.67$ and $\kappa = 0.57$, respectively). There also was almost perfect intraobserver and interobserver agreement in the measurement of displacement at the fracture site during both rounds 1 and 2. Intraobserver reliability for treatment decision was substantial, $\kappa = 0.74$ and $\kappa = 0.80$, respectively, during round 1 and 2. However, interobserver agreement for treatment decision was moderate ($\kappa = 0.48$) and fair ($\kappa = 0.36$), respectively, during round 1 and 2. Surgeons indicated that they would like to order CT scans for 66%

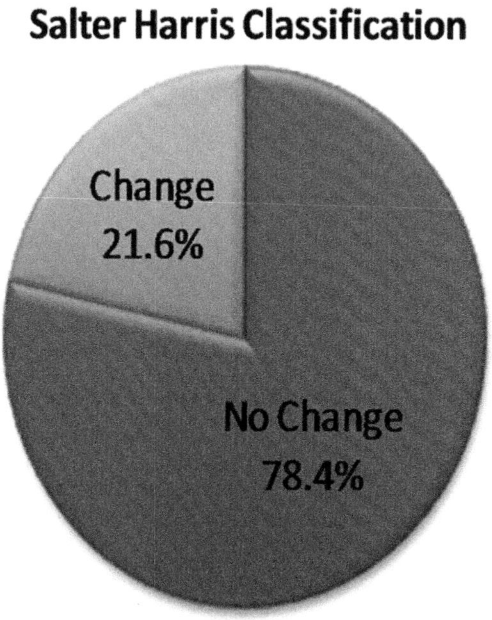

FIGURE 1.—Changes in Salter Harris Classification from round 1 (plain x-ray) to round 2 (x-ray+ computed tomography). (Reprinted from Thawrani D, Kuester V, Gabos PG, et al. Reliability and necessity of computerized tomography in distal tibial physeal injuries. *J Pediatr Orthop.* 2011;31:745-750, with permission from Lippincott Williams & Wilkins.)

of the time in round 1, but the interobserver agreement as to who would best benefit from the CT was only fair ($\kappa = -0.23$). The main purpose of ordering the CT was to delineate fracture anatomy (55% of the time) and the observers felt CT would add to their treatment decision only 26% of the time. During round 2, 75% of time surgeons felt that CT scan was useful. CT was thought to be most useful in guiding screw placement (56% of the time) and not as useful (28% of time) for treatment decision making.

Conclusions.—Addition of CT in complex distal tibial physeal fractures did not increase interobserver reliability to classify the fracture or the treatment decision. Surgeons reported that the CT was most useful to plan screw placement and changed their treatment decision in about a fifth of the cases (Figs 1 and 2, Tables 1 and 2).

▶ Computed tomography (CT) scans are commonly ordered after radiographic identification of a physeal fracture in the ankle. This well-conceived study attempts to clarify the benefit in diagnosis and treatment decisions. The inter- and intrarater reliability of fracture classification is quite strong with both diagnostic techniques. The addition of the CT scan did lead to changes in treatment decisions in both directions in a few cases; however, the CT scan was mostly useful in planning lag screw placement in the epiphysis. I am doubtful that this research will result in large decreases in overall use of CT scans in this clinical setting. Appropriate reading of the conclusions should make us all more thoughtful about which fractures/patients should have the CT scan and restrict

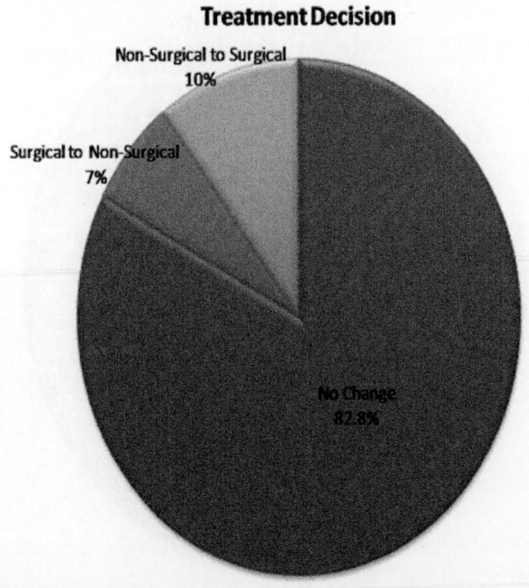

FIGURE 2.—Changes in treatment decision (surgical or nonsurgical) from round 1 (plain x-ray) to round 2 (x-ray+computed tomography). (Reprinted from Thawrani D, Kuester V, Gabos PG, et al. Reliability and necessity of computerized tomography in distal tibial physeal injuries. *J Pediatr Orthop.* 2011;31:745-750, with permission from Lippincott Williams & Wilkins.)

TABLE 1.—Intraobserver Reliability and Interobserver Agreement for Plain x-ray Images

	Intraobserver Reliability			Interobserver Agreement		
Variables	κ Coefficient	P	Interpretation	κ Coefficient	P	Interpretation
Salter Harris classification	0.76	<0.001	Substantial	0.64	<0.001	Substantial
Displacement	0.92	<0.001	Almost perfect	0.95	<0.001	Almost perfect
Order computed tomography based on x-ray	0.53	<0.001	Moderate	0.23	<0.001	Fair
Treatment	0.74	<0.001	Substantial	0.48	<0.001	Moderate

TABLE 2.—Intraobserver Reliability and Interobserver Agreement for Combined x-ray and CT Images

	Intraobserver Reliability			Interobserver Agreement		
Variables	κ Coefficient	P	Interpretation	κ Coefficient	P	Interpretation
SH Classification	0.80	<0.001	Substantial	0.57	<0.001	Substantial
Displacement	0.90	<0.001	Almost perfect	0.94	<0.001	Almost perfect
CT was useful	0.72	<0.001	Substantial	0.09	<0.02	Slight
Treatment	0.80	<0.001	Substantial	0.36	<0.001	Moderate

CT indicates computed tomography.

the use of this diagnostic technique where there is a good chance that treatment will be impacted.

M. F. Swiontkowski, MD

Syndesmotic Fixation in Supination-External Rotation Ankle Fractures: A Prospective Randomized Study

Pakarinen HJ, Flinkkilä TE, Ohtonen PP, et al (Oulu Univ Hosp Finland)
Foot Ankle Int 32:1103-1109, 2011

Background.—This study was designed to assess whether transfixion of an unstable syndesmosis is necessary in supination-external rotation (Lauge-Hansen SE/Weber B)-type ankle fractures.

Methods.—A prospective study of 140 patients with unilateral Lauge-Hansen supination-external rotation type 4 ankle fractures was done. After bony fixation, the 7.5-Nm standardized external rotation (ER) stress test for both ankles was performed under fluoroscopy. A positive stress examination was defined as a difference of more than 2 mm side-to-side in the tibiotalar or tibiofibular clear spaces on mortise radiographs. If the stress test was positive, the patient was randomized to either syndesmotic transfixion with 3.5-mm tricortical screws or no syndesmotic fixation. Clinical outcome was assessed using the Olerud-Molander scoring system, RAND 36-Item Health Survey, and Visual Analogue Scale (VAS) to measure pain and function after a minimum 1-year of followup.

Results.—Twenty four (17%) of 140 patients had positive standardized 7.5-Nm ER stress tests after malleolar fixation. The stress view was positive three times on tibiotalar clear space, seven on tibiofibular clear space, and 14 times on both tibiotalar and tibiofibular clear spaces. There was no

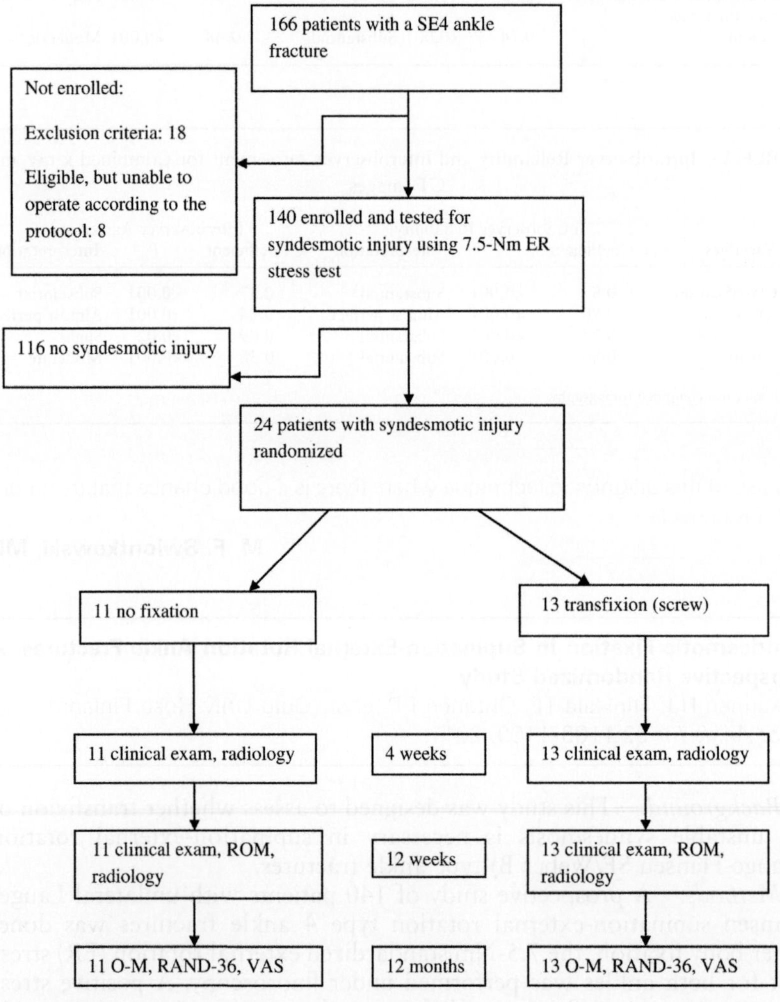

Footnotes:

SE4, supination-external rotation type 4; ER, external rotation; VAS, visual analogue scale; O-M, Olerud-Molander.

FIGURE 1.—Flowchart of the study. (Reprinted from Pakarinen HJ, Flinkkilä TE, Ohtonen PP, et al. Syndesmotic fixation in supination-external rotation ankle fractures: a prospective randomized study. *Foot Ankle Int.* 2011;32:1103-1109. Copyright © 2011 by the American Orthopaedic Foot and Ankle Society, Inc., originally published in Foot & Ankle, International 32:1103-1109 and reproduced here with permission.)

TABLE 2.—Syndesmotic Fixation and Self-Reported Disability at 1 Year

	Screw	No Fixation	Difference Between Means	95% CI for the Difference Lower	95% CI for the Difference Upper	*p*
Olerud–Molander score	79.6 (15.5)	83.6 (13.1)	4.0	−8.2	16.3	0.50
VAS pain	25.5 (25.4)	11.3 (12.5)	−14.2	−31.2	3.3	0.38
VAS function	22.6 (24.6)	14.9 (15.0)	−7.8	−25.5	9.9	0.37
Rand-36 physical function	0.9 (0.2)	1.0 (0.2)	0.1	−0.1	0.3	0.23
Rand-36 pain	0.9 (0.4)	1.1 (0.2)	0.2	−0.1	0.5	0.32

VAS = visual analogue scale. The values of the Rand-36 are ratios of the study group compared age—(10 years interval) and sex adjusted general Finnish population. Values are presented as mean, standard deviation (SD), and 95% confidence interval (95% CI).

significant difference between the two randomization groups with regards to Olerud–Molander functional score, VAS scale measuring pain and function, or RAND 36-Item Health Survey pain or physical function at 1 year.

Conclusion.—Relevant syndesmotic injuries are rare in supination–external rotation ankle fractures, and syndesmotic transfixion with a screw did not influence the functional outcome or pain after the 1-year followup compared with no fixation (Fig 1, Table 2).

▶ This is a well-conceived randomized clinical trial examining the impact of screw stabilization versus expectant observation for the clinical situation of a wide medial clear space or distal tib-fib space on stress testing after internal fixation of a Weber B ankle fracture. The situation is rare, with a 17% occurrence on standardized intraoperative radiographic testing after fixation of the distal fibular fracture. The postoperative treatment was standardized with weight bearing as tolerated in short leg casts for 1 month. The surprising finding is that there is no functional outcome difference at 1 year between these cohorts. This is a relatively short-term outcome when the possible impact of stabilization of the syndesmosis is a reduced risk of degenerative arthritis of the ankle in the longer term. Until we see no radiographic or functional outcome differences at 5 and 10 years, I would not recommend a change in clinical practice.

M. F. Swiontkowski, MD

Does Adding Computed Tomography Change the Diagnosis and Treatment of Tillaux and Triplane Pediatric Ankle Fractures?

Liporace FA, Yoon RS, Kubiak EN, et al (UMDNJ – New Jersey Med School, Newark; NYU Hosp for Joint Diseases; The Univ of Utah, Salt Lake City; et al)
Orthopedics 35:e208-e212, 2012

Computed tomography (CT) has been deemed a necessary part of management for Tillaux and triplane pediatric ankle fractures. However, no previously published study has attempted to quantify its usefulness in

TABLE 2.—Treatment Plan Based on Radiographic Evaluation

	%		
	Plain Radiographs	Plain Radiographs+CT	*P*
Nonoperative	52	39	.033
Operative	48	61	
CRPP	15	19	
ORIF	33	42	

Abbreviations: CRPP, closed reduction with percutaneous pinning; CT, computed tomography; ORIF, open reduction internal fixation.

changing management. Six third-party, blinded orthopedic surgeons (F.A.L., E.N.K., D.M.P., K.J.K., D.S.F., K.A.E.) were randomly assigned to evaluate 24 pediatric Tillaux or triplane fractures with plain radiographs; after 6 months, they were again randomly assigned to evaluate the 24 radiographs plus CT scans, totaling 144 third-party, blinded evaluations. Intra- and interobserver agreements were assessed via correlation coefficient analysis. Evaluation of CT scans changed the original diagnosis of fracture type from Tillaux to triplane fracture in 7 (4.9%) of 144 evaluations. Inter- and intraobserver agreements regarding primary treatment plans did not significantly differ between radiographs and radiographs plus CT scans (0.5 vs 0.4, respectively; $P>.05$). The addition of CT did not significantly change the impression of the amount of displacement per case. By adding CT, more patients who were assigned nonoperative management were reassigned to operative treatment ($P=.033$). Adding CT, although it may influence the decision to operate on Tillaux and triplane fractures, may not be as useful as previously thought (Table 2).

► Fractures involving the growth plate of the distal tibia are common in adolescents where the physis has started to close. This carefully designed study confirms excellent intrarater and interrater reliability among 6 reviewers classifying radiographs and CT scans. CT imaging rarely alters a treatment decision made based on plain radiographs. CT imaging also does not significantly alter the treatment plan when it relates to open reduction and fixation versus closed reduction and fixation although the addition of CT results in an increase in recommendations for operative management. However, the fact that percutaneous lag screw fixation is minimally invasive and has a low rate of complications may cause clinicians to continue to use CT to evaluate the magnitude of articular gapping in these injuries.

M. F. Swiontkowski, MD

Foot and Ankle Fractures

Increased rates of wound complications with locking plates in distal fibular fractures

Schepers T, Van Lieshout EMM, De Vries MR, et al (Reinier de Graaf Groep Delft, The Netherlands; Univ Med Ctr Rotterdam, The Netherlands)
Injury 42:1125-1129, 2011

Introduction.—There is a growing use of locking compression plates in fracture surgery. The current study was undertaken to investigate the wound complication rates of locking versus non-locking plates in distal fibular fractures.

Patients and Methods.—During a 6-year study period all consecutive, closed distal fibular fractures treated with either a locking or a non-locking plate were included and retrospectively analysed for complication related to the fibula.

Results.—A total of 165 patients received a one-third tubular plate and 40 patients were treated with a locking plate. The two groups were comparable with respect to patient characteristics (age, gender, smokers and diabetics), injury characteristics (affected side, fracture dislocations, number of fractured malleoli and classification) and operation characteristics (surgical delay and duration, use of a tourniquet and plate length). The wound complication rate was 5.5% in the conventional plating group, and 17.5% in the locking plate group ($p = 0.019$). This difference was largely due to an increase in major complications, for which removal of the plate was necessary ($p = 0.008$).

Conclusion.—There is a significant increase in wound complications in distal fibular fractures treated with a locking compression plate. In light of the current study, we would caution against the application of the

TABLE 2.—Surgical Details on Both Plate Groups

	Overall Population	One-Third Tubular Plate	Locking Plate	*p*-Value
Operation delay (days)	7 (1–11)	7 (1–11)	7.5 (1–11)	0.655[c]
Operation time (min)	60 (49–76)	60 (49–78)	60 (52.5–74)	0.686[c]
Tourniquet (%)	90 (43.9)	77 (46.7)	13 (32.5)	0.050[b]
Plate length (holes)	7 (6–7)	7 (6–7)	7 (6–7)	0.588[c]
Operated by resident (%)	66.3	63.0	80.0	0.105[b]
Reduction accuracy (%)				
Anatomical	187 (91.2)	153 (92.7)	34 (85)	0.128[a]
Zero to 2 mm	18 (8.8)	12 (7.3)	6 (15)	
More than 2 mm	0 (0)	0 (0)	0 (0)	

Data is presented as number with the percentage between brackets (categoric data) or as mean with the P_{25} and P_{75} between brackets (numeric data).
[a]Data were analysed using the Fisher's exact test.
[b]Data were analysed using the Chi-square test.
[c]Data were analysed using the Mann–Whitney *U*-test.

TABLE 3.—Complication-Rates Between Both Patient Groups

	Overall Population (n = 205)	One-Third Tubular Plate (n = 165)	Locking Plate (n = 40)	p-Value
Wound complication (%)	16 (7.8)	9 (5.5)	7 (17.5)	0.019[a]
Complication type (%)				
Minor	10 (4.9)	7 (4.2)	3 (7.5)	0.008[b]
Major	6 (2.9)	2 (1.2)	4 (10)	
Plate removal (%)	56 (27.3)	45 (27.3)	11 (27.5)	1.000[a]
Plate removal (months)	8.8 (5.2–13.7)	10 (5.6–14.0)	7.8 (5.0–8.8)	0.117[c]

Data is presented as number with the percentage between brackets (categoric data) or as mean with the P_{25} and P_{75} between brackets (numeric data).
[a]Data were analysed using the Fisher's exact test.
[b]Data were analysed using the Chi-square test.
[c]Data were analysed using the Mann–Whitney *U*-test.

currently used locking compression plates in the treatment of distal fibular fractures (Tables 2 and 3).

▶ This retrospective case-controlled cohort series raises concerns regarding the routine use of locking plates for distal fibular fractures. With this nonrandomized design, it is entirely possible that selection bias (more comminuted fractures receiving the locking plates) is the explanation for the findings of the increased minor and major wound complication rates, as well as the nonsignificant rate of poor reductions. The findings may well be attributable to the plate design used in this study (thicker than the second-generation one third tubular locking designs). Nevertheless, with these findings and the added expense of the locking plates, they should be used only in rare circumstances for highly comminuted fractures in patients with poor bone density.

M. F. Swiontkowski, MD

Medial Joint Space Widening of the Ankle in Displaced Tillaux and Triplane Fractures in Children

Gourineni P, Gupta A (Advocate Hope Children's Hosp, Oak Lawn, IL; Univ of Illinois, Chicago)
J Orthop Trauma 25:608-611, 2011

Objectives.—Tillaux and Triplane fractures occur in children predominantly from external rotation mechanism. We hypothesized that in displaced fractures, the talus would shift laterally along with the distal fibula and the distal tibial epiphyseal fragment increasing the medial joint space.

Design.—Consecutive cases evaluated retrospectively.

Setting.—Level I and Level II centers.

Patients.—Twenty-two skeletally immature patients with 14 displaced Triplane fractures and eight displaced Tillaux fractures were evaluated for medial joint space widening.

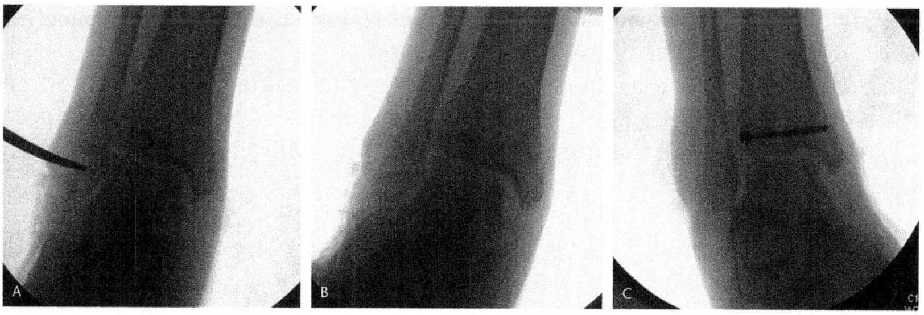

FIGURE 2.—(A) Anteroposterior radiograph of a Tillaux fracture showing slight medial joint space widening. (B) Intraoperative external rotation anteroposterior stress fluoroscopy showed further widening of the medial space. (C) Intraoperative fluoroscopic mortise view after closed reduction and screw fixation. (Reprinted from Gourineni P, Gupta A. Medial joint space widening of the ankle in displaced tillaux and triplane fractures in children. *J Orthop Trauma.* 2011;25:608-611, with permission from Lippincott Williams & Wilkins.)

TABLE 1.—Information on All Patients*

Patient No.	Age (years)	Intervention	TS	SS	MSW Pre	Fracture Gap on CT	MSW Post	MSW Final	Complications
					Triplane Fractures				
1	13	ORIF	1	1	0	—	0	0	
2	15	ORIF	3	0	2	2	0	0	
3	14	ORIF	1	1	2	2	0	0	
4	11	ORIF	2	0	0	3	0	0	
5	14	ORIF	1	0	1	1	0	0	
6	11	CRIF	1	1	2	2	0	0	
7	15	ORIF	2	1	9	—	0	0	
8	14	CRIF	1	1	2	2	0	0	
9	12	ORIF	2	0	3	—	0	0	
10	14	ORIF	1	0	1	1	0	0	Achilles contracture
11	12	ORIF	2	0	2	2	0	0	
12	14	ORIF	2	1	2	—	0	0	
13	13	ORIF	1	1	2	—	0	0	Broken screw
14	15	ORIF	2	0	3	3	0	0	
					Tillaux Fractures				
15	11	ORIF	1	0	1	1	0	0	
16	14	ORIF	1	0	2	2	0	0	Achilles contracture
17	14	ORIF	1	0	3	—	0	0	
18	12	ORIF	1	0	1	1	0	0	
19	14	CRIF	0	2	2	2	0	0	Broken screw
20	14	CRIF	1	1	0	4	0	0	Pin removal
21	14	CRIF	0	1	2	2	0	0	
22	10	ORIF	1	0	1	1	0	0	

TS, tibial screw; SS, syndesmotic screw; MSW Pre, medial joint space widening prereduction; MSW Post, medial joint space widening postreduction; MSW Final, medial joint space widening at final clinic visit; CT, computed tomography; ORIF, open reduction and internal fixation; CRIF, closed reduction and internal fixation.
*All measurements are in millimeters.

Intervention.—Measurement of fracture displacement and medial joint space widening before and after intervention.

Results.—Thirteen Triplane and six Tillaux fractures (86%) showed medial space widening of 1 to 9 mm and equal to the amount of fracture displacement. Reduction of the fracture reduced the medial space to normal. There were no known complications.

Conclusions.—Medial space widening of the ankle may be a sign of ankle fracture displacement. Anatomic reduction of the fracture reduces the medial space and may improve the results in Tillaux and Triplane fractures (Fig 2, Table 1).

▶ This is an interesting cohort study that brings to our attention the important feature of medial joint space widening on triplane or Tillaux fractures. If that space is asymmetric and wide, it seems to be a clear indicator of displacement as confirmed by computed tomography (Table 1). Recognizing this sign can, therefore, prompt the treating surgeon to percutaneous reduction and lag screw fixation to assure long-term favorable clinical and functional outcomes.

M. F. Swiontkowski, MD

Operative Fixation of Unstable Ankle Fractures in Patients Aged Over 80 Years

Shivarathre DG, Chandran P, Platt SR (Wirral Univ Hosps NHS Trust, UK)
Foot Ankle Int 32:599-602, 2011

Introduction.—Controversy exists regarding the surgical treatment of unstable ankle fractures in the very elderly age group of over 80 years. However, the literature regarding the prognosis of surgery in this elderly group is limited. The purpose of our study was to evaluate the results of patients above 80 years old who underwent operative fixation for unstable ankle fractures.

Materials and Methods.—Ninety-two consecutive patients, 80 females and 12 males, above 80 years of age had open reduction and internal fixation for unstable ankle fractures during the period of January 1998 to August 2007. The data was collected retrospectively from the case records and radiographs. The complications were noted and the risk factors for poor outcome were analyzed. The average age was 85.2 (range, 80.1 to 95.1) years. The minimum duration of followup was 9 months, with an average of 15 (range, 9 to 28) months.

Results.—The most common fracture pattern was Danis-Weber B type. The superficial wound infection rate was 7% (6 cases) and the deep infection rate was 4.6% (4 cases). The 30 day postoperative mortality was 5.4% (five cases). Eighty-six percent (75 out of 87 cases) were able to return back to their pre injury mobility at the last followup. Diabetes, dementia, peripheral vascular disease and smoking were found to be statistically significant risk factors associated with wound complications.

Conclusion.—The results of operative fixation of unstable ankle fractures were encouraging with good functional recovery and return to pre injury mobility status in most cases (Tables 1 and 2).

▶ This is a large series of older patients with displaced ankle fractures that underwent operative treatment. There are few reports of patient cohorts older

TABLE 1.—Fracture Pattern ($n = 92$)

Gustilo Anderson	**Number of patients**
Closed	90
Grade 1 open	2
Danis-Weber	**Number of patients (%)**
Type B	77 (83.7)
Type C	14 (15.2)
Isolated lateral malleolus	4 (4.5%)
Isolated medial malleolus	1 (1.1%)
Bimalleolar	70 (76%)
Trimalleolar	16 (17.4%)

TABLE 2.—ASA Grade & Medical Comorbities ($n = 92$)

ASA grade	
Grade 2	58 (63%)
Grade 3	30 (32.6%)
Grade 4	4 (4.4%)
Associated co-morbidities	
Vascular disease	18
Diabetes	8
Peripheral Neuropathy	2
Dementia	10
Smokers	10
Multiple (more than 3 systems involved)	14

than 80 years of age that are this large. The findings regarding risk factors for poor results being diabetes, smoking, peripheral vascular disease, and dementia are not surprising. We should all use these data to reinforce the risks of operative therapy in these older patients in shared decision making with patients and families. What is encouraging is the favorable rate of return to baseline function in 86% of cases. These results are far superior to those of other fractures in the lower extremity in this age group. We should be encouraged to counsel patients that operative indications should be standardized based on the fracture pattern and displacement and that age should not be a major consideration.

M. F. Swiontkowski, MD

Closed Intramedullary Screw Fixation for Nonunion of Fifth Metatarsal Jones Fracture

Habbu RA, Marsh RS, Anderson JG, et al (Orthopaedic Associates of Michigan, Grand Rapids)
Foot Ankle Int 32:603-608, 2011

Background.—Nonunion following a proximal fifth metatarsal metaphyseal-diaphyseal or Jones fracture can cause considerable pain with high morbidity and loss of work. Treatment should aim for early union, thus

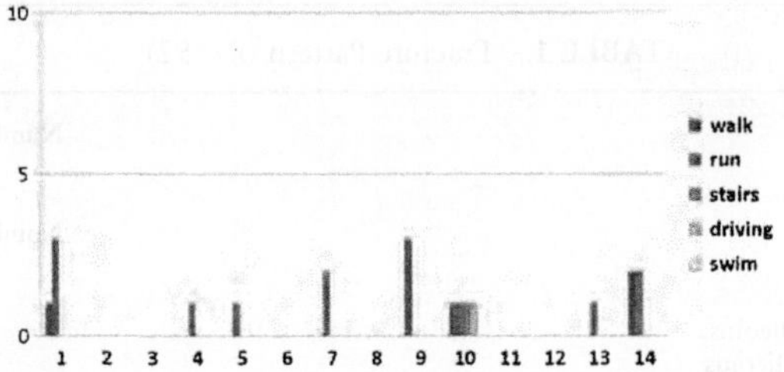

FIGURE 6.—Graph for followup pain levels of the study group. (Reprinted from Habbu RA, Marsh RS, Anderson JG, et al. Closed intramedullary screw fixation for nonunion of fifth metatarsal Jones fracture. *Foot Ankle Int.* 2011;32:603-608, Copyright 2011, with permission from the American Orthopaedic Foot & Ankle Society.)

TABLE 1.—Effect of Other Variables on Followup Pain Scores

	ρ	p Value
BMI	−0.05	>0.05
Age	−0.3	>0.05
Duration since injury	−0.2	>0.05
Early FWB	0.1	>0.05
Time to union	0.05	>0.05

allowing early return to activity. The present study evaluated the outcomes and the time required for union following closed intramedullary screw fixation for this condition.

Materials and Methods.—Between January 2005 to August 2009, 14 patients were diagnosed with nonunion following a Jones fracture. Mean age at surgery was 49 years. Mean duration from injury to surgery was 28 weeks. All nonunions were fixed with a single intramedullary screw inserted from the base of the fifth metatarsal without opening the nonunion site. Serial postoperative radiographs were evaluated to determine union. Time required for return to activity was determined. Outcome was assessed with help of pain scores. Mean followup was 27 months.

Results.—Union was achieved in all 14 patients with one delayed union. Mean time to union was 13.3 (range, 8 to 20) weeks. All patients were able to start unassisted full weightbearing without pain at mean 10.2 weeks. Overall pain score improved from a preoperative mean of 5.4 to postoperative mean of 1.0. Complications included one deep infection, one delayed wound healing and one sural neuroma.

Conclusion.—Closed intramedullary screw fixation achieved an excellent union rate when used in the treatment of nonunion of a Jones fractures (Fig 6, Table 1).

► Nonunion of a Jones fracture was a fairly common condition in times past but is becoming increasingly rare as early fixation moves toward becoming the standard management in younger active patients. When it does occur, most surgeons now recommend percutaneous intramedullary screw fixation. This retrospective cohort study confirms that this procedure can be recommended for patients with this condition with a high level of confidence for fracture healing and improvement in pain and function (Fig 6). Healthy active patients have the most predictable results (Table 1).

M. F. Swiontkowski, MD

Complications of Syndesmotic Screw Removal

Schepers T, Van Lieshout EMM, de Vries MR, et al (Reinier de Graaf Groep, Delft, The Netherlands; Erasmus MC, Rotterdam, The Netherlands)
Foot Ankle Int 32:1040-1044, 2011

Background.—Currently, the metallic syndesmotic screw is the gold standard in the treatment of syndesmotic disruption. Whether or not this screw needs to be removed remains debatable. The aim of the current study was to determine the complications which occur following routine removal of the syndesmotic screw following operative treatment of unstable ankle fractures.

Methods.—This was a retrospective study with consecutive cases in a Level-2 Trauma center. All patients with routine removal of a syndesmotic screw, following the treatment of an unstable ankle fracture, between January 1, 2004 and November 30, 2010 were included. Complications recorded were: 1) minor or major wound infection following removal of the syndesmotic screw, 2) recurrent syndesmotic diastasis, and 3) unnecessary removal of a broken screw, not recognized during preoperative planning prior to surgery.

Results.—A total of 76 patients were included. A wound infection occurred in 9.2% (N=7) of which 2.6% (N=2) were deep infections requiring reoperation. Recurrent syndesmotic diastasis was found in 6.6% (N=5) of patients, and in 6.6% (N=5) screws were broken at the time of implant removal. In the group with recurrent diastasis the screws were removed significantly earlier compared with the group without recurrent diastasis (Mann- Whitney U-test; $p = 0.011$) and the group with screw breakage had their screws significantly longer in place compared with the group without breakage ($p = 0.038$).

Conclusion.—A total of 22.4% complications occurred upon routine removal of the syndesmotic screw. Removal might therefore be considered only in selected cases with complaints, after a minimum of eight to twelve weeks and using antibiotic prophylaxis during removal (Fig 2).

▶ The subject of syndesmosis screw management remains an important and active area for clinical research in orthopedic surgery. This cohort study focuses on complications surrounding the removal of these screws. Based on the 22% complication rate and 6.6% rate of recurrent syndesmosis widening, routine removal cannot be recommended. This would be an important topic for an

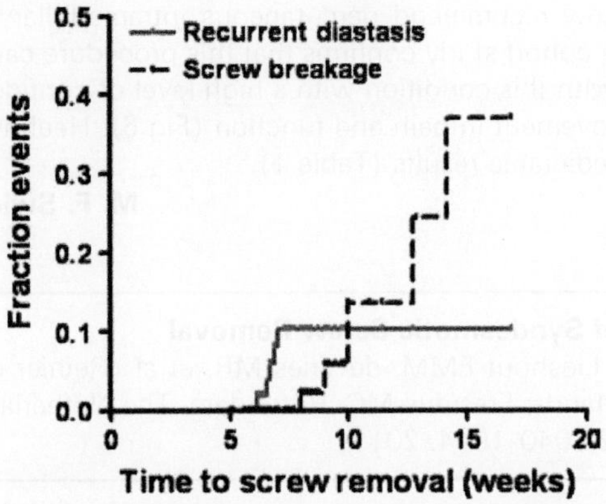

FIGURE 2.—Kaplan-Meier plot showing the correlation between the time the syndesmotic screw was in place and the number of adverse events: recurrent diastasis (solid line) and screw breakage (dotted line). (Reprinted from Schepers T, Van Lieshout EMM, de Vries MR, et al. Complications of syndesmotic screw removal. Copyright © 2011 by the American Orthopaedic Foot and Ankle Society, Inc., originally published in *Foot Ankle Int.* 2011;32:1040-1044 and reproduced here with permission.)

adequately powered controlled trial standardized around removal versus leaving the syndesmosis screw in place and accepting a degree of screw breakage and lucency around the screw. Of course, elements such as 3 versus 4 cortex screws and screw type would need to be standardized. In one of the radiographs in this article, a cancellous screw with smaller core diameter and suboptimal fatigue properties is shown—cortical screws are most certainly a better choice.

M. F. Swiontkowski, MD

Tibia

Injury to the infrapatellar branch of the saphenous nerve, a possible cause for anterior knee pain after tibial nailing?

Leliveld MS, Verhofstad MHJ (St Elisabeth Hosp, Tilburg, The Netherlands)
Injury 43:779-783, 2012

The purpose of this study was to determine the long-term incidence of infrapatellar nerve damage after tibial nailing and its relation to anterior knee pain. We retrospectively evaluated 71 patients in whom 72 isolated tibial shaft fractures were treated with an intramedullary nail. The mean follow-up time was 84 months. Twenty-seven patients (38%) complained of chronic anterior knee pain. Infrapatellar nerve damage was found in 43 patients (60%). Of the 27 patients with knee pain, 21 (78%) had sensory deficits in the distribution area of the infrapatellar nerve, compared to 22 of the 45 patients (49%) without knee pain ($p = 0.025$). Patient and fracture characteristics showed no significant differences between the two groups. At time of follow-up a total of 33 nails were removed of which twelve were taken out because of knee pain. The pain persisted in seven of these twelve patients (58%).

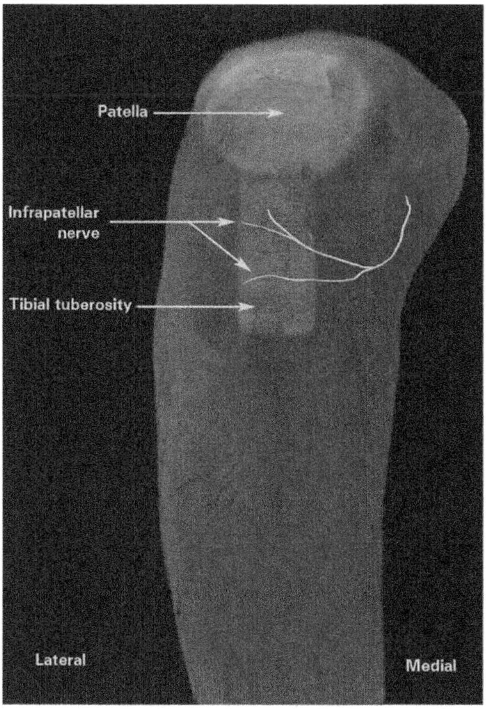

FIGURE 1.—The infrapatellar branch of the saphenous nerve is exclusively sensory and runs subcutaneously medial and almost perpendicular to the patellar tendon just caudal to the patella. (Reprinted from Leliveld MS, Verhofstad MHJ. Injury to the infrapatellar branch of the saphenous nerve, a possible cause for anterior knee pain after tibial nailing? *Injury.* 2012;43:779-783, Copyright 2012, with permission from Elsevier.)

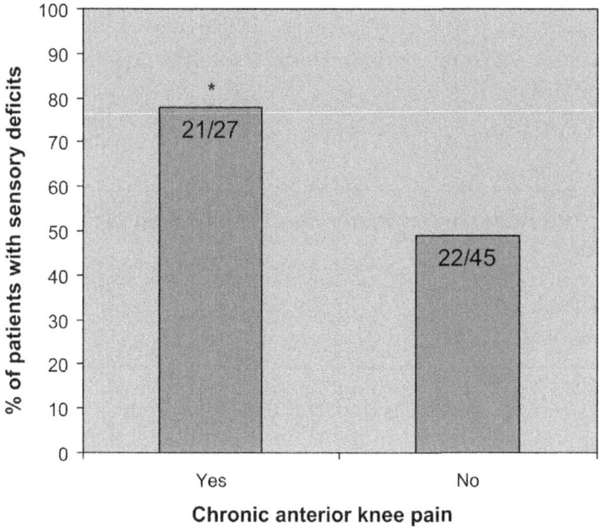

FIGURE 2.—Significantly more sensory deficits were found in patients with chronic anterior knee pain (*0.025). (Reprinted from Leliveld MS, Verhofstad MHJ. Injury to the infrapatellar branch of the saphenous nerve, a possible cause for anterior knee pain after tibial nailing? *Injury.* 2012;43:779-783, Copyright 2012, with permission from Elsevier.)

TABLE 3.—Comparative Analysis of Patients with and Without Chronic Anterior Knee Pain

Clinical Characteristics	Chronic Anterior Knee Pain Yes ($n = 27$)		No ($n = 45$)		p Value
Mean AKPS score	75.41 ± 15.67		86.56 ± 15.46		0.004
	n	%	n	%	
Patellar tendon approach					
Medial parapatellar	10	37	16	36	1.000
Transpatellar	17	63	29	64	
Nail prominence	9	33	10	26	0.408
Nail removal	19	70	14	31	0.002
Kneeling pain	23	85	21	47	0.001

The incidence of iatrogenic damage to the infrapatellar nerve after tibial nailing is high and lasting. Injury to this nerve appears to be associated with anterior knee pain after tibial nailing (Figs 1 and 2, Table 3).

▶ Anterior knee pain occurs in approximately 50% of patients undergoing intramedullary nail placement for tibia fractures. This retrospective review focuses on the possibility that this pain is related to injury to the infrapatellar branch of the saphenous nerve. The theory is highly plausible given the variable course of this nerve (Fig 1). The association of hypesthesia with the knee pain seems to be variable. If this was the major associated issue with knee pain, one would expect that nail removal would not produce improvement, and this was the case in this study. Regardless of the strength of the association, it would seem prudent to place incisions proximal just off the inferior pole of the patella and limit the distal extent. I suspect that knee pain is multifactorial, and in a significant number of cases, the infrapatellar branch is part of the cause. Other factors would be fat pad scarring, capsular scaring, and injury to the ligaments stabilizing the menisci.

M. F. Swiontkowski, MD

Evaluation of Popliteal Artery Injury Risk With Locked Lateral Plating of the Tibial Plateau

Dee M, Sojka JM, Daccarett MS, et al (Nebraska Med Ctr, Omaha, NE; Univ of Kansas Med Ctr)
J Orthop Trauma 25:603-607, 2011

Objectives.—This study was undertaken to determine if there is increased likelihood of popliteal artery injury as one places a fixed-angle lateral proximal tibia locking plate with posterior plate lift off and or anterior plate translation from the ideal position.

Methods.—A Synthes (Synthes USA, West Chester, PA) 3.5-mm and 4.5-mm lateral proximal tibia locking plate was placed consecutively on each of six specimens in the straight lateral (SL) position. Screw position

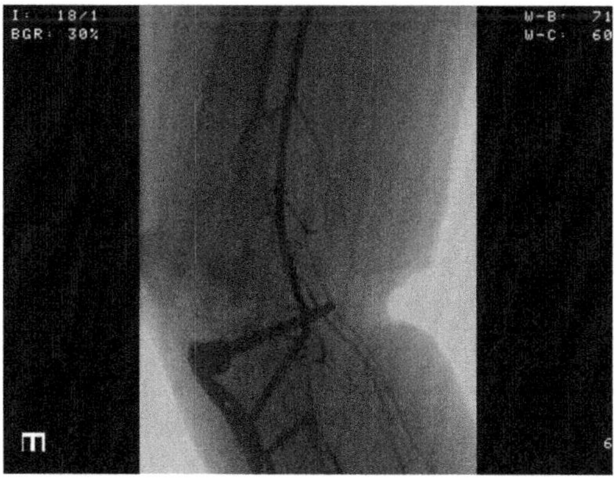

FIGURE 1.—Example of posterior most screw of proximal tibial lateral locking plate injuring the popliteal artery. This case represents a legal review by one of the senior authors. (Reprinted from Dee M, Sojka JM, Daccarett MS, et al. Evaluation of popliteal artery injury risk with locked lateral plating of the tibial plateau. *J Orthop Trauma.* 2011;25:603-607, with permission from Lippincott Williams & Wilkins.)

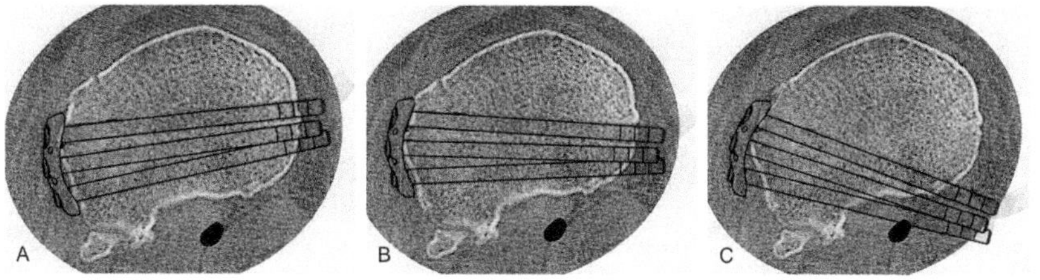

FIGURE 5.—Axial cut computed tomographic scan with schematic representation of the 4.5-mm proximal tibia lateral locking plate with the plate in the straight lateral position (A), 5-mm anterior translated position (B), and the 5-mm anterior translated 6-mm posterior liftoff position (C). (Reprinted from Dee M, Sojka JM, Daccarett MS, et al. Evaluation of popliteal artery injury risk with locked lateral plating of the tibial plateau. *J Orthop Trauma.* 2011;25:603-607, with permission from Lippincott Williams & Wilkins.)

with respect to the medial cortex was recorded as well as the distance of the posterior most screw tip to the popliteal artery. Next a 3-mm shim was placed under the posterior edge of the same plate to mimic posterior plate lift off (LO) followed by placement of a 6-mm shim. The same experiment was repeated with the plate translated 5 mm anteriorly (AT).

Results.—The popliteal artery was injured in zero of six specimens using the 3.5-mm plate. The popliteal artery was injured in six of six specimens using the 4.5-mm plate in the 5-mm AT 6-mm LO position, five of six with 5-mm AT and 3-mm LO, two of six with only 5-mm AT, four of six with SL and 6-mm LO, two of six with SL and 3-mm LO, and zero of six with SL.

Conclusion.—The Synthes 4.5-mm plate can put the popliteal artery at risk with as little as 3-mm posterior liftoff in the intended straight lateral position or with 5-mm anterior plate translation with no posterior liftoff. Therefore, placement of the 4.5-mm plate in the proper position and confirmation of its position with a true lateral radiograph is paramount to avoid injury to the popliteal artery (Figs 1 and 5).

▶ This is a practical anatomic exercise based on a vascular injury that occurred in the course of clinical care. The take-home message is simple: be sure that the plate stays completely on the lateral surface of the proximal tibia when using 4.5-mm locking plates. Hopefully, these findings will be widely disseminated to prevent future patient vascular injury.

M. F. Swiontkowski, MD

Knee Pain Correlates With Union After Tibial Nailing

Ryan SP, Tornetta P III, Dielwart C, et al (Boston Univ Med Ctr, MA)
J Orthop Trauma 25:731-735, 2011

Objectives.—The purpose of this study is to evaluate the change in quantitatively scored knee pain during union.

Design.—This is a retrospective review of prospectively collected data over a 15-year period.

Setting.—Academic medical center.

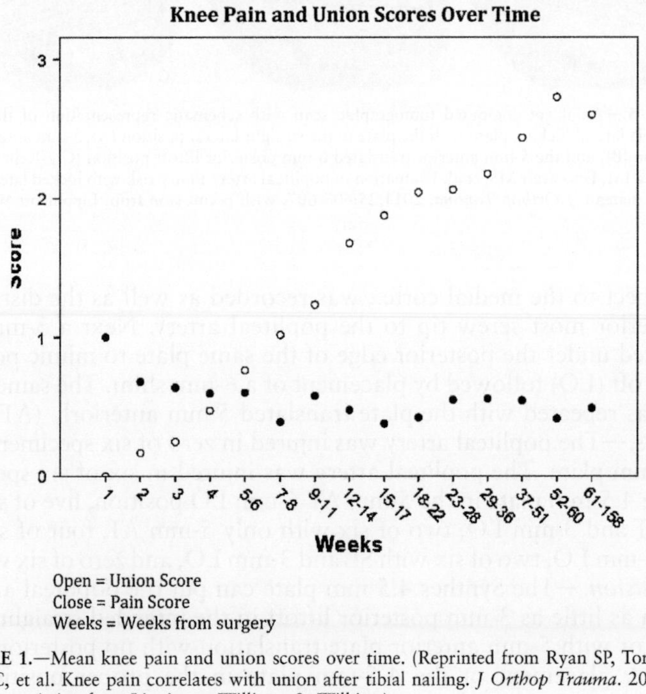

FIGURE 1.—Mean knee pain and union scores over time. (Reprinted from Ryan SP, Tornetta P III, Dielwart C, et al. Knee pain correlates with union after tibial nailing. *J Orthop Trauma.* 2011;25:731-735, with permission from Lippincott Williams & Wilkins.)

Patients.—All patients treated with an intramedullary nail were evaluated for knee pain and union. Four hundred twenty-eight patients with 443 tibia fractures were included.

Intervention.—All tibia fractures were treated with an intramedullary nail.

Outcomes.—Patient-based knee pain was scored from 0 to 3. Fracture union was also graded using a modified Hammer score based on cortical bridging and remodeling.

Results.—We found a significant inverse association between pain and union score ($P < 0.01$). In contradistinction, there was not a correlation between time from surgery and pain ($P = 0.13$). Because union score and time were related, a model was created with both parameters. This model demonstrated a statistical correlation with union score ($P < 0.01$), but not for time from surgery ($P = 0.18$).

Conclusions.—We postulated that knee pain may correlate with either union or time from surgery. We found a statistically significant, negative correlation between knee pain and fracture union. There was no such association between pain and time from surgery (Figs 1 and 2).

▶ For the past decade, there has been a significant focus on the issue of knee pain following intramedullary nail fixation of tibial fractures. The question of patellar tendon splitting versus a medial approach to insert the nail has been

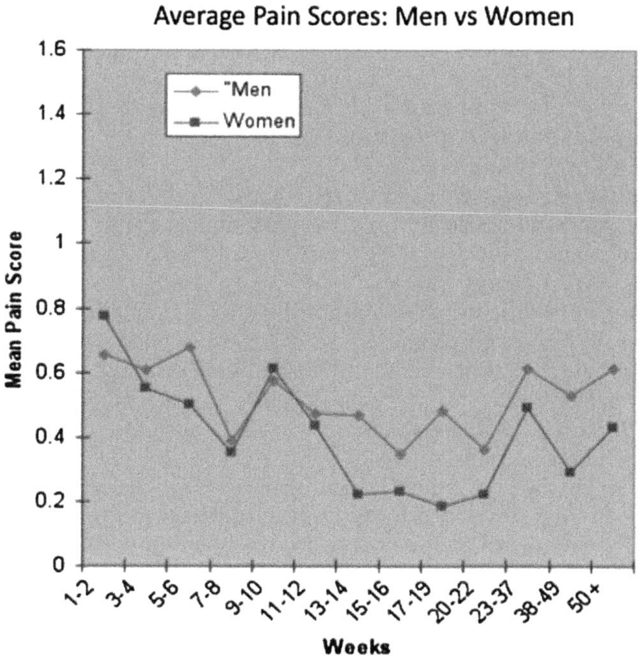

FIGURE 2.—Knee pain during healing (men versus women). (Reprinted from Ryan SP, Tornetta P III, Dielwart C, et al. Knee pain correlates with union after tibial nailing. *J Orthop Trauma*. 2011;25:731-735, with permission from Lippincott Williams & Wilkins.)

exhaustively studied, but the issue of knee pain over time following operative management of these fractures has not been as carefully studied. This well-done prospective cohort study evaluates the relation of knee pain to time since surgery as well as fracture union in patients treated with intramedullary nails. There is no relation to time since surgery, but there is a fairly strong relationship of pain with fracture union. This makes clinical sense because the loading of the implant decreases as fracture union progresses. The lack of relationship over time is a bit more puzzling. It seems to indicate that factors other than fracture union also play a role. This may include fat pad irritation, prominence of proximal tibial locking bolts, capsular scarring, and undetermined patient factors.

M. F. Swiontkowski, MD

Randomized, Prospective Comparison of Plate versus Intramedullary Nail Fixation for Distal Tibia Shaft Fractures

Vallier HA, Cureton BA, Patterson BM (Dept of Orthopaedic Surgery, Cleveland, OH)

J Orthop Trauma 25:736-741, 2011

Objectives.—Malalignment has been frequently reported after intramedullary stabilization of distal tibia fractures. Nails have also been associated with knee pain in several studies. Historically, plate fixation has resulted in increased risks of infection and nonunion. Our purposes were to compare plate and nail stabilization for distal tibia shaft fractures by assessing complications and secondary procedures. We hypothesized that nails would be associated with more malalignment and nonunion.

Design.—Randomized, prospective study.

Setting.—Level I trauma center.

Patients/Participants.—One hundred four skeletally mature patients with extra-articular distal tibia shaft fractures with a mean age of 38 years (range, 18–95 years) and mean Injury Severity Score of 13.5 (range, 9–50). The majority had high-energy injuries.

Intervention.—Patients were randomized to a reamed intramedullary nail ($n = 56$) or a large fragment medial plate ($n = 48$). Forty fractures (39%) were open. Twenty-eight (27%) had concomitant fibula fractures that were stabilized.

Main Outcome Measurements.—Malunion, nonunion, infection, and secondary operations.

Results.—The two treatment groups were evenly matched with respect to age, gender, Injury Severity Score, fracture pattern, and presence of open fracture. Six patients (5.8%) developed deep infection with equal numbers in the two groups. Eighty-three percent of infections occurred after open fracture ($P < 0.001$). Four patients (7.1%) developed nonunion after nailing versus two (4.2%) after plating ($P = 0.25$) with a trend for nonunion in patients who had distal fibula fixation (12% versus 4.1%, $P = 0.09$). All nonunions occurred after open fracture ($P = 0.0007$); the primary union rate for closed fractures was 100%. Primary angular malalignment of 5°

or greater occurred in 13 patients with nails (23% of all nails) and four with plates (8.3% of all plates; $P = 0.02$ for plates versus nails). Six additional patients experienced malalignment after immediate weightbearing against medical advice. Valgus was the most common deformity ($n = 16$). Malunion was more common after open fracture (55%, $P = 0.04$). Eighty-five percent of patients with malalignment after nailing did not have fibula fixation. Eleven patients underwent 15 secondary procedures after plating, five of which were for prominent implant removal. This was not significantly different from patients treated with nailing: 10 patients had 14 procedures and five for prominent implant removal.

Conclusions.—High primary union rates were noted after surgical treatment of distal tibia shaft fractures with both nonlocked plates and reamed intramedullary nails. Rates of infection, nonunion, and secondary procedures were similar. Open fractures had higher rates of infection, nonunion, and malunion. Intramedullary nailing was associated with more malalignment versus plating. Fibula fixation may facilitate reduction of the tibia at the time of surgery. The effect of fibula fixation on tibia healing deserves further study. Economic assessment and functional outcomes data for this population will help to enhance our treatment decision-making (Fig 1, Table 1).

▶ This randomized controlled trial focused on the incidence of fracture healing complications, including malalignment, in distal tibia fractures treated with

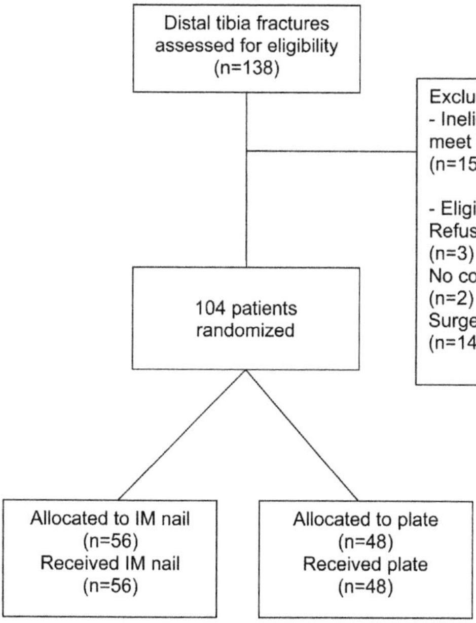

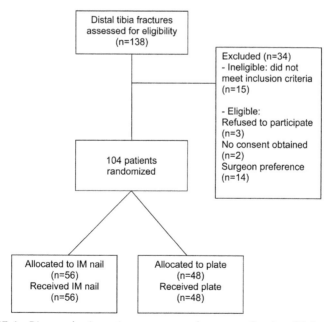

FIGURE 1.—Diagram showing patient assessment and treatment allocation. IM, intramedullary. (Reprinted from Vallier HA, Cureton BA, Patterson BM. Randomized, prospective comparison of plate versus intramedullary nail fixation for distal tibia shaft fractures. *J Orthop Trauma*. 2011;25:736-741, with permission from Lippincott Williams & Wilkins.)

TABLE 1.—Demographic Information

	Plate	Nail	Total	*P*
Male	40	45	85	0.80
Female	8	11	19	0.80
Mean age (years)	38.5	38.1	38.3 ± 13	1.0
Mean ISS	14.7	12.6	13.5 ± 6.7	0.93
Mechanism of Injury				
Motor vehicle collision	8	11	19	0.80
Motorcycle accident	12	15	27	1.0
High-energy fall	6	7	13	1.0
Low-energy fall	9	16	25	0.26
Crush	12	5	17	0.14
Other	1	2	3	1.0
OTA classification[17]				
42-A	31	32	63	0.57
42-B	10	17	27	0.37
42-C	7	7	14	0.78
Open fracture	19	21	40	0.84
Closed fracture	29	35	64	0.84

ISS, Injury Severity Score[18]; OTA, Orthopaedic Trauma Association.
Editor's Note: Please refer to original journal article for full references.

intramedullary nails versus plates. The majority of these fractures were high energy with nearly 40% of presenting as open fractures. The cohorts were equivalent as expected with a randomized design. The outcomes are similar for the 2 treatment approaches with more malalignment in nailed fractures. However, most of this malalignment was associated with failure to plate the fibula, which provides improved alignment of the distal tibia fragment. With that caveat, equal clinical results can be obtained with either approach. Plating the fibula is helpful with either management strategy.

M. F. Swiontkowski, MD

Pulsed Electromagnetic Field Stimulation for Acute Tibial Shaft Fractures: A Multicenter, Double-Blind, Randomized Trial

Adie S, Harris IA, Naylor JM, et al (Liverpool Hosp, New South Wales, Australia)
J Bone Joint Surg Am 93:1569-1576, 2011

Background.—Tibial shaft fractures are sometimes complicated by delayed union and nonunion, necessitating further surgical interventions. Pulsed electromagnetic field stimulation is an effective treatment for delayed unions and nonunions, but its efficacy in preventing healing complications in patients with acute fractures is largely untested. The purpose of this pragmatic trial was to determine whether adjuvant pulsed electromagnetic field therapy for acute tibial shaft fractures reduces the rate of surgical revision because of delayed union or nonunion.

TABLE 2.—Secondary Operations for Delayed Union or Nonunion within Each Time Point Following Injury

	Secondary Operations for Delayed Union or Nonunion (*No. of Patients*)						
	Active (N = 106)	Placebo (N = 112)	*P* Value	Risk Ratio* (95% CI)	Absolute Risk Reduction† (95% CI)	Relative Risk Reduction† (95% CI)	Number Needed to Harm
3 months	6 (5.7%)	5 (4.5%)	0.69	1.01 (0.95 to 1.08)	−0.01 (−0.08 to 0.05)	−0.27 (−1.76 to 1.15)	84
6 months	12 (11.3%)	10 (8.9%)	0.56	1.03 (0.94 to 1.12)	−0.02 (−0.11 to 0.06)	−0.27 (−1.21 to 0.65)	42
12 months	16 (15.1%)	15 (13.4%)	0.72	1.02 (0.91 to 1.14)	−0.02 (−0.11 to 0.08)	−0.13 (−0.84 to 0.57)	59

*Adjusted results presented.
†A negative effect implies an increase in risk.

Methods.—In a double-blind randomized trial involving six metropolitan trauma hospitals, 259 participants with acute tibial shaft fractures (AO/OTA type 42) were randomized by means of external allocation to externally identical active and inactive pulsed electromagnetic field devices. Participants were instructed to wear the device for ten hours daily for twelve weeks. Management was otherwise unaltered. The primary outcome was the proportion of participants requiring a secondary surgical intervention because of delayed union or nonunion within twelve months after the injury. Secondary outcomes included surgical intervention for any reason, radiographic union at six months, and the Short Form-36 Physical Component Summary and Lower Extremity Functional Scales at twelve months. Main analyses were by intention to treat.

Results.—Two hundred and eighteen participants (84%) completed the twelve-month follow-up. One hundred and six patients were allocated to the active device group, and 112 were allocated to the placebo group. Compliance was moderate, with 6.2 hours of average daily use. Overall, sixteen patients in the active group and fifteen in the inactive group experienced a primary outcome event (risk ratio, 1.02; 95% confidence interval, 0.95 to 1.14; $p = 0.72$). According to per-protocol analysis, there were six primary events (12.2%) in the active, compliant group and twenty-six primary events (15.1%) in the combined placebo and active, noncompliant group (risk ratio, 0.97; 95% confidence interval, 0.86 to 1.10; $p = 0.61$). No between-group differences were found with regard to surgical intervention for any reason, radiographic union, or functional measures.

Conclusions.—Adjuvant pulsed electromagnetic field stimulation does not prevent secondary surgical interventions for delayed union or nonunion and does not improve radiographic union or patient-reported functional outcomes in patients with acute tibial shaft fractures (Tables 2, 5, and 7).

▶ This is a long-sought randomized, controlled trial focused around the use of pulsed electromagnetic fields for enhancing union of tibial fractures. One of the nice features of this trial is that tibia fractures treated with intramedullary nails, plates, and casts were included. We can safely conclude that pulsed electromagnetic fields do not favorably impact the rate of secondary procedures to

TABLE 5.—Per-Protocol Analysis Comparing Patients who Actually Received the Prescribed Dose of Pulsed Electromagnetic Fields (Compliant Patients in Active Group) Versus Patients in Placebo Group

	Active Compliant (N = 49)	Placebo (N = 112)	*P* Value	Risk Ratio* (95% CI)
Secondary operations to promote union *(no. of patients)*	6 (12.2%)	15 (13.4%)	0.84	0.91 (0.38 to 2.22)
Total secondary operations *(no. of patients)*	17 (34.7%)	30 (26.8%)	0.18	1.30 (0.79 to 2.12)

*Adjusted results presented.

TABLE 7.—Radiographic Union at Each Time Point Following Injury

	Active		Placebo			
	No. of Patients	No. of Patients with Union	No. of Patients	No. of Patients with Union	*P* Value	Risk Ratio (95% CI)
3 months	52	12 (23%)	59	11 (19%)	0.57	1.24 (0.60 to 2.56)
6 months	44	29 (66%)	49	35 (71%)	0.57	0.92 (0.70 to 1.22)

gain union of tibial diaphyseal fractures, nor does it limit the incidence of delayed unions.

M. F. Swiontkowski, MD

Cigarette smoking influences the clinical and occupational outcome of patients with tibial shaft fractures

Moghaddam A, Zimmermann G, Hammer K, et al (Berufsgenossenschaftliche Unfallklinik Ludwigshafen, Germany; Theresienkrankenhaus Mannheim, Germany; et al)

Injury 42:1435-1442, 2011

Tibial shaft fracture is one of the most common types of bone fracture in young patients. In this prospective clinical cohort study, we investigated the effects of cigarette smoking on the clinical, functional, psychosocial and occupational outcomes after isolated lower-leg fracture.

We examined 85 patients, including 61 men and 24 women, with a collective mean age of 46 years (range: 18–84 years). Thirty-nine patients had never smoked (G1) and 45 patients were current or previous smokers (G2).

The G2 group displayed a significantly increased risk for delayed union or nonunion (G1 = 3 patients, G2 = 18 patients; $P = 0.0007$) and increased time required for fracture healing (mean times: G1 = 11.9 weeks, G2 = 17.4 weeks; $p = 0.003$) and a markedly increased time out of work (mean times: G1 = 16.1 weeks, G2 = 21.5 weeks; $p = 0.1177$ (not significant)). The 18 negatively affected patients in G2 displayed a significant increase in the time required for fracture healing and time out of work (26 weeks ($p = 0.02$) and 31 weeks ($p = 0.03$), respectively). G2 group members had a 3- to 18-fold higher risk of impaired bone healing. The mean Short Form 36 (SF-36) was similar in both groups. The physical-function scores were G1 = 49.6 and G2 = 48.6; the mental scores were G1 = 52.7 and G2 = 52.8.

These findings indicate that smoking significantly increases the risk of impaired fracture healing, which has clinical and occupational consequences for the affected patients. Based on our data, we developed a score to estimate the individual risk of impaired fracture healing. These types of patients must be informed and closely monitored to determine the need

TABLE 3.—Treatment of the Fracture

Characteristic	Total ($N=85$)	Nonsmokers (G1) ($N=39$)	Current and Previous Smokers (G2) ($N=46$)
Time between injury and surgery			
Days	0.8 days	0.9 days	0.6 days
Within 6 h	64 (79%)	29 (76.3%)	35 (81%)
Treatment			
Intramedullary nailing	58 (68.2%)	30 (76.9%)	28 (60.1%)
Osteosynthesis plate	15 (17.6%)	5 (12.8%)	10 (21.7%)
External fixation	8 (9.4%)	3 (7.7%)	5 (10.8%)
Cast	4 (4.7%)	1 (2.6%)	3 (6.5%)
Fibula fracture	71 (83.5%)	34 (87.2%)	37 (80.4%)
Fibula stabilisation	38/71 (53.5%)	18/34 (52.9%)	20/37
Urgent fasciotomy	17 (20%)	9 (23.1)	8 (17.4%)
Removal of the implant			
Yes	49 (60.5%)	25 (65.8%)	24 (55.8%)
No	32 (39.5%)	13 (34.2%)	19 (44.2%)
Time to implant removal	18 months	19 months	18 months
Number of surgeries[a]	2.8 (3; 1–6)[b]	2.8 (2; 1–6)[b]	2.8 (3; 1–6)[b]

[a]Including implant removal surgery.
[b]Average (median; minimum–maximum).

TABLE 4.—Outcome A

Characteristic	Total ($N=85$)	Non-smokers (G1) ($N=39$)	Current and Previous Smokers (G2) ($N=46$)
Hospital stay in days (primary care)	17.7 (15; 5–53)[a]	17 (15; 7–34)[a]	18 (15; 5–53)[a]
Complication			
Yes	31 (36.5%)	9 (23.1%)	22 (47.8%)
No	54 (63.5%)	30 (76.9%)	24 (52.2%)
Bone healing			
On time (within four months)	64 (75.3%)	36 (92.3%)	28 (60.9%)
Impaired*	21 (24.7%)	3 (7.7%)	18 (39.1%)
Weeks until fracture healing **	14.9 (12; 8–63)[a]	11.9 (11; 8–32)[a]	17.4 (14; 8–63)[a]
Delayed union	12 (14.1%)	3 (7.7%)	9 (19.6%)
Nonunion	9 (10.6%)	0	9 (19.6%)
Nonunion with no previous history of fracture to the affected tibia	5 (5.9%)	0	5 (10.9%)
Nonunion with previous history of fracture to the affected tibia	4 (4.7%)	0	4 (8.7%)
Fasciotomy (postoperative)	6 (7.1%)	3 (7.9%)	3 (6.5%)
Infection			
Superficial	3 (3.5%)	1 (2.6%)	2 (4.3%)
Deep	3 (3.5%)	2 (5.1%)	1 (2.2%)
Arterial patency available?			
Dorsalis pedis artery	82 (97%)	38 (97.4%)	44 (95.7%)
Tibialis posterior artery	79 (93%)	37 (94.8%)	42 (91.3%)

Time until fracture healing in 18 patients in G2 with impaired bone healing was 26 ± 13.9 (21; 16–63 weeks) compared to 11 ± 2.5 (11; 8–19 weeks) in patients with proper bone healing ($p=0.02$). Level of significance α was set to 5%.
[a]Average (median; minimum–maximum).
*$p=0.0007$.
**$p=0.0032$ level of significance α was set to 5%.

TABLE 8.—Statistical Retest of the Entire Population With Regard to Impaired Fracture Healing

Effect	Odds Ratio	95% Confidence	Pr > ChiSq	
Gender (m/f)	0.52	0.13	2.07	0.351
Soft-tissue damage (y/n)	3.42	0.81	14.39	0.093
Fasciotomy (y/n)	2.09	0.56	7.76	0.273
Smoking (y/n)[a]	**18.46**	**3.45**	**98.86**	**0.0007**
Fracture form[b]				
42 A vs. 43 A	3.99	0.32	49.85	0.757
Fracture form[b]				
42 B vs. 43 A	3.21	0.24	43.51	–
Fracture form[b]				
42 C vs. 43 A	3.93	0.18	86.84	–
Age	0.96	0.91	1.01	0.126

Level of significance α was set to 5%.
Editor's Note: Please refer to original journal article for full references.
[a]Current and previous smokers (G2) vs. nonsmokers (G1).
[b]According to AO-classification[31].

for timely re-intervention with additional therapy, such as BMP s or ultrasound (Tables 3, 4 and 8).

▶ The issue of the impact of smoking on fracture healing and complications is highly clinically relevant. This cohort study documents this impact in isolated tibia fractures. The study was not ideally conducted with a substantial issue of detection bias, particularly because the determination of fracture healing was likely not preformed with the assessors blinded to the smoking history of the patient. Some of the outcomes measures were not validated. It is not surprising that the SF-36 data did not show a significant difference at final follow-up because this instrument has some issues with floor effects with lesser degrees of lower-extremity functional impairment. Nevertheless, this study provides another important source of information of substantial use to clinicians and patients. The time out of work is a complex outcome measure that may be related to functional demand as well as other psychosocial impact factors that accompany a lifestyle, which include smoking. Smoking has a definite negative impact on fracture healing and functional outcome that is certainly multifactorial.

M. F. Swiontkowski, MD

Factors Influencing Functional Outcomes After Distal Tibia Shaft Fractures

Vallier HA, Cureton BA, Patterson BM (Case Western Reserve Univ School of Medicine, Cleveland, OH)
J Orthop Trauma 26:178-183, 2012

Objectives.—Surgical treatment of displaced distal tibia fractures yields reliable results with either plate or nail fixation. Comparative studies suggest more malalignment and nonunions with nails. Some studies have reported knee pain after tibial nailing. However, plates may be associated with soft tissue complications, such as infections or wound-healing problems. The purpose of this study was to assess functional outcomes after distal tibia shaft fractures treated with a plate or a nail. We hypothesized that tibial nails would be associated with more knee pain and that plates would be associated with pain from implant prominence, each of which would adversely affect functional outcome scores.

Design.—Randomized prospective study.

Setting.—Level 1 trauma center.

Patients/Participants.—One hundred four patients with extra-articular distal tibia shaft fractures (OTA 42), mean age of 38 years (range, 18–95), and mean Injury Severity Score of 14.3 (range, 9–50).

Intervention.—Patients were randomized to treatment with a reamed intramedullary nail (n = 56) or standard large fragment medial plate (n = 48).

Main Outcome Measurements.—Ability to work was evaluated after a minimum of 12 months, with mean of 22 months. Foot Function Index (FFI) and Musculoskeletal Function Assessment (MFA) questionnaires were completed.

Results.—Mean MFA was 27.5, and mean total FFI was 0.26; $P < 0.0001$ versus an uninjured reference population. Sixty-one of 64 patients (95%) employed at the time of injury had returned to work, although 31% had modified their work duties because of injury. Three patients were unable to find work. None reported unemployment secondary to their tibial fracture. Forty percent of all patients described some persistent ankle pain, and 31% had knee pain after nailing, versus 32% and 22%, respectively after plating. Both knee and ankle pain were present in 27% with nails and 15% with plates ($P = 0.08$), and rates of implant removal were similar after nails versus plates. Patients with malunion ≥5 degrees were more likely to report knee or ankle pain (36% vs 20%, $P < 0.05$). Except 1 patient with knee pain when kneeling, none reported modifying activity because of persistent knee or ankle pain, although knee and ankle pain were more frequent in the unemployed ($P = 0.03$). Unemployed patients requested implant removal more frequently (24% vs 9.2%, $P = 0.07$) and continued to report pain afterward. Although FFI and MFA scores were not related to plate or nail fixation, open fracture, fracture pattern, multiple injuries, Injury Severity Score, or age, both MFA and FFI scores were worse when knee pain or ankle pain was present (all *P*s < 0.004) and in patients who remained unemployed ($P < 0.0001$). All 4 patients with work-related injuries had returned to employment but had worse FFI scores ($P = 0.01$).

Conclusions.—Mean MFA and FFI scores suggest substantial residual dysfunction after distal tibia fractures when compared with an uninjured population. Mild ankle or knee pain was reported frequently after plate or nail fixation but was not limiting to activity in most. Angular malunion was associated with both knee and ankle pain, and there was a trend toward more patients with knee and ankle pain after tibial nailing. No patients reported unemployment because of their tibia fracture, but

TABLE 2.—Comparison of Plate and Nail Treatment Groups

	Plate (n = 41)	Nail (n = 45)	Total	*P*
Malunion, %	9 (22)	11 (24)	20 (23)	0.39
≥5 degrees	9	11	20	
≥10 degrees	2	2	4	
Secondary procedures, %	11 (27)	11 (24)	22 (26)	0.40
For complications	7	5	12	0.21
Prominent implant removal	4	6	10	0.30
Ankle pain, %	13 (32)	18 (40)	31 (36)	0.21
Knee pain, %	9 (22)	14 (31)	23 (27)	0.17
Both ankle and knee pain, %	6 (15)	12 (27)	18 (21)	0.08
Ongoing pain medication, %	4 (9.8)	8 (18)	12 (14)	0.14
OTC	3	4	7	
Narcotic	1	2	3	
NSAID	0	2	2	
Ambulatory aids	0	0	0	

Data are presented at a mean of 22-month follow-up.
NSAID, nonsteroidal anti-inflammatory drug; OTC, over-the-counter (nonprescription) medication.

TABLE 3.—Functional Outcome Scores as Measured by FFI or MFA Questionnaires

	FFI				
Tibia Treatment	Pain	Disability	Activity	Total	MFA
Plate (n = 41)	0.31 (0–0.97)	0.23 (0–0.96)	0.20 (0–0.69)	0.23 (0–0.79)	28.0 (1–66)
Nail (n = 45)	0.35 (0–0.87)	0.30 (0–0.83)	0.21 (0–0.67)	0.29 (0–0.75)	27.0 (2–71)
Total	0.33	0.29	0.21	0.26	27.5

Mean scores and range are presented. FFI subscores for pain, disability, and activity are included.

unemployed people described knee and ankle pain more frequently and had the worst functional outcome scores (Tables 2 and 3).

▶ This is a fairly well done controlled trial comparing the functional outcomes from distal tibia fixation with plate versus intramedullary nail. There were no essential differences in knee or ankle pain at follow-up and no differences in patient function as measured by validated patient reported outcome measures. This is a single center trial with highly skilled and experienced orthopedic trauma surgeons. The take-home message is that malunion is associated with pain and functional disability and that both are possible with either plate or nail treatment of distal tibia fractures. The surgeon contributes to at least 90% of the result, with the implant choice having a minor impact. Skilled surgeons can achieve good results with either approach. The disability may be more related to the injury and musculotendinous atrophy from the lack of weight bearing. Focus in the future should be on methods to lessen the impact of these factors.

M. F. Swiontkowski, MD

Recombinant Human Bone Morphogenetic Protein-2: A Randomized Trial in Open Tibial Fractures Treated with Reamed Nail Fixation

Aro HT, Govender S, Patel AD, et al (Turku Univ Hosp, Finland; Univ of Kwazulu-Natal, Durban, South Africa; Norfolk and Norwich Univ Hosp, UK; et al)
J Bone Joint Surg Am 93:801-808, 2011

Background.—Recombinant human bone morphogenetic protein-2 (rhBMP-2) improves healing of open tibial fractures treated with unreamed intramedullary nail fixation. We evaluated the use of rhBMP-2 in the treatment of acute open tibial fractures treated with reamed intramedullary nail fixation.

Methods.—Patients were randomly assigned (1:1) to receive the standard of care consisting of intramedullary nail fixation and routine soft-tissue management (the SOC group) or the standard of care plus an absorbable collagen sponge implant containing 1.5 mg/mL of rhBMP-2 (total, 12.0 mg) (the rhBMP-2/ACS group). Randomization was stratified by fracture severity. The absorbable collagen sponge was placed over the fracture at wound closure. The primary efficacy end point was the proportion of subjects with a healed fracture as demonstrated by radiographic and clinical assessment thirteen and twenty weeks after definitive wound closure.

Results.—Two hundred and seventy-seven patients were randomized and were the subjects of the intent-to-treat analysis. Thirteen percent of the fractures were Gustilo-Anderson Type IIIB. The proportions of patients with fracture-healing were 60% and 48% at week 13 ($p = 0.0541$) and 68% and 67% at week 20 in the rhBMP-2/ACS and SOC groups, respectively. Twelve percent of the subjects underwent secondary procedures in each group; more invasive procedures (e.g., exchange nailing) accounted for 30% of the procedures in the rhBMP-2/ACS group and 57% in the SOC group ($p = 0.1271$). Infection was seen in twenty-seven (19%) of the patients in the rhBMP-2/ACS group and fifteen (11%) in the SOC group ($p = 0.0645$; difference in infection risk = 0.09 [95% confidence interval, 0.0 to 0.17]). The adverse event incidence was otherwise similar between the treatment groups.

Conclusions.—The healing of open tibial fractures treated with reamed intramedullary nail fixation was not significantly accelerated by the addition of an absorbable collagen sponge containing rhBMP-2 (Tables 1 and 2).

► The use of recombinant human bone morphogenetic protein-2 (rhBMP-2) has accelerated based on the findings of the BESTT trial published nearly a decade ago. This investigative team was comprised of multiple individuals who participated in that trial, and they demonstrated a dose-dependent decrease in the need for secondary intervention to gain fracture union in a population of 450 patients with open tibia fractures. This trial had a different end point—fracture union. Fracture union was defined differently in this trial (2 cortices) in contrast to the BESTT trial (3 cortices). It is this critical distinction that may explain the differences in the findings of the 2 trials (Table 3 in the original article). The event rate in both the experimental and treatment groups was low in this study, indicative of expert surgical

TABLE 1.—Patient Demographics and Fracture Classification

	rhBMP-2/ACS (N = 139)	SOC (N = 138)
Age		
Mean *(yr)*	39.5	37.5
≥65 yr *(no. [%])*	9 (6)	9 (7)
Male sex *(no. [%])*	113 (81)	111 (80)
No tobacco use *(no. [%])*	73 (53)	76 (55)
Intraoperative Gustilo-Anderson classification *(no. [%])*		
Stratum A		
I	41 (29)	46 (33)
II	51 (37)	45 (33)
IIIA	26 (19)	27 (20)
Stratum B: IIIB	18 (13)	18 (13)
Missing	3 (2)	2 (1)

TABLE 2.—Prevalence of Local Adverse Events

	rhBMP-2/ACS (N = 139) *(No. [%])*	SOC (N = 138) *(No. [%])*
Infection	27 (19)	15 (11)
Deep	12 (9)	3 (2)
Superficial	15 (11)	12 (9)
Hardware failure	24 (17)	21 (15)
Peripheral edema	36 (26)	39 (28)
Heterotopic ossification/soft-tissue calcification	12 (9)	8 (6)
Pain (new or increased)	88 (63)	80 (58)
Delayed union*	9 (6)	16 (12)
Nonunion*	1 (1)	5 (4)

*Delayed union and nonunion were defined as adverse events separate from the primary assessment of healing. Subjects with a fracture not classified as healed might not have had an adverse event recorded as a delayed union or nonunion. Furthermore, subjects with delayed union recorded as an adverse event might have also have been reported to have nonunion later in the trial.

treatment as well as the potential for the subjects in this trial to represent lower-energy injuries. Further studies of the impact of rhBMP-2 are required for both high-energy fractures and ununited fractures, for which its off-label use continues.

M. F. Swiontkowski, MD

Knee

Infection After Spanning External Fixation for High-Energy Tibial Plateau Fractures: Is Pin Site–Plate Overlap a Problem?

Laible C, Earl-Royal E, Davidovitch R, et al (NYU Hosp for Joint Diseases)
J Orthop Trauma 26:92-97, 2012

Objectives.—The purpose of this study was to determine whether overlap between temporary external fixator pins and definitive plate fixation correlates with infection in high-energy tibial plateau fractures.

Design.—Retrospective chart and radiographic review.

Setting.—Academic medical center.

Patients.—Seventy-nine patients with unilateral high-energy tibial plateau fractures formed the basis of this report.

Intervention.—Placement of knee-spanning external fixation followed by delayed internal fixation for high-energy tibial plateau fractures treated at our institution between 2000 and 2008.

Methods.—Demographic patient information was reviewed. Radiographs were reviewed to assess for the presence of overlap between the temporary external fixator pins and the definitive plate fixation. Fisher exact and *t* test analyses were performed to compare those patients who had overlap and those who did not and were used to determine whether this was a factor in the development of a postoperative infection.

Main Outcome Measurements.—Development of infection in those whose external fixation pin sites overlapped with the definitive internal fixation device compared with those whose pin sites did not overlap with definitive plate and screws.

Results.—Six knees in six patients developed deep infections requiring serial irrigation and débridement and intravenous antibiotics. Of these six infections, three were in patients with closed fractures and three in patients with open fractures. Two of these six infections followed definitive plate fixation that overlapped the external fixator pin sites with an average of 4.2 cm of overlap. In the four patients who developed an infection and had no overlap, the average distance between the tip of the plate to the first external fixator pin was 6.3 cm. There was no correlation seen between infection and distance from pin to plate, pin–plate overlap distance, time in the external fixator, open fracture, classification of fracture, sex of the patient, age of the patient, or healing status of the fracture.

Conclusion.—Fears of definitive fracture fixation site contamination from external fixator pins do not appear to be clinically grounded. When needed, we recommend the use of a temporary external fixation construct with pin placement that provides for the best reduction and stability of the fracture, regardless of plans for future surgery.

▶ The issue of pin site contamination of the operative site in patients requiring temporary external fixation has been a topic of concern for a decade or so since this temporizing maneuver has become the standard. This retrospective review confirms that this is not a valid concern. Of course, these pins were applied in high-volume centers with supervision of very experienced surgeons, so thermal necrosis of bone and soft tissue tension were minimized. This information can be used to reassure patients undergoing staged reconstructions of highly displaced tibial plateau fractures.

M. F. Swiontkowski, MD

Weight-bearing-induced displacement and migration over time of fracture fragments following split depression fractures of the lateral tibial plateau: A case series with radiostereometric analysis

Solomon LB, Callary SA, Stevenson AW, et al (Royal Adelaide Hosp and Univ of Adelaide, Australia)

J Bone Joint Surg [Br] 93-B:817-823, 2011

We investigated the stability of seven Schatzker type II fractures of the lateral tibial plateau treated by subchondral screws and a buttress plate followed by immediate partial weight-bearing. In order to assess the stability of the fracture, weight-bearing inducible displacements of the fracture fragments and their migration over a one-year period were measured by differentially loaded radiostereometric analysis and standard radiostereometric analysis, respectively. The mean inducible craniocaudal fracture fragment displacements measured −0.30 mm (−0.73 to 0.02) at two weeks and 0.00 mm (−0.12 to 0.15) at 52 weeks. All inducible displacements were elastic in nature under all loads at each examination during follow-up. At one year, the mean craniocaudal migration of the fracture fragments was −0.34 mm (−1.64 to 1.51).

Using radiostereometric methods, this case series has shown that in the Schatzker type II fractures investigated, internal fixation with subchondral screws and a buttress plate provided adequate stability to allow immediate post-operative partial weight-bearing, without harmful consequences.

▶ This is a well done study using a radiostereometric (RSA) technique to evaluate tibial plateau fracture stability in the postoperative period under conditions of immediate partial weight bearing. RSA has been long used in the investigation of total joint arthroplasty to understand component stability and is well validated. The implications are that we are too cautious in advising patients RE weightbearing after fixation of tibial plateau fracture fixation. Several areas of caution are advisable. First, we do not understand the loads that these patients actually put on their knee; they may have limited weightbearing that is substantially more significant than the investigators considered. Second, these are a highly selected group of patients, likely with outstanding anatomic reductions. The conclusions may not apply to less well-reduced fractures. In general, however, the conclusions are valid given these caveats. I agree that we are far too conservative in general in advising our patients RE weightbearing after fractures in the lower extremity. This is an area that is wide open for additional well-designed controlled trials.

M. F. Swiontkowski, MD

Upper Extremity

Volar Locking Plates Versus K-Wire Fixation of Dorsally Displaced Distal Radius Fractures—A Functional Outcome Study

Hull P, Baraza N, Gohil M, et al (Worcester Acute Hosps NHS Trust and Warwick Univ Med School, Coventry, UK; Dept of Trauma and Orthopaedic, Birmingham, West Midlands, UK; Dept of Trauma and Orthopaedic, Hollywood, Worcestershire, UK; et al)
J Trauma 70:E125-E128, 2011

Background.—Fractures of the distal radius are common. As the population of the western world ages, their incidence is set to increase further. There are various methods of treating these fractures, but optimal management remains controversial. In the United Kingdom, the most common surgical treatment of closed distal radius fractures is by Kirschner-wires (K-wires) or volar locking plate. In this study, we compared long-term functional outcomes of volar locking plates with those of K-wires.

Methods.—A retrospective comparative study of 71 patients with dorsally displaced distal radius fractures treated contemporaneously in two independent hospitals was performed. One group was treated with a volar locking plate (n = 36) and the other group with manipulation and K-wire fixation (n = 35). There was no difference between the two groups in terms of demographics or grade of fracture. Outcome was measured 15 months to 27 months post surgery using the Disabilities of the Arm, Shoulder and Hand score and the Patient-Rated Wrist Evaluation score.

Results.—We found no statistical difference between the two groups in the Patient-Rated Wrist Evaluation score or Disabilities of the Arm, Shoulder and Hand score at 1 year to 2 years postsurgery.

Conclusion.—We have been unable to demonstrate a clinically relevant advantage of using volar locking plates over K-wires at 1 year to 2 years postoperatively (Tables 4 and 6).

▶ This retrospective cohort study compares the long-term outcomes of distal radius fractures fixed with K-wires versus plate and screw constructs. No differences were identified. This fits with other prospective studies that have confirmed

TABLE 4.—Intra-Articular Fractures: (Universal Grades 3 or 4) Functional Outcome Scores

	Locking Plate Group (n = 18)	K-Wire Group (n = 18)	p*
PRWE pain	13.3 (0–35)	13.8 (0–45)	0.691
PRWE function	11.3 (0–32)	10.1 (0–47)	0.714
Final PRWE	24.6 (0–67)	23.8 (0–85)	0.727
DASH	22.9 (0–63)	20.2 (0–86)	0.486

*p-values from Wilcoxon-Mann-Whitney two-sample rank-sum tests; group means were considered to differ significantly if $p < 0.05$.

TABLE 6.—Postoperative Complications

	Locking Plate Group (n = 36)	K-Wire Group (n = 35)	p^*
Numbness/tingling, n (%)	12 (33)	4 (11)	0.054
Superficial infection (scar or wire), n (%)	2 (6)	4 (11)	0.644

*p-Values from binomial tests of proportions; proportions were considered to differ significantly if $p < 0.05$.

early benefit to open reduction internal fixation with less immobilization required and earlier return to function. Both factors are important to discuss with patients when electing how best to manage displaced distal radius fractures in adults.

M. F. Swiontkowski, MD

Three- and Four-part Fractures Have Poorer Function Than One-part Proximal Humerus Fractures

Ong C, Bechtel C, Walsh M, et al (NYU Hosp for Joint Diseases)
Clin Orthop Relat Res 469:3292-3299, 2011

Background.—Locking plates have become a commonly used fixation device in the operative treatment of three- and four-part proximal humerus fractures. Examining function in patients treated nonoperatively and operatively should help determine whether and when surgery is appropriate in these difficult-to-treat fractures.

Questions/Purposes.—We compared functional scores, ROM, and radiographs in patients with one-part proximal humerus fractures treated nonoperatively to those in patients with displaced three- and four-part proximal humerus fractures treated with open reduction and internal fixation using locking plates.

TABLE 3.—Functional and Radiographic Outcomes

Variable	Nonoperative Cohort (One-Part Proximal Humerus Fractures)	Operative Cohort (Three- or Four-Part Proximal Humerus Fractures)	p Value
ROM			
Forward elevation (°)	147.0 (33.5)	133.9 (32.8)	0.08
External rotation (°)	40.4 (17.1)	41.5 (19.7)	0.81
Functional score (points)			
SF-36 (physical)	81.5 (13.7)	67.9 (24.5)	< 0.001
SF-36 (mental)	83.1 (9.4)	74.0 (22.1)	0.0085
ASES	91.7 (11.4)	74.5 (20.5)	< 0.001
Radiographs			
Fracture union	100% (28% with minimal displacement < 5 mm)	100% (8% with displacement resulting in screw penetration)	

Values are expressed as mean, with SD in parentheses; ASES = American Shoulder and Elbow Surgeons.

TABLE 4.—Complications and Select Patient and Surgical Variables

Patient	Sex	Age (Years)	Smoker	Neer Classification	SF-36 Score (Points) (Physical/Mental/Total)	ASES Score (Points)	ROM (FE/ER) (°)	Complication Type
1	Female	83	No	Three-part	13/25/17	12	90/30	Screw cutout, osteonecrosis
2	Male	58	No	Four-part	85/84/87	82	60/10	Heterotopic ossification
3	Male	61	No	Four-part	64/88/75	63	100/10	Greater tuberosity malunion, postoperative infection
4	Male	46	Yes	Three-part	13/25/17	12	90/30	Hardware failure
5	Female	71	No	Three-part	57/68/57	72	110/30	Screw cutout
6	Female	69	No	Three-part	40/36/36	48	110/5	Screw cutout
7	Female	61	No	Three-part	39/76/54	62	170/40	Postoperative infection
8	Female	74	No	Three-part	46/66/52	62	95/30	Screw cutout
9	Male	57	No	Four-part	65/89/76	75	110/30	Postoperative infection

ASES = American Shoulder and Elbow Surgeons; FE = forward elevation; ER = external rotation.

Patients and Methods.—We retrospectively reviewed 142 patients with proximal humerus fractures treated with a standardized treatment algorithm over a 6-year period. Three- and four-part fractures were treated surgically while one-part fractures were treated nonoperatively. Functional scores, ROM, and radiographs were used to evaluate outcomes. American Shoulder and Elbow Surgeons and SF-36 scores were obtained at 12 months. Of the 142 patients, 101 (51 with three- or four-part fractures and 50 with one-part fractures) had a minimum followup of 12 months (average, 19 months; range, 12–64 months).

Results.—The fractures united in all patients. At 1 year, the patients with one-part fractures had better SF-36 physical and mental scores and American Shoulder and Elbow Surgeons scores than the three- and four-part fractures. Both groups had similar shoulder ROM. Nine patients treated operatively had complications, four of which were related to screw penetration into the joint.

Conclusions.—Patients with three- and four-part fractures should be advised of the likelihood of persistent functional impairment and a relatively higher risk of complications when treated operatively with locked plates.

Level of Evidence.—Level III, therapeutic study. See Guidelines for Authors for a complete description of levels of evidence (Tables 3 and 4).

▶ This carefully preformed retrospective cohort study confirms a principle long understood in regard to proximal humerus fractures: the higher the degree of comminution as defined by Neer's system, the worse the functional outcome. The added benefit of this investigation is that it confirms the principle in operatively treated proximal humerus fractures (Table 3). The complications occurred in patients with 3- and 4-part fractures (Table 4). This information is important to share with patients to adjust expectations appropriately and increase motivation for postoperative rehabilitation.

M. F. Swiontkowski, MD

Excessive Complications of Open Intramedullary Nailing of Midshaft Clavicle Fractures With the Rockwood Clavicle Pin

Mudd CD, Quigley KJ, Gross LB (Saint Louis Univ School of Medicine, MO; The Orthopedic Ctr of Saint Louis, Chesterfield, MO)

Clin Orthop Relat Res 469:3364-3370, 2011

Background.—Intramedullary clavicle fixation is a potential alternative to plate fixation. Previous studies documenting the complication rates of intramedullary clavicle fixation have demonstrated variable rates of soft tissue complications and fracture healing.

Questions/Purposes.—We asked the following questions: (1) Does use of the Rockwood Clavicle Pin (DePuy Orthopaedics Inc, Warsaw, IN) predispose patients to soft tissue complications requiring additional surgery or a high infection risk? (2) Does the Rockwood Clavicle Pin provide a truly minimally invasive insertion technique and reliable fracture fixation?

Patients and Methods.—We retrospectively evaluated 18 patients (mean age, 31 years) who sustained a closed midshaft fracture of the clavicle treated with open intramedullary nailing with a Rockwood Clavicle Pin. We determined the incidence of complications and rate of fracture healing.

Results.—Fourteen complications occurred in 10 patients. Five patients experienced a complication with fracture healing, including three nonunions. Nine patients experienced complications relating to soft tissue, including infection, skin necrosis, or posterior pain from pin prominence.

Conclusions.—The Rockwood Clavicle Pin remains a historically relevant method of clavicle fixation. However, due to an unacceptably high rate of nonunion, repeat operation, and soft tissue complications, we do not recommend this device for treating middiaphyseal clavicle fractures.

Level of Evidence.—Level IV, therapeutic study. See Guidelines for Authors for a complete description of levels of evidence (Table 2).

▶ This cohort series of patients treated with the Rockwood pin points out the high complication rate with intramedullary devices. The use of intramuscular (IM) devices should be restricted to middle one-third fractures with relatively

TABLE 2.—Soft Tissue and Osseous Complications

Patient	Age (Years)	Sex	Soft Tissue Complications	Osseous Complications
1	18	Female	Posterior skin necrosis requiring operative débridement	None
2	21	Male	Posterior pin prominence with pain, transient axillary sensory neuropathy	None
3	22	Male	Posterior pain necessitating premature pin removal	Secondary alteration in reduction after pin removal
4	24	Male	None	None
5	27	Male	None	None
6	27	Male	None	None
7	28	Male	None	Atrophic nonunion, posterior pin migration with loss of reduction, reoperation with bone grafting and PDGF
8	29	Male	None	None
9	30	Male	None	None
10	32	Male	Anterior medial skin necrosis	Medial pin migration, reoperation, chronic fibrous nonunion
11	32	Male	Posterior skin necrosis with exposed pin requiring débridement	Secondary alteration in reduction after pin removal
12	32	Female	Anterior wound infection requiring premature pin removal	Secondary alteration in reduction after pin removal
13	32	Male	None	None
14	33	Female	Posterior pain	Delayed union
15	41	Male	Staphylococcus aureus wound infection requiring premature pin removal	Secondary alteration in reduction after pin removal, infected nonunion, ORIF × 2
16	44	Male	Posterior pain necessitating premature pin removal	None
17	47	Male	None	None
18	47	Female	None	None

PDGF = platelet-derived growth factor; ORIF = open reduction and internal fixation.

simple fracture patterns managed by surgeons experienced in the use of IM devices for clavicle fixation. The bone is curved in 2 planes, which makes the use of straight devices difficult. Good bone quality with excellent reduction is a requirement for the use of these devices.

M. F. Swiontkowski, MD

Distal Radioulnar Joint Instability (Galeazzi Type Injury) After Internal Fixation in Relation to the Radius Fracture Pattern

Korompilias AV, Lykissas MG, Kostas-Agnantis IP, et al (Univ of Ioannina School of Medicine, Greece; Univ of Athens School of Medicine, Greece)

J Hand Surg 36A:847-852, 2011

Purpose.—The purpose of this study was to classify Galeazzi type injuries and determine the association of residual instability after rigid fixation with the fracture pattern of the shaft of the radius, using a system that is based on anatomic landmarks of the radial shaft.

Methods.—The clinical records of 95 patients (72 men and 23 women) with Galeazzi type injuries requiring open reduction and internal fixation of the fractures were retrospectively reviewed. The mean follow-up was 6.8 years (range, 18 mo to 11 y) after injury. Sixty-nine fractures occurred in the distal third of the radial shaft (type I), 17 fractures were in the middle third (type II), and 9 fractures were in the proximal third of the shaft of the radius (type III). Gross instability of the distal radioulnar joint (DRUJ) was determined intraoperatively by manipulation after radial fixation as compared to the uninjured side.

Results.—Forty patients had DRUJ instability after internal fixation and were treated with temporary pinning with a K-wire placed transversely proximal to the sigmoid notch. Distal radioulnar joint instability after internal fixation was recorded in 37 type I fractures, 2 type II fractures, and 1 type III fracture.

Conclusions.—Distal radioulnar joint instability following radial shaft fracture fixation is significantly higher in patients with type I fractures than in patients with type II or type III fractures. The location of the radius fracture can be sufficiently used for preoperative estimation of percentage chance of potential DRUJ instability after fracture fixation.

► All orthopedic surgeons are trained to evaluate the stability of the distal radioulnar joint with isolated fractures of the radius. This retrospective review simply points out that the risk is markedly increased with fractures in the distal third of the radial shaft but can occur in more proximal fractures. Vigilance for all radial shaft fractures with regard to distal radioulnar joint stability evaluation remains the take-home message.

M. F. Swiontkowski, MD

Clinical Results of Volar Locking Plate for Distal Radius Fractures: Conventional versus Minimally Invasive Plate Osteosynthesis

Zenke Y, Sakai A, Oshige T, et al (Kagawa Rosai Hosp, Jyotocho, Marugame, Japan; Univ of Occupational and Environmental Health, Kitakyushu, Japan)

J Orthop Trauma 25:425-431, 2011

Objectives.—The purpose of this study was to compare the postoperative radiologic and clinical outcomes of conventional plate osteosynthesis (C) with minimally invasive plate osteosynthesis (M) using a transverse skin incision without cutting the pronator quadratus muscle for distal radius fractures.

Design.—Retrospective consecutive cohort with prospective data collection.

Setting.—One community teaching hospital. Surgical treatment was performed by a single surgeon.

Patients.—Sixty-six patients (C group, 36; M group, 30) underwent open reduction and internal fixation of dorsally displaced distal radius fractures with the volar locking plating system from June 2006 to August 2008. Their mean age was 63.5 years and the mean follow-up period was 22.7 months.

Main Outcome Measures.—Radiologic parameters (volar tilt, radial inclination, ulnar variance), range of motion, grip strength, and Disability of the Arm, Shoulder, and Hand score were evaluated at each examination. The visual analog scale of wrist pain and evaluations of cosmetic problems were assessed at the final follow-up.

Results.—The groups did not differ significantly in all main outcomes. In the M group, the mean values of the Disability of the Arm, Shoulder, and Hand score at 2 weeks postoperatively ($P = 0.06$) and visual analog scale ($P = 0.07$) were lower and the mean value of the patient's satisfaction score of cosmetic problems ($P = 0.08$) was higher than those in the C

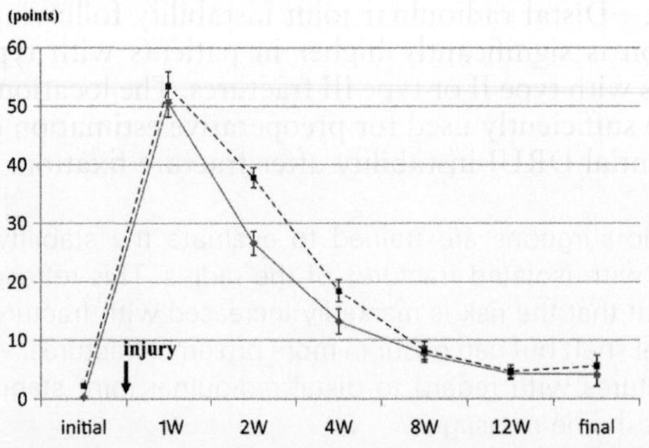

FIGURE 4.—Sequential changes in the score for Disability of the Arm, Shoulder, and Hand. W, weeks; dotted line, conventional group; solid line, minimally invasive plate osteosynthesis group. (Reprinted from Zenke Y, Sakai A, Oshige T, et al. Clinical results of volar locking plate for distal radius fractures: conventional versus minimally invasive plate osteosynthesis. *J Orthop Trauma.* 2011;25:425-431, with permission from Lippincott Williams & Wilkins.)

TABLE 1.—Characteristics of Patients

	Conventional Group	MIPO Group	Total
Number of patients	36	30	66
Mean age (years)	64.7 ± 17.8	62.1 ± 15.6	63.5
Sex, male/female	9/27	10/20	19/47
Injured side, right/left	19/17	12/18	31/35
Mean period from injury to surgery (days)	1.4 ± 1.5	2.5 ± 2.6	1.9
Mean follow-up period (months)	23.9 ± 9.9	21.0 ± 7.3	22.7
OTA classification (23-), A2/A3/C1/C2	12/13/2/9	7/10/5/8	19/23/7/17

Data are mean ± standard deviation.
MIPO, minimally invasive plate osteosynthesis; OTA, Orthopaedic Trauma Association.

TABLE 4.—Complications

	Conventional Group	MIPO Group
Case (%)	3 (8.3)	1 (3.3)
Details	EPL tendon rupture Incomplete palsy of the superficial branch of the median nerve Loosening of a cortical screw	The distal locking pin protruded into the wrist joint
Reoperation	None Neurolysis None	Removal of pins and plate at 6 months after surgery

MIPO, minimally invasive plate osteosynthesis; EPL, extensor pollicis longus.

TABLE 5.—Range of Motion and Grip Strength at Final Follow-Up

	Conventional Group	MIPO Group
Range of motion (degrees) (extension/flexion)	68.3 ± 5.6/86.0 ± 6.7	67.2 ± 6.7/86.5 ± 6.7
Range of motion (degrees) (pronation/supination)	88.8 ± 3.4/88.2 ± 5.7	88.9 ± 3.2/88.6 ± 4.3
Grip strength, percent of the opposite uninjured side	96.2 ± 14.0	94.2 ± 12.8

Data are mean ± standard deviation.
MIPO, minimally invasive plate osteosynthesis.

group, but no statistically significant differences were apparent in these values.

Conclusion.—No significant differences were found between the minimally invasive plate osteosynthesis and conventional plating for distal radius fractures based on the data from postoperative radiologic and clinical outcomes (Fig 4, Tables 1, 4, 5).

▶ This consecutive series study attempts to document the benefits of a limited surgical exposure for fixation of distal radius fractures using locked plates. It is a well-conducted, nonrandomized study that fails to confirm any patient benefit

(Tables 4 and 5) in either complications or functional outcome. The additional risk of a limited surgical incision in terms of a major neurologic or tendon injury is definitely not worth it for surgical management of this fracture with locked plates.

M. F. Swiontkowski, MD

Proximal Humerus Fractures in the Elderly Can Be Reliably Fixed With a "Hybrid" Locked-plating Technique

Barlow JD, Sanchez-Sotelo J, Torchia M (Mayo Clinic, Rochester, MN)
Clin Orthop Relat Res 469:3281-3291, 2011

Background.—Controversy exists regarding the best treatment of proximal humerus fractures in the elderly. Recent studies of open reduction and internal fixation have demonstrated high complication rates.

Questions/Purposes.—We asked whether (1) open reduction and internal fixation could be performed with low rates of immediate and delayed complications, (2) reduction of these fractures could be maintained over time by evaluating long-term radiographs and visual analog pain scores, and (3) 6-week immobilization would lead to disabling stiffness by evaluating postoperative motion and functional scores.

Patients and Methods.—We retrospectively reviewed all 35 patients older than 75 years with displaced proximal humerus fractures treated using a "hybrid" technique between 2002 and 2008. All patients were immobilized for 6 weeks after surgery. Thirteen of the 35 patients either died or developed severe dementia during followup. The analysis included 22 patients followed a minimum of 1 year (mean, 3 years; range, 1–6.7 years).

Results.—There were no early or late reoperations in this series. An acceptable reduction was achieved in 89% of the shoulders and maintained over time. All fractures healed. Osteonecrosis was noted on radiographs in 11% of the shoulders. Six weeks of immobilization did not lead to disabling stiffness. At most recent followup, mean active elevation was 141°, mean active internal rotation L1, mean active external rotation 36°, and mean American Society of Shoulder and Elbow Surgeons score 68.

Conclusions.—Utilizing this approach, open reduction and internal fixation followed by 6-week immobilization results in a low rate of reoperation and good functional outcomes for elderly patients with proximal humerus fractures.

Level of Evidence.—Level IV, therapeutic study. See Guidelines for Authors for a complete description of levels of evidence (Table 1).

▶ With the explosion in the use of open reduction and internal fixation (ORIF) for the management of proximal humerus fractures, the question of how elderly patients fare with this more aggressive treatment is highly relevant. This highly skilled and ethical group of surgeons looked retrospectively at the outcomes of ORIF of the proximal humerus in patients older than 75 years. The results are highly encouraging with active forward flexion of more than 140° and minimal

TABLE 1.—ROM in Operative and Nonoperative Extremities at Final Followup

ROM	Operative Extremity Mean	Operative Extremity SD	Contralateral Extremity Mean	Contralateral Extremity SD
Elevation	141°	47°	172°	25°
Abduction	132°	46°	163°	32°
Internal rotation	L1	2 levels	T8	2 levels
External rotation	36°	24°	47°	22°

pain (Table 1, Fig 4 in the original article). The question remains "how much better an outcome is this than conservative treatment for these fractures in this age group?" I suspect that this group of surgeons chose patients with high activity levels and higher functional demands than many 75 year olds. This is a question that will only be answered with an adequately powered multi-center randomized, controlled trial. I believe that the results will favor ORIF in the higher functional demand older patient, but the study needs to be done.

M. F. Swiontkowski, MD

Removal of Locked Volar Plates After Distal Radius Fractures

Gyuricza C, Carlson MG, Weiland AJ, et al (Hosp for Special Surgery, NY)
J Hand Surg 36A:982-985, 2011

Purpose.—We present our experience with removal of locked volar distal radius plates and screws and note the indications for removal, types of plates removed, completeness of hardware removal, and complications occurring during plate removal.

Methods.—We reviewed all distal radial volar locking plates removed at our institution from 2004 to 2009. A total of 28 patients operated on by 5 hand surgeons were identified. We gathered information regarding the incidence of successful removal of hardware and operative findings in cases of difficult removal of hardware.

Results.—A total of 28 patients (16 women, 12 men) underwent removal of locked volar distal radius plates from 2004 to 2009. The mean length of implantation was 63 weeks (range, 3—223 wk). Reasons for removal of hardware included tenosynovitis, tendon rupture, pain, and prominent or intra-articular hardware. Of 28 cases of locked volar plate removal, 2 had complications. In the first case, a screw was cross-threaded in an earlier generation DVR Hand Innovations plate implanted in 2003. The plate and screw were removed by rotating them out as 1 unit. In the second case, in which the current generation DVR Hand Innovations plate was implanted in 2007, the recess in the screw head had been stripped on insertion. The plate was cut and the remaining fragment of plate and screw were removed together. Despite these difficulties, hardware was successfully removed completely in 28 patients.

Conclusions.—This case series highlights the result that all removals of locked volar plates were successful. There were 2 complications, and strategies for removal are described.

Type of Study/Level of Evidence.—Therapeutic IV.

▶ This is an important retrospective cohort report that describes a large referral center's experience with removing locked volar distal radius plates. The indications and results are important additions to the literature, given the increasing use of these implants in the management of distal radius fractures for both extra as well as intra-articular fractures. It is interesting to note that removal of the locked pegs is more difficult than that of locked screws. This does make sense because there are no threads to keep the screw head turning as it is backed out with the screw driver. This series assures us that, in the rare case in which these plates need to be removed, it can be done successfully.

M. F. Swiontkowski, MD

Closed Reduction and Early Mobilization in Fractures of the Humeral Capitellum

Puloski S, Kemp K, Sheps D, et al (Univ of Calgary, Alberta, Canada; Univ of Alberta, Edmonton, Canada)

J Orthop Trauma 26:62-65, 2012

Seven consecutive patients with an isolated fracture of the humeral capitellum were treated by a single surgeon at a Level II care facility according to a simple treatment algorithm. Closed reduction was attempted in all cases

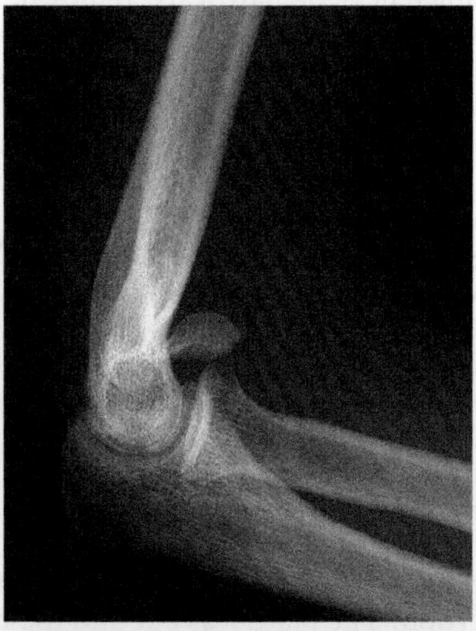

FIGURE 1.—Lateral elbow radiograph showing the typical Type 1 displaced capitellar fracture with the Hahn-Steinthal fragment. (Reprinted from Puloski S, Kemp K, Sheps D, et al. Closed reduction and early mobilization in fractures of the humeral capitellum. *J Orthop Trauma*. 2012;26:62-65, with permission from Lippincott Williams & Wilkins.)

using a standard technique. After reduction, the arm was splinted at 90° of flexion and mobilized at 14 days. All patients completed a clinical and radiographic follow-up consisting of a radiographic evaluation of reduction, elbow range of motion, Disabilities of the Arm, Shoulder and Hand Questionnaire, and a subjective rating of patient satisfaction. None of the patients required conversion to open reduction internal fixation or excision. Disabilities of the Arm, Shoulder and Hand Questionnaire scores ranged from 6 to 13 points (out of 100; mean, 9). The mean flexion/extension arc of motion obtained was 126° with minimal loss of rotation. Patient satisfaction was rated as excellent in five patients and good in two. All fractures appeared united at the most recent clinical and radiographic review. Closed reduction and early mobilization appears to be a safe and effective method of treating displaced fractures of the humeral capitellum with clinical results comparable to that of open reduction internal fixation (Figs 1-3, Table 1).

▶ This is a small cohort study of a relatively rare fracture with good follow-up. It demonstrated that isolated fractures of the capitellum can be treated with closed reduction, short-term immobilization, and active range of motion with the expectation of good functional outcome. The caveat is that the closed reduction must be held to an anatomic standard. With slight malreduction, open reduction

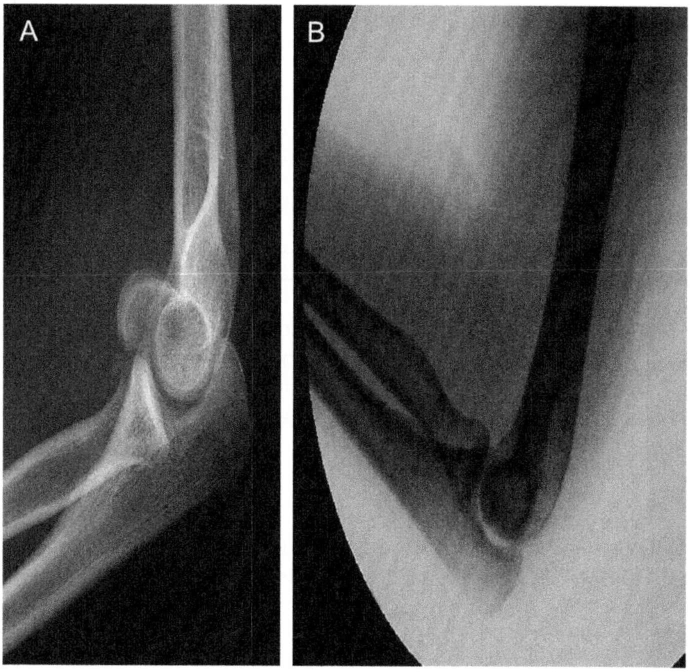

FIGURE 2.—Lateral radiograph of displaced fracture of the humeral capitellum (A). The fracture is reduced anatomically with closed manipulation and the elbow is splinted at 90° after confirmation with intraoperative fluoroscopy (B). (Reprinted from Puloski S, Kemp K, Sheps D, et al. Closed reduction and early mobilization in fractures of the humeral capitellum. *J Orthop Trauma.* 2012;26:62-65, with permission from Lippincott Williams & Wilkins.)

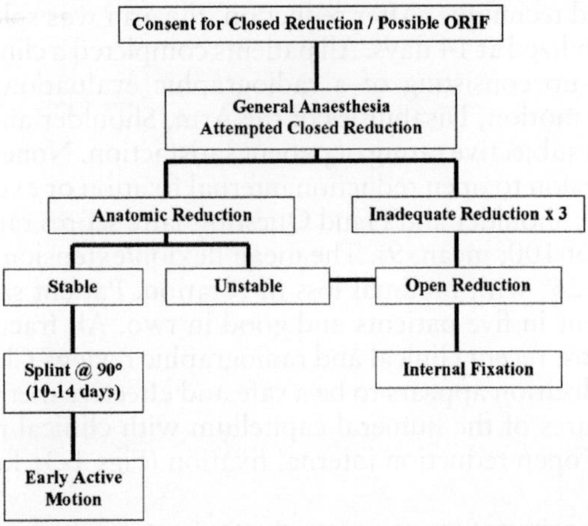

FIGURE 3.—Treatment algorithm for Type I capitellar fracture as suggested by the authors. (Reprinted from Puloski S, Kemp K, Sheps D, et al. Closed reduction and early mobilization in fractures of the humeral capitellum. *J Orthop Trauma*. 2012;26:62-65, with permission from Lippincott Williams & Wilkins.)

TABLE 1.—Patient Demographics and Clinical Results

Case No.	Age (yr)	Side	Dominant Hand	DASH Score	Flexion Arc, Range (Degrees)	Rotation	Overall Satisfaction
1	41	Right	Right	13	0–145	Full	Good
2	30	Left	Left	8	0–135	Full	Excellent
3	44	Left	Right	12	45–125	10 Loss	Good
4	19	Left	Right	6	0–135	5 loss	Excellent
5	38	Right	Right	8	0–140	Full	Excellent
6	18	Right	Right	10	10–130	Full	Excellent
7	22	Left	Right	0	5–140	Full	Excellent

ROM, range of motion; DASH, Disabilities of the Arm, Shoulder and Hand Questionnaire.

internal fixation is indicated (Fig 3). This article should influence the management of these injuries toward an initial attempt at a closed reduction with a CT follow-up to assess the accuracy of the reduction and short-term immobilization if the reduction is anatomic or within a millimeter or two.

M. F. Swiontkowski, MD

Surgical Treatment With an Angular Stable Plate for Complex Displaced Proximal Humeral Fractures in Elderly Patients: A Randomized Controlled Trial

Fjalestad T, Hole MØ, Hovden IAH, et al (Oslo Univ Hosp Ullevål HF, Norway; et al)
J Orthop Trauma 26:98-106, 2012

Objective.—The objective of the study was to evaluate functional outcome, patient self-assessment, and radiographic outcome at 1 year in displaced three- and four-part proximal humeral fractures (OTA group 11-B2 and 11-C2).

Design.—Randomized controlled trial.

Setting.—Academic medical center.

Patients/Participants.—Fifty patients aged 60 years or older with displaced three- or four-part proximal humeral fractures and no previous shoulder injuries were randomized either to surgical treatment or to conservative closed treatment. Twenty-five patients were included in each group. Forty-eight patients completed 12-month follow-up. Two surgical patients died within 3 months.

Intervention.—The surgically treated group had a standardized surgical treatment with open reduction and internal fixation using an angular stable plate and cerclages. Instructed physical therapy started the third postoperative day. The conservative treatment group had a standardized nonoperative treatment that included closed reduction if displacement between the head and metaphyseal shaft fragment exceeded 50% of the diaphyseal diameter. Physical therapy started on the fifteenth postoperative day.

Main Outcome Measurements.—The main outcome was the mean difference in Constant score between the injured and noninjured shoulder at

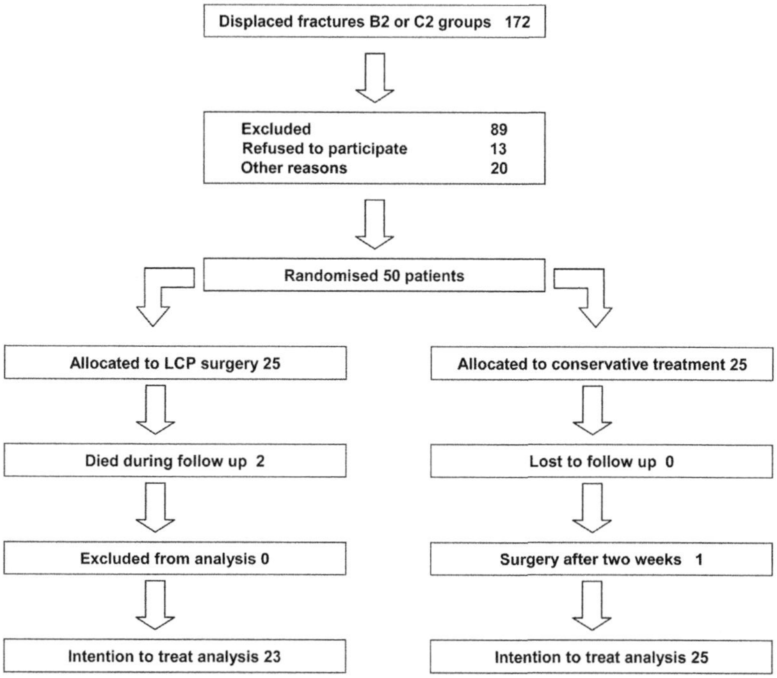

FIGURE 1.—Patients admitted in the hospital with proximal humeral fractures classified as OTA group 11-B2 and 11-C2 during the inclusion period. (Reprinted from Fjalestad T, Hole MØ, Hovden IAH, et al. Surgical treatment with an angular stable plate for complex displaced proximal humeral fractures in elderly patients: a randomized controlled trial. *J Orthop Trauma.* 2012;26:98-106, with permission from Lippincott Williams & Wilkins.)

TABLE 2.—Functional Rating at Follow-Ups*

Constant Mean (SD)	3 Months CSD3	6 Months CSD6	12 Months CSD12	12 Months ACS12	Difference 12 Months CSD12	ACS12
Surgical	52.6 (12.8)	45.6 (15.5)	35.2 (17.2)	74.4 (29.4)	2.4 ($P = 0.62$)	0.0 ($P = 0.99$)
Conservative	47.1 (16.9)	40.5 (18.9)	32.8 (16.2)	74.4 (22.9)		

SD, standard deviation.
*Constant score difference (CSD) and adjusted Constant score (ACS) at 12 months.

TABLE 3.—Mean Subscores for the Injured Shoulder at 12 Months (No Adjustment for Age and Gender)

Subscores CS	Pain	ADL 1	ADL 2	ROM	Strength	CS Total (95% CI)
Surgical	11.1	5.5	7.7	17.0	10.9	52.3 (43.2–61.2)
Conservative	11.7	5.2	8.7	18.2	9.9	52.2 (44.6–59.7)

Best scores: Pain = 15 points; ADL 1 (activity of daily living) = 10 points; ADL 2 (positioning of the arm) = 10 points; ROM (range of movement) = 40 points; Strength = 25points; Best score Total = 100 points.
CS, Constant score; CI, confidence interval.

12 months. The secondary outcomes were patient self-assessment (American Shoulder and Elbow Surgeons score) and radiographic ratings at 12 months.

Results.—At 12 months, mean Constant scores favored conservative treatment by 2.4 points (nonsignificant; $P = 0.62$). There was no significant difference in mean patient self-assessment. However, radiographic outcomes were significantly better for surgically treated patients.

Conclusion.—There is no evidence of a difference in functional outcome at 1-year follow-up between surgical treatment and conservative treatment of displaced proximal humeral fractures in elderly patients (Fig 1, Tables 2 and 3).

▶ This is a very well conducted surgical trial comparing operative fixation with a standard locking plate with conservative treatment in older patients with 3- and 4-part proximal humerus fractures. All confounding variables were addressed in the analyses, and there were no clinically relevant differences between the 2 cohorts. The fact that the radiographic outcomes were consistently better in the operative cohort confirms that the surgical care was appropriate. The closed reduction rule of greater than 50% of diaphyseal displacement in the conservative cohort is clinically appropriate. The fact that the Constant score at 1 year favored the nonoperative group should give us pause in the trajectory favoring open reduction and internal fixation for these fractures. The low functional demand of this patient population is probably the overwhelming reason for these results; however, the needs of this elderly patient group should dominate our thinking. After reading this article, I personally will be less inclined to recommend operative intervention for elderly patients.

M. F. Swiontkowski, MD

Functional and Quality-of-Life Results of Displaced and Nondisplaced Proximal Humeral Fractures Treated Conservatively

Torrens C, Corrales M, Vilà G, et al (Hosp del Mar., Barcelona, Spain)

J Orthop Trauma 25:581-587, 2011

Objectives.—Functional and quality-of-life outcomes of conservatively treated proximal humeral fractures.

Design.—Prospective study.

Setting.—University orthopedic department at a hospital.

Patients/Participants.—Seventy consecutive patients between the ages of 60 and 85 years.

Intervention.—Conservative treatment.

Main Outcome Measurements.—Functional outcome measured according to the Constant score, quality of life assessed using EuroQol-5D, and fracture pattern analyzed with x-ray and computed tomography scan.

Results.—All fractures consolidated uneventfully with no loss of reduction in either group. Four-part fractures obtained the worst functional results (33.66) followed by three-part fractures (54.64) and finally two-part fractures (65.88 and 71). Mild pain was expected in three- and four-part fractures, whereas two-part fractures achieved near complete pain relief. Nondisplaced fractures obtained a final Constant score of 73.58 and displaced fractures a score of 59.41 with significant differences in all Constant score items with the exception of external rotation. Although patients older than 75 years scored lower (54.63) than those younger than 75 years (70.83), there was no difference in the quality-of-life perception.

TABLE 2.—Descriptive of the Constant Score and EuroQol 5D in Patients Younger Than 75 Years and Older Than 75 Years

	75 Years or Younger		Older Than 75 Years		
	Mean	SD	Mean	SD	Significance
Pain affected side	12.11	3.34	10.71	4.64	$P = 0.26$
Pain nonaffected	14.11	2.20	14.13	2.45	$P = 0.81$
ADL affected side	18.74	2.62	14.83	5.89	$P = 0.001$
ADL nonaffected	19.73	1.51	19.39	2.91	$P = 0.98$
AE affected side	7.57	1.62	5.83	2.12	$P = 0.001$
AE nonaffected	8.62	1.52	7.65	2.46	$P = 0.11$
ABD affected side	7.52	1.74	5.75	2.06	$P = 0.001$
ABD nonaffected	8.58	1.63	7.74	2.43	$P = 0.16$
ER affected side	7.17	1.81	5.25	3.27	$P = 0.017$
ER nonaffected	8.58	1.68	7.57	2.48	$P = 0.09$
IR affected side	6.78	1.99	6.25	2.06	$P = 0.33$
IR nonaffected	8.00	1.70	7.57	1.47	$P = 0.16$
Strength affected side	11.06	5.37	6.09	5.00	$P = 0.001$
Strength nonaffected	12.55	5.34	9.81	4.34	$P = 0.54$
Constant affected side	70.83	13.48	54.63	20.67	$P = 0.002$
Constant nonaffected	80.22	11.20	73.30	15.07	$P = 0.01$
VAS tarif	0.63	0.20	0.54	0.25	$P = 0.37$

SD, standard deviation; ADL, activities of daily living; AE, anterior elevation; ABD, abduction; ER, external rotation; IR, internal rotation; VAS, visual analog scale.

TABLE 4.—Descriptive of the Constant Score and EuroQol 5D in Displaced Fractures

	2-Part SN Mean	2-Part GT-Dislocation Mean	3-Part GT Mean	4-Part Mean
Age	70.88	69.83	76.88	75.66
Pain affected side	11.76	13.33	9.44	7
Pain nonaffected	15	13	14.44	11.66
ADL affected side	17.52	19	16.11	8
ADL nonaffected	20	20	20	16
AE affected side	7.17 (91°–120°)	7.66 (61°–90°)	5.33 (91°–120°)	4.33 (61°–90°)
AE nonaffected	8.87 (121°–150°)	7.66 (91°–120°)	7.77 (91°–120°)	7 (91°–120°)
ABD affected side	7.05 (91°–120°)	7.66 (61°–90°)	5.33 (91°–120°)	4 (61°–90°)
ABD nonaffected	8.87 (121°–150°)	7.66 (121°–150°)	8 (91°–120°)	6.66 (91°–120°)
ER affected side	6.47	6.33	6	4.33
ER nonaffected	9.25	7.2	8	7.33
IR affected side	6.94	7	5.55	4
IR nonaffected	8.62	7.6	7.11	6.66
Strength affected side	8.94	10	6.82	2.66
Strength nonaffected	12.12	12	11.03	6.33
Constant affected side	65.88	71	54.64	33.66
Constant nonaffected	82.82	75	76.14	60
VAS tarif	0.63	0.58	0.55	0.30

ADL, activities of daily living; AE, anterior elevation; ABD, abduction; ER, external rotation; IR, internal rotation; VAS, visual analog scale; SN, surgical neck; GT, greater tuberosity.

Conclusion.—Conservative treatment of proximal humeral fractures in those patients older than age 75 years provides good pain relief with limited functional outcome. Despite limited functional outcome, this appears to have no effect on the quality-of-life perception in the population studied. Four-part fractures present the worst results and treatment options may need to be discussed with the patient to adjust treatment to patient expectations (Tables 2 and 4).

▶ This is a carefully conducted prospective study evaluating the functional outcomes of proximal humerus fractures in patients older than 60 years treated with conservative methods in a standard fashion. We learn that age and fracture severity are important predictors of patient outcome, both of which make intuitive sense. There seems to be little controversy that the majority of these fractures heal with conservative care. The issue that needs further clarity is whether open reduction and internal fixation with locked plates improve the outcomes for the more severe fractures. The authors attempt to give us some sense of this critical comparison in their discussion of other published data with operative treatment, but this question can only be answered with a large multicenter controlled trial in which patients who refuse randomization are followed with the same functional outcome instruments and at the same time intervals.

M. F. Swiontkowski, MD

Distraction Plating for the Treatment of Highly Comminuted Distal Radius Fractures in Elderly Patients

Richard MJ, Katolik LI, Hanel DP, et al (Duke Univ Med Ctr, Durham, NC; The Philadelphia Hand Ctr, PA; Univ of Washington, Seattle)

J Hand Surg 37A:948-956, 2012

Purpose.—To evaluate internal distraction plating for the management of comminuted, intra-articular distal radius fractures in patients greater than 60 years of age at two level 1 trauma centers. We specifically desired to determine whether patients would have acceptable results from the clinical standpoint of range of motion, Disabilities of the Arm, Shoulder, and Hand (DASH) score, and the radiographic measurements of ulnar variance, radial inclination, and palmar tilt. Our hypothesis was that distraction plating of comminuted distal radius fractures in the elderly would result in acceptable outcomes regarding range of motion, DASH score, and radiographic parameters and would, thereby, provide the upper extremity surgeon with another option for the treatment of these fractures.

Methods.—A retrospective review was performed on 33 patients over 60 years of age with comminuted distal radius fractures treated with internal distraction plating at two level 1 trauma centers. Patients were treated with internal distraction plating across the radiocarpal joint. At the time of final follow-up, radiographs were evaluated for ulnar variance, radial inclination, and palmar tilt. Range of motion, complications, and DASH scores were also obtained.

Results.—We treated 33 patients (mean age, 70 y) with distraction plating for comminuted distal radius fractures. At final follow-up, all fractures had healed, and radiographs demonstrated mean palmar tilt of 5°and mean positive ulnar variance of 0.6 mm. Mean radial inclination was 20°. Mean values for wrist flexion and extension were 46°and 50°, respectively.

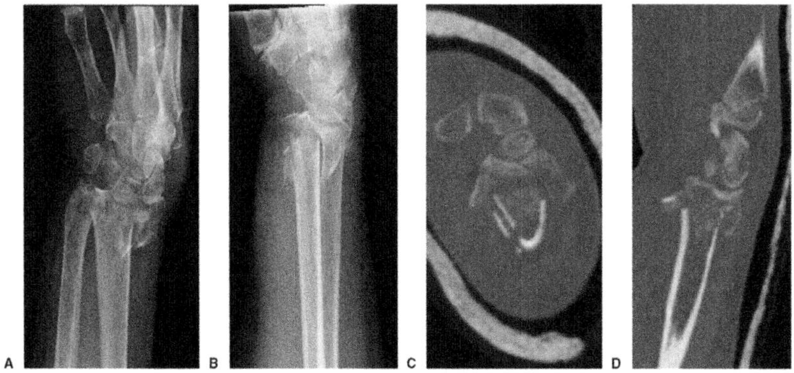

FIGURE 1.—**A** Posteroanterior and **B** lateral radiographs and **C** coronal and **D** sagittal computed tomography scan of a 67-year-old woman who sustained a comminuted distal radius fracture in a fall. (Reprinted from Richard MJ, Katolik LI, Hanel DP, et al. Distraction plating for the treatment of highly comminuted distal radius fractures in elderly patients. *J Hand Surg*. 2012;37A:948-956, Copyright 2012, with permission from the American Society for Surgery of the Hand.)

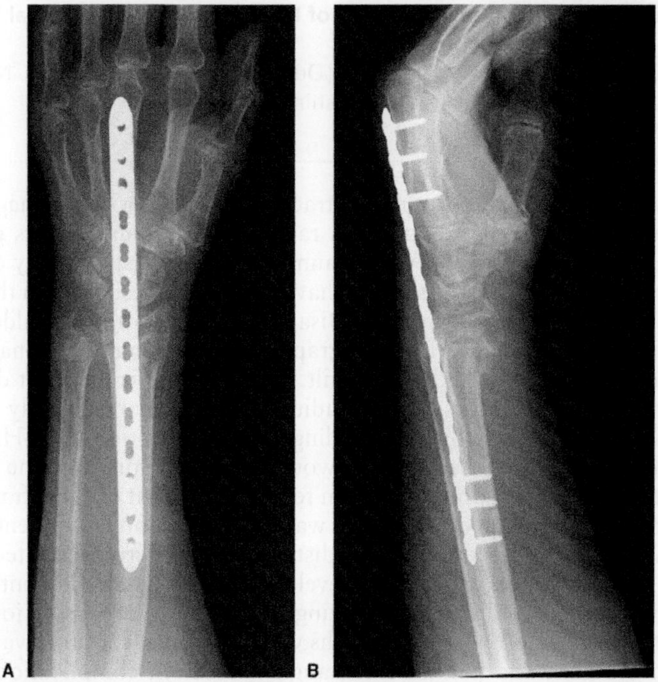

FIGURE 2.—Immediate A postoperative posteroanterior and B lateral radiographs that demonstrate placement of a 14-hole, small-fragment locking compression plate. Note that 3 bicortical screws were placed in the radial diaphysis and 3 bicortical screws were placed into the third metacarpal. (Reprinted from Richard MJ, Katolik LI, Hanel DP, et al. Distraction plating for the treatment of highly comminuted distal radius fractures in elderly patients. *J Hand Surg*. 2012;37A:948-956, Copyright 2012, with permission from the American Society for Surgery of the Hand.)

Mean pronation and supination were 79° and 77°, respectively. At final follow-up, the mean DASH score was 32.

Conclusions.—In the elderly, distraction plating is an effective method of treatment for comminuted, osteoporotic distal radius fractures.

Type of Study/Level of Evidence.—Therapeutic IV (Figs 1-3, Table 1).

▶ Distraction plating is a relatively new concept for highly comminuted distal radius fractures. It is essentially the concept of moving external fixation into the subcutaneous space to avoid the problems with pin track infection and to increase patient acceptability. This retrospective review, with all the issues of selection and detection bias that surround this experimental design, confirms that the clinical and radiographic results are acceptable. This technique should be considered in the older patient population where this fracture pattern is more common. Although it involves a second procedure to remove the distraction plate and there are concerns with the effects of overdistraction on metacarpophalangeal and interphalangeal motion, the long-term results seem to indicate that it is worth these concerns.

M. F. Swiontkowski, MD

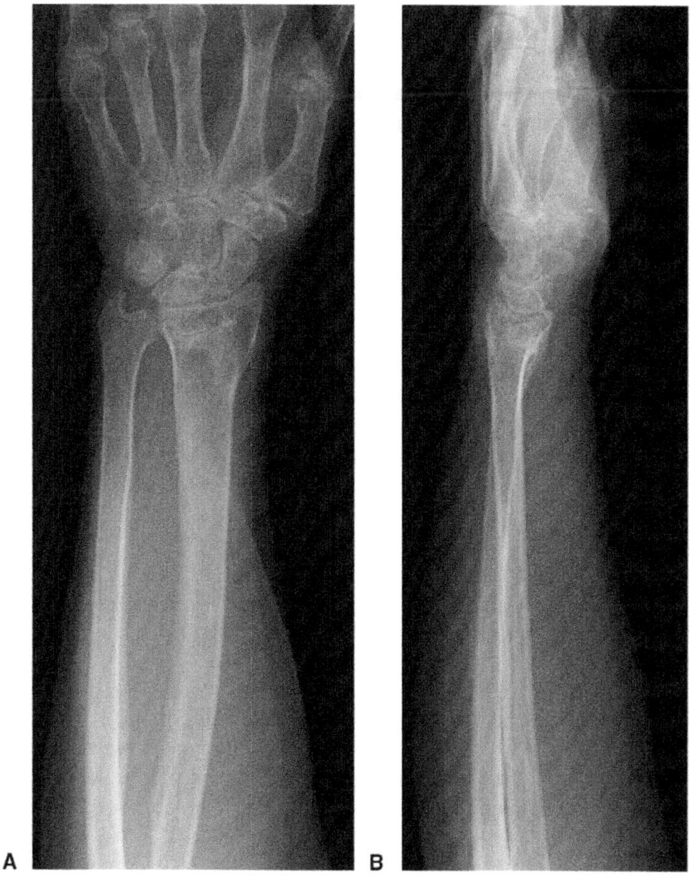

FIGURE 3.—A Posteroanterior and B lateral x-rays taken 1 year after the original surgery. The dorsal plate has been removed. (Reprinted from Richard MJ, Katolik LI, Hanel DP, et al. Distraction plating for the treatment of highly comminuted distal radius fractures in elderly patients. *J Hand Surg*. 2012;37A: 948-956, Copyright 2012, with permission from the American Society for Surgery of the Hand.)

TABLE 1.—Patient Demographic Information

Number of patients included in the study	33
Average age (y)	70
Sex	
M	10
F	23
Mechanism of injury	
Fall	23
Motor vehicle collision	8
Crush	1
Car colliding with pedestrian	1
Fracture	
Open	7
Closed	26
Supplemental K-wire fixation	7
Average follow-up duration (wk)	47
Average time of plate removal (d)	119

A Systematic Review of Outcomes and Complications of Treating Unstable Distal Radius Fractures in the Elderly

Diaz-Garcia RJ, Oda T, Shauver MJ, et al (The Univ of Michigan Health System, Ann Arbor)

J Hand Surg 36A:824-835, 2011

Purpose.—As the population in developed countries continues to age, the incidence of osteoporotic distal radius fractures (DRFs) will increase as well. Treatment of DRF in the elderly population is controversial. We systematically reviewed the existing literature for the management of DRFs in patients aged 60 and over with 5 common techniques: the volar locking plate system, nonbridging external fixation, bridging external fixation, percutaneous Kirschner wire fixation, and cast immobilization (CI).

Methods.—We reviewed articles retrieved from MEDLINE, Embase, and CINAHL Plus that met predetermined inclusion and exclusion criteria in 2 literature reviews. Outcomes of interest included wrist arc of motion, grip strength, functional outcome measurements, radiographic parameters, and the number and type of complications. We statistically analyzed the data using weighted means and proportions based on the sample size in each study.

Results.—We identified 2,039 papers and selected 21 papers fitting the inclusion criteria in the primary review of articles with a mean patient age of 60 and older. Statistically significant differences were detected for wrist arc of motion, grip strength, and Disabilities of the Arm, Shoulder, and Hand score, although these findings may not be clinically meaningful. Volar tilt and ulnar variance revealed significant differences among groups, with CI resulting in the worst radiographic outcomes. The complications were significantly different, with CI having the lowest rate of complications, whereas the volar locking plate system had significantly more major complications requiring additional surgical intervention.

Conclusions.—This systematic review suggests that despite worse radiographic outcomes associated with CI, functional outcomes were no different from those of surgically treated groups for patients age 60 and over. Prospective comparative outcomes studies are necessary to evaluate the rate of functional recovery, cost, and outcomes associated with these 5 treatment methods (Tables 5, 7, and 8).

► This very well done meta-analysis focuses on the management of distal radius fractures in patients over the age of 60. The search strategy was comprehensive,

TABLE 5.—Grip Strength at Final Follow-Up (Weighted Mean)

Grip Strength (% Compared With Contralateral)	VLPS (n = 235)	Non-BrEF (n = 28)	BrEF (n = 138)	PKF (n = 95)	CI (n = 220)	*P* Value
Primary literature review	81	69	84	74	85	.707
Secondary literature review	76			83	84	<.001

TABLE 7.—Radiographic Parameters at Final Follow-Up (Weighted Mean)

	VLPS	Non-BrEF	BrEF	PKF	CI	*P* Value
Volar tilt (°)						
Primary literature review	3.9 (n = 235)	6.5 (n = 81)	−0.8 (n = 169)	3.7 (n = 52)	−11 (n = 220)	.018
Secondary literature review	3.1 (n = 94)		0.3 (n = 35)	0.5 (n = 49)	−11 (n = 168)	<.001
Radial inclination (°)						
Primary literature review	13.4 (n = 149)	13.7 (n = 53)	13.9 (n = 113)	21 (n = 52)	14.8 (n = 137)	.182
Secondary literature review	22.8 (n = 94)		19.5 (n = 35)	21 (n = 49)	18.0 (n = 168)	<.001
Ulnar variance (mm)						
Primary literature review	1.5 (n = 53)	1.0 (n = 53)	1.1 (n = 81)	3.0 (n = 27)	3.6 (n = 143)	<.001
Secondary literature review	1.5 (n = 53)		2.4 (n = 35)	3.0 (n = 49)	3.6 (n = 143)	<.001

The *P* values were calculated using ANOVA. Significant difference (95% confidential level using Tukey-style multiple comparisons test) was found between treatment groups for the following variables in the primary literature review: volar tilt—VLPS/CI, non-BrEF/CI; ulnar variance—VLPS/BrEF, VLPS/CI, non-BrEF/CI. Significant difference (95% confidential level using Tukey-style multiple comparisons test) was found between treatment groups for the following variables in the secondary literature review: Volar tilt—VLPS/CI, BrEF/CI, PKF/CI; radial inclination—all groups were significantly different; ulnar variance—all groups were significantly different except for BrEF/CI. The non-BrEF could not be compared via ANOVA in the secondary literature review with the other groups because only 1 paper was present for analysis.

TABLE 8.—Summary of Complications

	VLPS	Non-BrEF	BrEF	PKF	CI	*P* Value
Minor Superficial infection	0	25	39	2	0	
Others	2	0	0	9	0	
Total (%)	2 (1%)	25 (31%)	39 (16%)	11 (8%)	0	<.001
Major not requiring surgery						
Nerve lesion	6	1	10	4	4	
CRPS	9	0	16	2	11	
Early hardware removal	0	0	6	3	0	
Others	3	0	2	0	0	
Total (%)	18 (6%)	1 (1%)	34 (14%)	9 (7%)	15 (7%)	<.001
Major requiring surgery						
Tendon rupture/adhesion	18	2	0	3	3	
Nerve lesion	2	0	2	0	0	
Infection	2	0	1	0	0	
Hardware loosening, failure, or removal	8	0	0	0	0	
Others	2	0	2	0	0	
Total (%)	32 (11%)	2 (3%)	5 (2%)	3 (2%)	3 (1%)	<.001

The *P* values were calculated using the chi-square test. Significant differences were found between the all treatment groups except the following pairs: major, not requiring surgery—PKF/CI; major, requiring surgery—non-BrEF/PKF, BrEF/PKF.

and high-quality techniques for identifying studies and including them in the analysis were utilized. Using all relevant clinical and functional outcomes, we can accept the conclusion that open reduction and internal fixation has the best radiographic outcomes with the highest complication rates and that closed reduction and casting have the worst radiographic outcomes with the lowest complication rates. The functional outcomes do not appear to be different. This may well be primarily influenced by the lower functional demand in this patient population. The authors appropriately call for more adequately powered head-to-head randomized clinical trials to definitively answer this question.

M. F. Swiontkowski, MD

Mini-C-Arm Fluoroscopy for Emergency-Department Reduction of Pediatric Forearm Fractures

Lee MC, Stone NE III, Ritting AW, et al (Connecticut Children's Med Ctr, Hartford; Maimonides Med Ctr, Brooklyn, NY; Univ of Connecticut Health Ctr, Farmington; et al)

J Bone Joint Surg Am 93:1442-1447, 2011

Background.—Reduction of pediatric forearm fractures with the patient under sedation in the emergency department is a common practice throughout the United States. We hypothesized that the use of a mini-c-arm fluoroscopy device as an alternative to routine radiographs for evaluation of fracture reduction would (1) allow a more anatomic fracture reduction, (2) decrease the number of repeat reductions or subsequent procedures, (3) reduce overall radiation exposure to the patient, and (4) decrease the orthopaedic consultation time in the emergency department.

Methods.—A retrospective cohort analysis of 279 displaced forearm and wrist fractures treated with closed reduction and casting with the patient under sedation in the emergency department of a level-I pediatric trauma center was performed, and the data were compared with historical controls. One hundred and thirteen fracture reductions were assessed with a mini-c-arm device, and 166 fracture reductions were evaluated with radiographs. All patients had radiographs of the injury. Blinded, independent reviewers graded the quality of reduction for residual angulation and translation of the reduced fracture. Radiation exposure was determined by the average number of radiographs made through either modality. Emergency department and outpatient charts were reviewed to determine the total orthopaedic consultation time and the need for repeat reductions or operative intervention.

Results.—Pediatric forearm fractures undergoing closed reduction with assistance of the mini c-arm had a significant improvement in reduction quality (average angulation [and standard deviation], 6° ± 4° vs. 8 ± 6°; $p = 0.02$), a decrease in repeat fracture reduction and need for subsequent operative treatment (two [2%] of 113 fractures vs. fourteen [8.4%] of 166 fractures; $p \leq 0.0001$), and a decrease in radiation exposure to the patient (mean, 14.0 ± 10.3 mrem vs. 50.0 ± 12.7 mrem). The average orthopaedic consultation time was decreased with use of a mini c-arm (28 ± 12 min vs. 47 ± 19 min, $p < 0.001$).

Conclusions.—Use of the mini c-arm to assist in the closed reduction of pediatric forearm and wrist fractures in the emergency department can

TABLE 2.—Reduction Quality

	Control Group	Mini-C-Arm Group	*P* Value
No. of patients with complete data	152	90	
Prereduction* (*deg*)			
Angulation	30 ± 13	28 ± 11	0.17
Translation	47 ± 42	48 ± 41	0.39
Postreduction* (*deg*)			
Angulation	8 ± 6	6 ± 4	0.02
Translation	20 ± 28	17 ± 25	0.15

*The values are given as the mean and the standard deviation.

TABLE 3.—Additional Reductions

Location of Fracture Reductions	Control Group* (N = 166)	Mini-C-Arm Group† (N = 113)	*P* Value
Emergency department	10*	1†	
Office	1‡	0	
Operating room	3§	1†	
Total	14	2	0.002

*The ten fractures included three distal radial fractures, four distal radial and ulnar fractures, and three radial and ulnar shaft fractures.

†Radial and ulnar shaft fracture.

‡Distal radial fracture.

§Two distal radial fractures and one radial and ulnar shaft fracture.

TABLE 4.—Average Radiation Exposure to the Patient

	Control Group (Radiographs)	Mini-C Arm Group (C-Arm Images)	*P* Value
No. of patients	152	90	
No. of reduction images*			
All fracture types	4.6 ± 1.2	5.2 ± 3.8	0.08
Distal radial fractures	4.8 ± 1.0	5.4 ± 4.8	0.08
Distal radial and ulnar fractures	4.8 ± 1.1	4.3 ± 2.5	0.11
Radial and ulnar shaft fractures	4.3 ± 1.3	5.8 ± 3.7	0.08
Radiation exposure for all fracture types† (*mrem*)	50.0 ± 12.7	14.0 ± 10.3	

*The values are given as the mean and the standard deviation.

†Mean radiation exposure = 11.0 mrem per traditional radiograph and 2.7 mrem per fluoroscopic image. Although the 700-msec snapshot mode was used for all mini-c-arm images, a 1000-msec (1-sec) exposure time was used to facilitate calculation and allow a more conservative estimate of radiation exposure.

improve the quality of the reduction, decrease the radiation exposure to the patient, and decrease the need for repeat fracture reduction or additional procedures. Mini-c-arm imaging can also decrease the average orthopaedic consultation time for fracture reduction (Tables 2-5).

▶ Pediatric forearm fractures are very common and often require reduction. This cohort study is designed to test the impact of a mini C-arm based in the

TABLE 5.—Time Efficiency

Interval	Control Group*	Mini-C-Arm Group*	*P* Value
Patient time in emergency department† (*min*)	252 ± 122	271 ± 86	0.10
Orthopaedic consultation time‡ (*min*)	47 ± 19	28 ± 12	<0.001
Time from beginning of consultation to discharge§ (*min*)	115 ± 85	107 ± 52	0.22

*The values are given as the mean and the standard deviation.
†Data were available for 148 patients in the control group and ninety-three in the mini-c-arm group.
‡Data were available for 150 and 104 patients, respectively.
§Data were available for 151 and eighty-four patients, respectively.

emergency department for orthopedic surgeon use in diagnosis and reduction versus the traditional management approach of multiple radiographs before and after reduction. This mini C-arm technique is faster and results in no greater radiation exposure for the patient (Tables 3 and 4). The quality of reductions is as good or better and the time spent in manipulation and evaluation of the reduction much less. This is a useful emergency department tool that results in improved outcomes for the patient and the surgeon. It is possible, however, that the favorable effects may be overstated because of the experimental design used with this study.

M. F. Swiontkowski, MD

Outcomes of Reduction More Than 7 Days After Injury in Supracondylar Humeral Fractures in Children

Silva M, Wong TC, Bernthal NM (Los Angeles Orthopaedic Hospital, CA; Univ of California, Los Angeles)
J Pediatr Orthop 31:751-756, 2011

Background.—Some slightly extended type II fractures initially treated with closed reduction and casting can displace during the first 2 weeks of follow-up. Although closed reduction and percutaneous pinning are desirable for displaced supracondylar humeral fractures treated acutely, there is little or no available information regarding the surgeon's ability to obtain a satisfactory reduction when such a procedure is performed more than a week after the original injury, or the clinical outcome of it.

Methods.—We reviewed the information on 143 type II pediatric supracondylar humeral fractures that were treated by closed reduction and percutaneous pinning. To determine the effect of late treatment, we compared a group of fractures that was treated within the first 7 days (group 1, n = 101) with a group that was treated >7 days after the injury (group 2, n = 42).

Results.—Mean time from presentation to surgery was 2.1 days (range, 0 to 5) and 9.8 days (range, 7 to 15) for fractures in groups 1 and 2, respectively. There was no need for an open reduction in either group. An

TABLE 1.—Outcome Measures

	Group 1 (<7 d) n = 101 (70.6%)	Group 2 (>7 d) n = 42 (29.4%)	*P*
Length of surgery (min) mean (95% CI)	43.7 (40.7-46.7)	41.9 (37.4-46.5)	0.25
Carrying angle (degrees) mean (95% CI)	6 (5-6)	7 (6-8)	0.002
Baumann angle (degrees) mean (95% CI)	17 (16-18)	18 (17-20)	0.13
Relative arc of motion (%) mean (95% CI)	98.1 (96.8-99.4)	98.3 (97.1-99.3)	0.44
Avascular necrosis (%)	0/101 (0%)	2/42 (4.8%)	0.08
Pin-site granuloma (%)	9/101 (8.9%)	0/42 (0%)	0.04
Unsatisfactory outcome (%)	12/101 (11.9%)	4/42 (9.5%)	0.47

TABLE 2.—95% Confidente Intervals for the Difference Between Group 1 and Group 2

	Mean Difference	95% CI of the Difference	SE	*P*
Length of surgery (min)	1.8	−3.6 to 7.3	2.8	0.25
Carrying angle (degrees)	−1.5	−2.5 to −0.5	0.5	0.002
Baumann angle (degrees)	−1.3	−3.6 to 1.0	1.2	0.13
Relative Arc of motion (%)	−0.2	−2.6 to 2.2	1.2	0.44
Avascular necrosis (%)	4.8	3.5 to 6.0	0.6	0.08
Pin-site granuloma (%)	−8.9	−11.8 to −5.9	1.5	0.04
Unsatisfactory outcome (%)	−2.4	−6.7 to 1.9	2.2	0.47

anatomic reduction was obtained in all fractures. There were no iatrogenic nerve injuries, vascular complications, or compartment syndromes in either group. Length of surgery was similar in both groups ($P = 0.3$). There were no significant differences in final carrying angle ($P = 0.2$) or range of motion of the treated elbow ($P = 0.21$). Avascular necrosis of the humeral trochlea was identified in 2 fractures that were treated surgically 8 days after the original injury (group 2).

Conclusions.—The results of this study suggest that it is possible to obtain an anatomic reduction of a type II pediatric supracondylar humeral fracture even after 7 days from the injury. Such a delay in surgery does not appear to lead to longer surgeries, a higher incidence of open reduction, or to alter the final alignment or range of motion of the elbow. However, the risk of developing an avascular necrosis of the humeral trochlea must be considered.

Level of Evidence.—II (Tables 1 and 2).

▶ Standard treatment for children with type 2 supracondylar fractures is cast immobilization when the anterior humeral line contacts the capitellum on the lateral radiograph. However, many surgeons fear displacement and, therefore, routinely insert percutaneous pins with the elbow in flexion. The question has repeatedly been asked as to whether the long-term results are compromised when displacement beyond the acceptable radiographic parameters is recognized late. This well-done cohort study confirms that when displacement is recognized within 7 days of presentation, the results of surgical reduction and pinning are equivalent to that treatment done emergently. The key point of this study is that surgeons need to see the patient within 5 to 7 days and obtain a high-quality lateral radiograph to be sure that no significant further displacement has occurred. If further extension has occurred, parents and patients can be reassured that the long-term results will not be compromised.

M. F. Swiontkowski, MD

A Prospective Randomized Controlled Trial Comparing Occupational Therapy with Independent Exercises After Volar Plate Fixation of a Fracture of the Distal Part of the Radius

Souer JS, Buijze G, Ring D (Massachusetts General Hosp, Boston)
J Bone Joint Surg Am 93:1761-1766, 2011

Background.—The effect of formal occupational therapy on recovery after open reduction and volar plate fixation of a fracture of the distal part of the radius is uncertain. We hypothesized that there would be no difference in wrist function and arm-specific disability six months after

TABLE 1.—Comparison of Cohorts at Three Months After Surgery

	Independent Exercise Group		Occupational Therapy Group		
	Mean	Standard Deviation	Mean	Standard Deviation	*P* Value
Wrist flexion-extension arc (*deg*)	111	22.4	104	22.9	0.10
Wrist flexion-extension arc (% *of value on uninjured side*)	81	10.7	87	10.6	0.98
Wrist flexion (*deg*)	57	14.9	54	14.5	0.25
Wrist flexion (% *of value on uninjured side*)	75	15.7	74	16.1	0.76
Wrist extension (*deg*)	54	12.7	51	13.0	0.12
Wrist extension (% *of value on uninjured side*)	87	15.9	83	13.3	0.07
Radial deviation (*deg*)	21	6.0	21	6.0	0.86
Radial deviation (% *of value on uninjured side*)	86	32.1	88	25.6	0.76
Ulnar deviation (*deg*)	33	10.7	33	10.9	0.90
Ulnar deviation (% *of value on uninjured side*)	83	18.2	82	26.7	0.66
Pronation (*deg*)	90	1.7	90	1.7	0.98
Pronation (% *of value on uninjured side*)	100	0.0	100	1.9	0.16
Supination (*deg*)	88	4.4	86	11.3	0.26
Supination (% *of value on uninjured side*)	99	4.9	99	22.5	0.90
Grip strength (*lb [kg]*)	55 (24.8)	22.6 (10.2)	45 (20)	17.4 (7.8)	<0.05*
Grip strength (% *of value on uninjured side*)	81	18.9	66	16.0	<0.05*
Pinch strength (*lb [kg]*)	14 (6.3)	4.3 (1.9)	13 (5.9)	4.1 (1.9)	0.11
Pinch strength (% *of value on uninjured side*)	90	23.7	80	22.7	<0.05*
Visual analog pain score (*points*)	1.2	0.6	1.3	0.9	0.35
DASH[†] (*points*)	13.1	12.1	13.3	9.5	0.91
Mayo wrist score (*points*)	77	8.8	74	11.4	0.10
Gartland and Werley score (*points*)	2	1.3	2	2.2	<0.05*

*The difference between the groups was significant ($p < 0.05$).
†DASH = Disabilities of the Arm, Shoulder and Hand questionnaire.

open reduction and volar plate fixation of a distal radial fracture between patients who receive formal occupational therapy and those with instructions for independent exercises.

Methods.—Ninety-four patients with an unstable distal radial fracture treated with open reduction and volar locking plate fixation were enrolled in a prospective randomized controlled trial comparing exercises done under the supervision of an occupational therapist with surgeon-directed independent exercises. The primary study question addressed combined wrist flexion and extension six months after surgery. Secondary study questions addressed wrist motion, grip strength, Gartland and Werley scores, Mayo wrist scores, and DASH (Disabilities of the Arm, Shoulder and Hand) scores at three months and six months after surgery.

Results.—There was a significant difference in the mean arc of wrist flexion and extension six months after surgery (118° versus 129°), favoring patients prescribed independent exercises. Three months after surgery, there was a significant difference in mean pinch strength (80% versus 90%), mean grip strength (66% versus 81%), and mean Gartland and Werley scores, favoring patients prescribed independent exercises. At six months, there was a significant difference in mean wrist extension (55° versus 62°), ulnar deviation (82% versus 93%), mean supination (84°

TABLE 2.—Comparison of Cohorts at Six Months After Surgery

	Independent Exercise Group		Occupational Therapy Group		
	Mean	Standard Deviation	Mean	Standard Deviation	*P* Value
Wrist flexion-extension arc (*deg*)	129	22.6	118	17.7	<0.05*
Wrist flexion-extension arc (*% of value on uninjured side*)	88	11.7	84	7.3	<0.05*
Wrist flexion (*deg*)	67	14.3	63	12.1	0.14
Wrist flexion (*% of value on uninjured side*)	88	15.5	85	10.9	0.26
Wrist extension (*deg*)	62	13.7	55	10.2	<0.05*
Wrist extension (*% of value on uninjured side*)	93	12.3	92	12.5	0.58
Radial deviation (*deg*)	25	7.6	23	7.4	0.1
Radial deviation (*% of value on uninjured side*)	93	23.7	97	23.9	0.31
Ulnar deviation (*deg*)	40	9.2	32	12.1	<0.05*
Ulnar deviation (*% of value on uninjured side*)	93	19.4	82	29.2	<0.05*
Pronation (*deg*)	90	1.9	90	1.7	0.68
Pronation (*% of value on uninjured side*)	99	2.1	100	1.9	0.65
Supination (*deg*)	90	0.9	84	13.1	<0.05*
Supination (*% of value on uninjured side*)	100	2.6	96	11.8	0.18
Grip strength (*lb [kg]*)	57 (25.7)	18.5 (8.3)	51 (23)	17.9 (8.1)	0.06
Grip strength (*% of value on uninjured side*)	92	19.8	81	16.4	<0.05*
Pinch strength (*lb [kg]*)	15 (6.8)	4.3 (1.9)	17 (7.7)	8.6 (3.9)	0.15
Pinch strength (*% of value on uninjured side*)	95	15.4	94	15.1	0.47
Visual analog pain score (*points*)	0.8	1.4	1.0	1.8	0.20
DASH† (*points*)	7.8	7.8	6.7	6.7	0.42
Mayo wrist score (*points*)	83.4	12.7	79.0	9.9	<0.05*
Gartland and Werley score (*points*)	0.9	1.2	1.1	1.3	0.38

*The difference between the cohorts was significant ($p < 0.05$).
†DASH = Disabilities of the Arm, Shoulder and Hand questionnaire.

versus 90°), mean grip strength (81% versus 92%), and mean Mayo score, favoring patients prescribed independent exercises. There were no differences in arm-specific disability (DASH score) at any time point.

Conclusions.—Prescription of formal occupational therapy does not improve the average motion or disability score after volar locking plate fixation of a fracture of the distal part of the radius (Tables 1 and 2).

▶ This is a well-conceived and conducted randomized, controlled trial focused on the impact of formal hand therapy on the ultimate pain and functional outcomes following volar plating of distal radius fractures. There is no advantage to patient self-directed therapy with instructions from the treating surgeon. This finding relates to the fact that with this treatment, the stability of the distal radius is optimally restored. Therefore, when self-instructed on which exercises to do at home, patients can follow through. Formal therapy following stabilization of distal radius fractures is unnecessary.

M. F. Swiontkowski, MD

External or internal fixation in the treatment of non-reducible distal radial fractures?: A 5-year follow-up of a randomized study involving 50 patients

Landgren M, Jerrhag D, Tägil M, et al (Lund Univ and Skåne Univ Hosp, Sweden)

Acta Orthop 82:610-613, 2011

Background and Purpose.—We have previously shown in a randomized study that in the first year after treatment, open reduction and internal fixation resulted in better grip strength and forearm rotation than closed reduction and bridging external fixation. In the present study, we investigated whether this difference persists over time.

Patients and Methods.—The 50 patients included in the original study (mean age 53 years, 36 women) were sent a QuickDASH questionnaire and an invitation to a radiographic and clinical examination after a mean of 5 (3–7) years.

Results.—All 50 patients returned the QuickDASH questionnaire and 45 participated in the clinical and radiographic examination. In the internal fixation group, the grip strength was 95% (SD 12) of the uninjured side and in the external fixation group it was 90% (SD 21) of the uninjured side ($p = 0.3$). QuickDASH score, range of motion, and radiographic parameters were similar between the groups.

Interpretation.—The difference originally found between internal and external fixation in distal radial fractures at 1 year regarding grip strength and range of motion was found to diminish with time. At 5 years, both groups had approached normal values (Tables 2 and 3).

▶ This is a longer-term follow-up of a randomized, controlled trial comparing open reduction and internal plate fixation of distal radius fractures with bridging

TABLE 2.—Radiographic Outcome

	O (n = 23)	C (n = 22)	p-Value
Radial inclination (°), mean (SD)	25 (4)	23 (5)	0.2
Ulnar variance (mm), mean (SD)	1.0 (2.1)	1.8 (2.1)	0.2
Dorsal angulation[a], mean (SD)	−4 (7)	−2 (9)	0.5
Osteoarthritis (n)	2	4	0.4
DRU joint incongruence (n)	0	4	0.05

[a]Negative values indicate palmar angulation.

TABLE 3.—Subjective Outcome: QuickDASH and SF-36

	O	C	p-Value
QuickDASH	15 (14)[a]	13 (16)[a]	0.6
	11 (0–46)[b]	3 (0–57)[b]	0.3
SF-36[b]			
Physical functioning	90 (60–100)	100 (5–100)	1.0
Role-physical	100 (25–100)	100 (0–100)	0.4
Bodily pain	84 (22–100)	100 (12–100)	0.2
General health	82 (52–100)	84 (30–100)	0.9
Vitality	80 (35–100)	85 (20–100)	0.7
Social functioning	100 (25–100)	100 (12–100)	0.8
Role-emotional	100 (32–100)	100 (0–100)	0.3
Mental health	88 (32–100)	90 (16–100)	0.6

[a]Mean (SD).
[b]Median (range).

external fixation. The functional and radiographic outcomes at this longer-term interval were essentially similar. The take-home message is that longer-term outcomes are equivalent. Surgeon skill and persistence in obtaining as anatomic reduction as possible seem to be the essential elements for a successful outcome in the management of distal radius fractures.

M. F. Swiontkowski, MD

Comparing Hook Plates and Kirschner Tension Band Wiring for Unstable Lateral Clavicle Fractures

Wu K, Chang C-H, Yang R-S (Far Eastern Memorial Hosp, Ban-Chaio, China; Natl Taiwan Univ & Hosp, Taipei City)
Orthopedics 34:e718-e723, 2011

The purpose of this study was to compare outcomes and complications of clavicular hook plate and Kirschner tension band wiring for fixation of unstable lateral clavicle fractures. The surgical outcomes of 92 consecutive patients (mean age, 49.30 ± 15.54 years) with unstable fractures of the lateral clavicle treated using AO clavicle hook plates were compared with

TABLE 2.—Comparison of Outcomes Between the 2 Groups

	Hook Plate Fixation (n=92)	K-wire Fixation (n=24)	*P* Value
Mean time to plate removal, mo	5.20±1.93	7.58±2.00	<.001[a,b]
Mean Constant-Murley score	90.43±4.7	85.63±5.38	<.001[a,b]
Mean follow-up, mo	22.76±2.22	25.67±2.75	<.001[a,b]
No. of complications	12	7	<.069[c]

[a]Independent 2-sample *t* test.
[b]Significant difference between the 2 groups: *P*<.05.
[c]Fisher's exact test.

those of 24 patients (mean age, 50.67 ± 17.58 years) treated using K-wire tension banding. Patients in the hook plate and K-wire groups were followed up for 22.76 ± 2.22 and 25.67 ± 2.75 months, respectively (*P*<.001). The time to hardware removal was significantly shorter (*P*<.001) in the hook plate group (5.20 ± 1.93 months) compared with the K-wire group (7.58 ± 2.00 months), whereas the Constant-Murley score was significantly higher (*P*<.001) in the hook plate group (90.43 ± 4.78) compared with the K-wire group (85.63 ± 5.38) at final follow-up. There were 12 complications in the hook plate group and 7 in the K-wire group (*P*=.069). Complications in the hook plate group included 7 periprosthetic fractures, 4 plate removals, and 1 plate malposition. Complications in the K-wire group included 3 K-wire migrations, 3 losses of reduction, and 1 wire breakage. We found that hook plate fixation of unstable lateral clavicle fractures was associated with statistically better shoulder function and earlier implant removal than K-wire tension band fixation, with an equivalent rate of complications. Our findings suggest that hook plates are useful for treating unstable lateral clavicular fractures (Table 2).

▶ This is a retrospective cohort study with all the attendant issues of variable surgeon expertise, important clinical differences in the patients in each cohort, detection and inclusion bias, and so on. The important information is the functional outcome data in the form of the Constant-Murley score, which could be used to preform a power calculation in planning for a randomized controlled trial. Although there is a statistically better functional outcome in patients with distal clavicle fractures treated with the hook plate compared with K-wires and tension band wire (TBW) loops, the limitations of the study design should prevent immediate use of this data in clinical decision making. One interesting note is that the hook plates were removed earlier than the K-wire/TBW implants. This may indicate important differences in the patient cohorts. Both implant choices are associated with significant irritation of the acromioclavicular joint and generally require implant removal. An issue that should not escape the orthopedic surgeon's notice is the 5 peri-implant fractures with the hook plate, a complication generally more severe than can occur with the K-wire/TBW approach. It is also possible to use the K-wire/TBW approach without crossing the AC joint, which can have advantages in mobilizing the shoulder postoperatively.

M. F. Swiontkowski, MD

Isolated fractures of the greater tuberosity of the proximal humerus: A long-term retrospective study of 30 patients

Mattyasovszky SG, Burkhart KJ, Ahlers C, et al (Johannes Gutenberg Univ Mainz, Germany)

Acta Orthop 82:714-720, 2011

Background and Purpose.—The diagnosis and treatment of isolated greater tuberosity fractures of the proximal humerus is not clear-cut. We retrospectively assessed the clinical and radiographic outcome of isolated greater tuberosity fractures.

Patients and Methods.—30 patients (mean age 58 (26–85) years, 19 women) with 30 closed isolated greater tuberosity fractures were reassessed after an average follow-up time of 3 years with DASH score and Constant score. Radiographic outcome was assessed on standard plain radiographs.

Results.—14 of 17 patients with undisplaced or slightly displaced fractures (≤5 mm) were treated nonoperatively and had good clinical outcome (mean DASH score of 13, mean Constant score of 71). 8 patients with moderately displaced fractures (6–10 mm) were either treated nonoperatively (n = 4) or operatively (n = 4), with good functional results (mean DASH score of 10, mean Constant score of 72). 5 patients with major displaced fractures (>10 mm) were all operated with good clinical results (mean DASH score of 14, mean Constant score of 69). The most common discomfort at the follow-up was an impingement syndrome of the shoulder, which occurred in both nonoperatively treated patients (n = 3) and operatively treated patients (n = 4). Only 1 nonoperatively treated patient developed a non-union. By radiography, all other fractures healed.

TABLE 1.—Overview of Clinical Evaluation Considering Fragment Displacement

	Degree of Fragment Displacement[a]			
Scores	None/Minor (n = 17)	Moderate (n = 8)	Major (n = 5)	p-Value
DASH score[b]				
75–100 (poor)	–	–	–	
50–74 (moderate)	1	–	1	
25–49 (good)	3	1	–	
<25 (excellent)	13	7	4	
Mean (SD)	13 (17)	10 (12)	14 (24)	0.9
95% CI	4 to 22	0 to 20	−16 to 44	
Constant score				
86–100 (excellent)	3	1	–	
71–85 (good)	7	5	3	
56–70 (moderate)	3	2	1	
< 55 (poor)	4	–	1	
Mean (SD)	71 (18)	72 (16)	69 (17)	1.0
95% CI	62 to 80	59 to 85	48 to 90	

[a]None/minor indicates displacement of ≤5 mm, moderate indicates displacement of 6–10 mm, and major indicates displacement of >10 mm.
[b]DASH: Disabilities of the Arm, Shoulder and Hand scale.

TABLE 2.—Active ROM at the Time of Follow-up Examination

	Degree of fragment displacement and ROM[a]			
	None/minor (n = 17)	Moderate (n = 8)	Major (n = 5)	p-value
Forward flexion	155 (105–170)	149 (100–170)	142 (130–155)	0.6
Abduction	147 (90–170)	142 (95–175)	146 (130–160)	0.9
External rotation	54 (30–70)	49 (30–70)	40 (20–60)	0.2
Internal rotation	72 (50–90)	69 (40–90)	68 (50–80)	0.8

[a]The range of motion (ROM) of the affected arm is presented as the mean value in degrees with the range in parentheses.

Interpretation.—We found that minor to moderately displaced greater tuberosity fractures may be treated successfully without surgery (Tables 1 and 2).

▶ This is a retrospective cohort study of a relatively rare clinical problem of an isolated greater tuberosity fracture. As would be expected with this study design, the fractures with lesser degrees of displacement were treated nonoperatively, whereas those with 5 mm or more of displacement were most often treated with operative reduction and displacement; those with a centimeter or more were always treated with surgery. The patients generally had good shoulder function; nonunion was rare and related to comminution in a patient treated nonoperatively. I agree with the authors' conclusion that these fractures, unless they exhibit marked displacement of a centimeter or more, can be treated conservatively with the expectation of a good functional outcome with a standard shoulder rehabilitation program.

M. F. Swiontkowski, MD

Can Complications of Titanium Elastic Nailing With End Cap for Clavicular Fractures Be Reduced?

Frigg A, Rillmann P, Ryf C, et al (Univ Hosp Basel, Switzerland; Davos Hosp, Switzerland)

Clin Orthop Relat Res 469:3356-3363, 2011

Background.—We found treatment of clavicular midshaft fractures using titanium elastic nails (TENs) in combination with postoperative free ROM was associated with a complication rate of 78%. The use of end caps reduced the rate to 60%, which we still considered unacceptably high. Thus, we explored an alternative approach.

Questions/Purposes.—We investigated whether (1) the complication rate could be reduced by cautious lateral advancement of the TENs, intraoperative oblique radiographs to rule out lateral perforation, and limited ROM postoperatively; (2) fluoroscopy time could be reduced; and (3) shoulder function would be reasonable.

Patients and Methods.—From March 2006 to December 2009, we treated 44 patients with midshaft clavicular fractures with TENs and end caps. In the first group (n = 15), the TEN was advanced laterally using an oscillating drill. The patients were permitted free ROM. In the second group (n = 29), the TEN was advanced by hand, conversion to open reduction followed two failed closed attempts and lateral perforation was checked with an intraoperative oblique radiograph. Furthermore, anteversion and abduction of the shoulder were limited to 90° for the first 6 weeks. Minimum followup was 12 months (mean, 16.7 months; range, 12–28 months).

Results.—The total complication rate was reduced from nine of 15 in the first group to five of 29 in the second group. Medial perforations ceased with the use of the end cap. Fluoroscopy time was reduced from a mean of 10 to 4 minutes by converting to open reduction after two failed closed attempts. All but three patients exhibited full shoulder ROM at three months and these three had a slight deficit of 10° to 20° in anteversion and/or abduction. At last followup, the mean American Shoulder and Elbow Surgeons score was 92 (range, 88–100) and the Disability of the Arm, Shoulder, and Hand score 1.4 (range, 0–12.5).

Conclusions.—Cautious insertion of the TENs, intraoperative oblique radiographs, and limiting the ROM for 6 weeks postoperatively reduced the complication rate. Using TENs with end caps for midshaft clavicular fractures is minimally invasive while associated with comparable complication rates and function to plate osteosynthesis.

Level of Evidence.—Level III, therapeutic study. See Guidelines for Authors for a complete description of levels of evidence (Tables 1 and 3).

▶ This is another cohort series confirming the high rate of complications with intramedullary devices for fixation of clavicle fractures. The authors document some improvements with an end cap and change in technique, which improved the rate of complications. However, the percentage of patients with complications remains fairly significant. The issue is a curved bone in 2 planes with

TABLE 1.—Overview of Complications Reported in the Literature Using TENs

Study	Number of Patients	Number of Complications	Type of Complications
Jubel et al. [8]	65	6 (9.2%)	Medial migration (n = 4), nonunion (n = 1), secondary shortening of 1.5 cm (n = 1)
Kettler et al. [10]	87	10 (11.5%)	Lateral (n = 3) and medial (n = 1) migration, nonunion (n = 2), secondary shortening of >1 cm (n = 2), malunion (n = 2)
Meier et al. [15]	14	4 (28.5%)	Medial migration (n = 1), medial skin irritation (n = 2), fracture dislocation (n = 1)
Müller et al. [16]	45	25 (55.5%)	Lateral (n = 2) and medial (n = 8) migration, TEN breakage (n = 2), wound infection (n = 1), secondary shortening of >4 mm (n = 12)
Walz et al. [26]	35	6 (22.2%)	Lateral (n = 1) and medial (n = 5) migration
Frigg et al. [2]	34	23 (70%)	Lateral (n = 7) and medial (n = 7) migration, TEN breakage (n = 1), TEN dislocation (n = 1) medial and lateral pain (n = 7)

TEN = titanium elastic nail.

Editor's Note: Please refer to original journal article for full references.

TABLE 3.—Summary of Complications and Perioperative Parameters

Variable	Group A (n = 15)	Group B (n = 29)	p Value
Complications (number of patients)			
Total	60%	17%	<0.001
Major	6/15 (40%)	3/29 (10%)	<0.001
Lateral perforation	4†	1	
Nail breakage	1†	0	
Nail dislocation	1†	0	
Subclavian vein thrombosis	0	1	
Nonunion	0	1	
Minor			
Medial or lateral pain	3/15 (20%)	2/29 (7%)	0.007
Operating time (minutes)*			
Total	37 ± 27 (10–105)	47 ± 19 (20–80)	0.16
Closed reduction	22 ± 13 (n = 6)	34 ± 13 (n = 15)	0.05
Open reduction	47 ± 29 (n = 9)	60 ± 15 (n = 14)	0.16
Fluoroscopy time (minutes)*			
Total	10.4 ± 7.9	4.0 ± 2.2	<0.001
Closed reduction	8.2 ± 11.2 (n = 6)	3.6 ± 1.8 (n = 15)	0.12
Open reduction	10.5 ± 6.5 (n = 9)	4.4 ± 2.6 (n = 14)	0.004
Visual analog scale (0–10)*			
Preoperative	6.1 (5–9)	5.7 (1–8)	0.08
Postoperative	2.3 (0–4)	1.5 (0–3)	0.32
6 weeks postoperatively†	1 (0–5)	1.7 (0–6)	0.27
3 months postoperatively†	0.1 (0–1)	0.6 (0–3)	0.07
ROM 3 months postoperatively†			
Anteversion free	100% (11/11)	97% (28/29)	0.53
Abduction free	91% (10/11)	97% (28/29)	0.47
Time to bony healing (months)*	3.2 ± 1.2 (1.5–5)	3.7 ± 1.7 (1.5–8)	0.32
Hardware removal (months)*	6 (3–12)	6 (2–13)	
ASES score (at final followup) (points)*,†	88 (0–100)	98 (88–100)	0.4
DASH score (at final followup) (points)*,†	1.5 (0–12.5)	1.3 (0–4.2)	0.87

*Values are expressed as mean or mean ± SD, with range in parentheses.
†numbers in Group A are reduced to n = 12 because three cases were converted to plating due to complications during the postoperative course; ASES = American Shoulder and Elbow Surgeons; DASH = Disability of the Arm, Shoulder, and Hand.

a small intramedullary canal. Using plate fixation translates the problem from reduction and placement of a straight device in a curved bone to contouring a plate to allow maintenance of reduction. Neither approach is without difficulty, but for surgeons who have not developed the expertise to use intramedullary devices in the clavicle, learning the plating technique will probably result in lower complication rates.

M. F. Swiontkowski, MD

A Prospective Randomized Trial Comparing Nonoperative Treatment with Volar Locking Plate Fixation for Displaced and Unstable Distal Radial Fractures in Patients Sixty-five Years of Age and Older

Arora R, Lutz M, Deml C, et al (Med Univ Innsbruck, Austria)
J Bone Joint Surg Am 93:2146-2153, 2011

Background.—Despite the recent trend toward the internal fixation of distal radial fractures in older patients, the currently available literature lacks adequate randomized trials examining whether open reduction and internal fixation (ORIF) with a volar locking plate is superior to nonoperative (cast) treatment. The purpose of the present randomized clinical trial was to compare the outcomes of two methods that were used for the treatment of displaced and unstable distal radial fractures in patients sixty-five years of age or older: (1) ORIF with use of a volar locking plate and (2) closed reduction and plaster immobilization (casting).

Methods.—A prospective randomized study was performed. Seventy-three patients with a displaced and unstable distal radial fracture were randomized to ORIF with a volar locking plate ($n = 36$) or closed reduction and cast immobilization ($n = 37$). The outcome was measured on the basis of the Patient-Rated Wrist Evaluation (PRWE) score; the Disabilities of the Arm, Shoulder and Hand (DASH) score; the pain level; the range of wrist motion; the rate of complications; and radiographic measurements including dorsal radial tilt, radial inclination, and ulnar variance.

Results.—There were no significant differences between the groups in terms of the range of motion or the level of pain during the entire follow-up period ($p > 0.05$). Patients in the operative treatment group had lower DASH and PRWE scores, indicating better wrist function, in the early postoperative time period ($p < 0.05$), but there were no significant differences between the groups at six and twelve months. Grip strength was significantly better at all times in the operative treatment group ($p < 0.05$). Dorsal radial tilt, radial inclination, and radial shortening were significantly better in the operative treatment group than in the nonoperative treatment group at the time of the latest follow-up ($p < 0.05$). The number of complications was significantly higher in the operative treatment group (thirteen compared with five, $p < 0.05$).

Conclusions.—At the twelve-month follow-up examination, the range of motion, the level of pain, and the PRWE and DASH scores were not different between the operative and nonoperative treatment groups. Patients in the operative treatment group had better grip strength through the entire time period. Achieving anatomical reconstruction did not convey any improvement in terms of the range of motion or the ability to perform daily living activities in our cohorts (Table 2).

▶ This well-done randomized clinical trial (RCT) examines the radiographic and functional outcomes of distal radius fractures in patients 65 years and older with operative management/volar plating versus closed reduction and casting. As has been the case with other RCTs, the early functional outcomes (6 and 12 weeks) were better in the operative cohort, but the long-term functional and clinical outcomes at 1 year were equivalent. The favorable radiographic outcomes in the operative and nonoperative cohorts speaks to the skill and precision of the surgeons treating these patients but were significantly better in the operative cohort. The only significant longer-term outcome of relevance to patients that was better in the operative cohort was grip strength. These data will be of great

TABLE 2.—Clinical Outcomes

	Operative Treatment Group	Nonoperative Treatment Group	*P* Value
6 weeks			
Extension* *(deg)*	46 ± 15 (76.1%)	45 ± 15 (75.4%)	0.67
Flexion* *(deg)*	44 ± 13 (72.3%)	41 ± 11 (72.7%)	0.42
Supination* *(deg)*	75 ± 18 (88.6%)	73 ± 16 (85.4%)	0.61
Pronation* *(deg)*	81 ± 9 (96.0%)	77 ± 16 (91.3%)	0.21
Ulnar deviation* *(deg)*	26 ± 8 (76.3%)	26 ± 11 (73.0%)	0.78
Radial deviation* *(deg)*	18 ± 8 (84.1%)	19 ± 8 (81.4%)	0.86
Grip strength* *(kg)*	14.1 ± 5.5 (60.3%)	10.7 ± 5.6 (54.9%)	0.01
Pain at rest† *(points)*	0.3 ± 0.8	0.3 ± 0.8	0.97
Pain under stress† *(points)*	2.0 ± 2.0	2.5 ± 2.1	0.24
DASH score† *(points)*	18.8 ± 17.9	34.4 ± 22.5	0.00
PRWE score† *(points)*	36.4 ± 28.7	64.9 ± 29.0	0.00
12 weeks			
Extension* *(deg)*	51 ± 13 (85.6%)	52 ± 9 (87.4%)	0.88
Flexion* *(deg)*	47 ± 12 (80.0%)	49 ± 11 (81.4%)	0.49
Supination* *(deg)*	80 ± 14 (93.4%)	80 ± 12 (95.7%)	0.96
Pronation* *(deg)*	81 ± 13 (94.8%)	81 ± 12 (96.5%)	0.81
Ulnar deviation* *(deg)*	30 ± 10 (91.7%)	28 ± 10 (79.5%)	0.38
Radial deviation* *(deg)*	20 ± 7 (82.2%)	20 ± 7 (89.0%)	0.94
Grip strength* *(kg)*	15.7 ± 6.2 (77.1%)	12.5 ± 4.4 (58.3%)	0.02
Pain at rest† *(points)*	0.2 ± 0.7	0.3 ± 0.8	0.78
Pain under stress† *(points)*	1.4 ± 2.0	1.8 ± 2.0	0.40
DASH score† *(points)*	13.3 ± 14.8	23.2 ± 19.3	0.02
PRWE score† *(points)*	33.7 ± 32.0	54.4 ± 31.8	0.01
6 months			
Extension* *(deg)*	55 ± 11 (91.1%)	55 ± 12 (94.6%)	0.99
Flexion* *(deg)*	51 ± 10 (88.4%)	48 ± 13 (83.1%)	0.28
Supination* *(deg)*	83 ± 9 (97.1%)	79 ± 12 (93.7%)	0.13
Pronation* *(deg)*	84 ± 8 (99.3%)	81 ± 14 (96.3%)	0.20
Ulnar deviation* *(deg)*	33 ± 9 (98.3%)	30 ± 10 (88.8%)	0.20
Radial deviation* *(deg)*	20 ± 7 (83.8%)	21 ± 12 (109.2%)	0.51
Grip strength* *(kg)*	19.8 ± 7.4 (88.4%)	16.1 ± 5.6 (79.0%)	0.02
Pain at rest† *(points)*	0.6 ± 1.3	0.3 ± 1.0	0.30
Pain under stress† *(points)*	1.3 ± 1.7	1.0 ± 1.6	0.43
DASH score† *(points)*	12.2 ± 14.4	12.4 ± 17.0	0.94
PRWE score† *(points)*	27.7 ± 32.0	31.4 ± 33.0	0.63
12 months			
Extension* *(deg)*	59 ± 10 (94.4%)	61 ± 7 (106.6%)	0.14
Flexion* *(deg)*	55 ± 11 (91.1%)	57 ± 10 (100.7%)	0.50
Supination* *(deg)*	85 ± 8 (99.6%)	85 ± 8 (100.4%)	0.99
Pronation* *(deg)*	84 ± 7 (99.4%)	85 ± 8 (100.8%)	0.53
Ulnar deviation* *(deg)*	35 ± 8 (101.6%)	35 ± 8 (102.4%)	0.88
Radial deviation* *(deg)*	24 ± 6 (98.0%)	25 ± 7 (114.9%)	0.52
Grip strength* *(kg)*	22.2 ± 6.3 (102.4%)	18.8 ± 5.8 (92.6%)	0.02
Pain at rest† *(points)*	0.1 ± 0.3	0.1 ± 0.5	0.80
Pain under stress† *(points)*	0.7 ± 1.0	0.6 ± 1.4	0.80
DASH score† *(points)*	5.7 ± 11.1	8.0 ± 9.3	0.34
PRWE score† *(points)*	12.8 ± 23.2	14.6 ± 22.8	0.73

*The values are given as the mean and the standard deviation, with the percentage of the value for the uninjured side in parentheses.
†The values are given as the mean and the standard deviation.

value to present to patients in the process of shared decision making in the older than 65 patient population.

M. F. Swiontkowski, MD

Retention of forearm plates: Risks and benefits in a paediatric population

Clement ND, Yousif F, Duckworth AD, et al (The Royal Hosp for Sick Children, Edinburgh, UK)

J Bone Joint Surg Br 94-B:134-137, 2012

Most surgeons favour removing forearm plates in children. There is, however, no long-term data regarding the complications of retaining a plate. We present a prospective case series of 82 paediatric patients who underwent plating of their forearm fracture over an eight-year period with a minimum follow-up of two years. The study institution does not routinely remove forearm plates. A total of 116 plates were used: 79 one-third tubular plates and 37 dynamic compression plates (DCP). There were 12 complications: six plates (7.3%) were removed for pain or stiffness and there were six (7.3%) implant-related fractures. Overall, survival of the plates was 85% at 10 years. Cox regression analysis identified radial plates (odds ratio (OR) 4.4, $p = 0.03$) and DCP fixation (OR 3.2, $p = 0.02$) to be independent risk factors of an implant-related fracture. In contrast ulnar plates were more likely to cause pain or irritation necessitating removal (OR 5.6, $p = 0.04$).

The complications associated with retaining a plate are different, but do not occur more frequently than the complications following removal of a plate in children (Table 1).

► The data on patient outcome following forearm plate removal are relatively rare. Clinical data on the indications for removal of forearm plates, especially in children, are even rarer. This cohort study provides information regarding both issues. A 7.3% complication rate from plate removal fits in with prior cohort studies on the topic in adults. Perhaps the most pertinent take-home message from this study is that if you leave forearm plates in as a practice, that will prove to be a sound decision in 85% of patients. Removing plates in 100% of adolescents to prevent the 15% complication rate does not seem prudent. The factor that is not considered in that practice decision is the potential negative impact of an 80-year exposure to nickel and chromium. This question must be answered in other investigations.

M. F. Swiontkowski, MD

TABLE 1.—Number of Late Complications and Mean Time of Occurrence From Fixation

Complication	Number (%)	Mean Time Incurred (mths) (Range)
Implant-related fracture	6 (*7.3*)	18.3 (10 to 34)
Pain/irritation	5 (*6.1*)	14.1 (10 to 26)
Screw extrusion	3 (*3.7*)	1.3 (1 to 3)
Stiffness	1 (*1.2*)	12.0
Total	15 (*18.3*)	

Closed Treatment of Overriding Distal Radial Fractures without Reduction in Children

Crawford SN, Lee LSK, Izuka BH (Univ of Hawaii Orthopaedics Residency Program, Honolulu; Children's Orthopaedics of Hawaii, Aiea)
J Bone Joint Surg Am 94:246-252, 2012

Background.—Traditionally, distal radial fractures with marked displacement and angulation have been treated with closed or open reduction techniques. Reduction maneuvers generally require analgesia and sedation, which increase hospital time, cost, patient risk, and the surgeon's time. In our study, a treatment protocol for pediatric distal radial fractures was used in which the fracture was left shortened in an overriding position and a cast was applied without an attempt at anatomic fracture reduction.

Methods.—Consecutive patients three to ten years of age presenting between 2004 and 2009 with a closed overriding fracture of the distal radial metaphysis were followed prospectively. Our protocol consisted of no analgesia, no sedation, and a short arm fiberglass cast gently molded to correct only angulation. Patients were followed for at least one year. All parents or guardians were given a questionnaire assessing their satisfaction with the treatment. Financial analysis was performed with use of Current Procedural Terminology codes and the average total cost of care.

Results.—Fifty-one children with an average age of 6.9 years were included in the study. Initial radial shortening averaged 5.0 mm. Initial sagittal and coronal angulation averaged 4.0° and 3.2°, respectively. The average duration of casting was forty-two days. Residual sagittal and coronal angulation at the time of final follow-up averaged 2.2° and 0.8°, respectively. All fifty-one patients achieved clinical and radiographic union with a full range of wrist motion. All parents and guardians answered the questionnaire and were satisfied with the treatment. Cost analysis demonstrated that closed reduction with the patient under conscious sedation or general anesthesia is nearly five to six times more expensive than the treatment used in this study. Adding percutaneous pin fixation increases costs nearly ninefold.

Conclusions.—This treatment protocol presents an alternative approach to overriding distal radial fractures in children and provides the orthopaedic

TABLE 1.—Radiographic Measurements After Initial Cast Application and at Final Follow-up

	Mean and Stand. Dev. (*deg*)	Range (*deg*)
Initial radiographs		
Sagittal angulation	4.0 ± 4.1	0-13
Coronal angulation	3.2 ± 3.1	0-10
Final radiographs		
Sagittal angulation	2.2 ± 2.7	0-10
Coronal angulation	0.75 ± 1.4	0-5

TABLE 2.—Treatment Cost by Common Procedural Terminology (CPT) Code

Treatment by CPT Code	Cost ($)
Office visit with application of short arm cast	1027
Emergency room with sedation, closed reduction, and casting	4846
Operating room with general anesthesia, closed reduction, and casting	6415
Operating room with general anesthesia, closed reduction with percutaneous pinning, and casting	8742

surgeon a simple, effective, and cost and time-efficient method of treatment (Tables 1 and 2).

▶ This is a well-performed cohort study assessing the results of treatment of pediatric forearm fractures in which initial shortening of the radius and ulna is accepted and closed manipulation performed in the office to correct angulatory malalignment. The results are surprising both in terms of the functional and radiographic outcomes. The follow-up is fairly comprehensive and is of adequate length to assure treating orthopedists and the patient's parents that the results will be more than satisfactory at 1 year after fracture. The cost estimates (Table 2) are worthy of mention.

M. F. Swiontkowski, MD

Radial Head and Neck Fractures

Early Radial Head Excision for Displaced and Comminuted Radial Head Fractures: Considerations and Concerns at Long-Term Follow-Up

Faldini C, Nanni M, Leonetti D, et al (Univ of Bologna, Italy)

J Orthop Trauma 26:236-240, 2012

Objectives.—The aim of this study is to retrospectively review the outcomes of patients with comminuted radial head fractures surgically treated with early radial head excision.

Design.—Retrospective follow-up study.

Setting.—University orthopaedic trauma center.

Patients.—Forty-two patients with unilateral, isolated, closed, displaced, or comminuted radial head fracture (Mason type 2-10, Type 3-32).

Intervention.—Early radial head excision.

Main Outcome Measurements.—Patients were clinically and radiographically evaluated at an average follow-up of 18 years. The uninjured contralateral limb was used as a comparison. Clinical evaluation was rated using the Broberg and Morrey system, the Disabilities of the Arm, Shoulder and Hand (DASH) questionnaire, and the visual analog scale (VAS) for pain.

Results.—At last follow-up, 36 patients had no complaints, whereas six admitted to occasional pain. The mean Broberg and Morrey score was

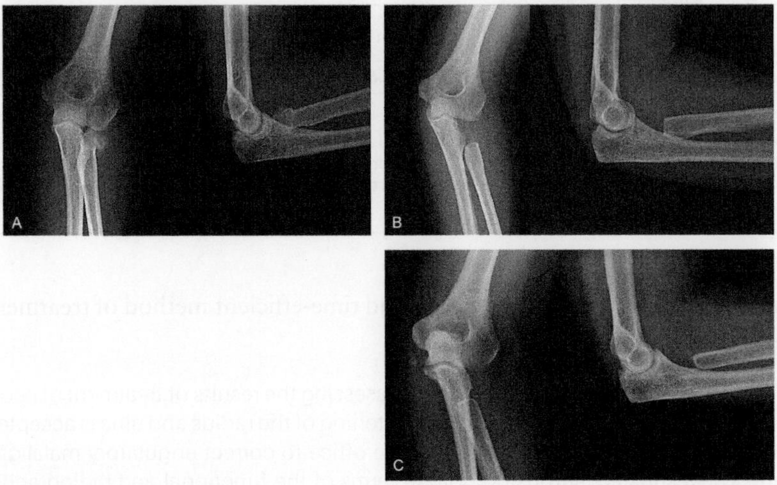

FIGURE 1.—Radiographic aspect of a Mason Type 3 radial head fracture in a 30-year-old man (A). Postoperative aspect after radial head excision (B). Radiographic aspect at 18-year follow-up: small periarticular ossifications are noticeable (C). Pain visual analog scale (VAS): 0; Broberg and Morrey score: 92; Disabilities of the Arm, Shoulder and Hand (DASH) score: 8. (Reprinted from Faldini C, Nanni M, Leonetti D, et al. Early radial head excision for displaced and comminuted radial head fractures: considerations and concerns at long-term follow-up. *J Orthop Trauma*. 2012;26:236-240, with permission from Lippincott Williams & Wilkins.)

91.2 ± 6.3, and the mean Disabilities of the Arm, Shoulder and Hand score was 10.1 ± 8.8.

Conclusion.—Early radial head excision represents a viable option in case of displaced and comminuted fractures. According to the results of this study, it demonstrated a high rate of good results and patient satisfaction, a quick recovery after surgery, and a low rate of complications with durable results at long-term follow-up.

Level of Evidence.—Therapeutic Level IV. See Instructions for Authors for a complete description of levels of evidence (Fig 1).

▶ This is a well-done, long-term, retrospective review of the results of radial head resection. It is perhaps the largest series of long-term results of radial head resection in the literature. The results are reassuring that this is a procedure that can be reliably selected and discussed with patients with Mason 3 fractures. For Mason 2 fractures, this series does not adequately address the question of whether this technique is superior to ORIF. Controlled trials are appropriate to answer the question for this fracture pattern.

M. F. Swiontkowski, MD

The Surgical Treatment of Isolated Mason Type 2 Fractures of the Radial Head in Adults: Comparison Between Radial Head Resection and Open Reduction and Internal Fixation

Zarattini G, Galli S, Marchese M, et al (Clinica Ortopedica dell'Università degli Studi di Brescia, Italy; et al)

J Orthop Trauma 26:229-235, 2012

Objectives.—To compare the outcomes of two different surgical treatments for the management of isolated closed Mason Type 2 radial head fractures.

Design.—Retrospective study. The Student *t* test and McPearson chi-square test were used to evaluate whether there was a significance difference between the groups.

Patients.—Fifty-nine patients with isolated Mason Type 2 radial head fractures.

Intervention.—Twenty-four patients treated with radial head excision (Group I) and 35 treated with open reduction and internal fixation (Group II).

Main Outcome Measurements.—Clinical outcomes were assessed using the Broberg and Morrey functional rating scores and the Disabilities of the Arm, Shoulder and Hand (DASH) questionnaire. Orthogonal radiographs were performed on both the elbow and the wrist; these were assessed for the presence of arthritis, heterotopic ossification, and the degree of proximal radial migration.

Results.—The length of postoperative follow-up was 157 ± 61.84 months (Group I) and 125 ± 39.09 months (Group II). The Broberg and Morrey functional rating score was 86.21 ± 6.10 points and 95.09 ± 4.78 points, respectively. The DASH score was 21.82 ± 6.01 points and 2.81 ± 2.73 points, respectively. Radiologically moderate or severe osteoarthritis was present in the elbows of nine patients in Group I and only two patients in Group II.

Conclusions.—Patients with isolated Mason Type 2 radial head fractures treated by open reduction and internal fixation (Group II) had less residual pain, greater range of motion, and better strength than patients treated by radial head excision (Group I). Additionally, Group II had a lower incidence of severe posttraumatic arthritis, which contributed to improved DASH and Broberg and Morrey functional scores. These results support open reduction and internal fixation as the treatment of choice for these fractures.

Level of Evidence.—Therapeutic Level III. See Instructions for Authors for a complete description of levels of evidence (Tables 1 and 2).

▶ This fairly well-done controlled trial confirms that salvage of the radial head for displaced Mason 2 radial head fractures is the strategy of choice. The length of follow-up in this study was more than adequate to confirm the clinical and radiologic outcomes for the 2 surgical strategies of excision versus open reduction and internal fixation (ORIF). Multiple outcome measures of elbow function

TABLE 1.—Pain Results, Arc of Motion, Valgus Deviation, Strength, and Functional Assessment Scores*

Measure	Group I	Group II
VAS result at elbow (points)	3.46 ± 2.55	1.20 ± 0.93
VAS result at wrist (points)	1.21 ± 2.02	0
Arc of elbow motion in flexion–extension	136.25° ± 15.41°	152.57° ± 8.52°
Arc of forearm rotation	163.54° ± 10.16°	172.29° ± 8.25°
Arc of wrist motion in flexion–extension	154.79° ± 8.66°	167.29° ± 8.86°
Grip strength of the injured arm (kg)	27.12 ± 8.05	35.12 ± 7.57
Broberg and Morrey functional rating score (points)	86.21 ± 6.10	95.09 ± 4.78
Definitive averaged DASH value (points)	21.82 ± 6.01	2.81 ± 2.73

VAS, visual analog scale; DASH, Disabilities of the Arm, Shoulder and Hand.
*The values are given as mean and standard deviation. $P < 0.05$ for all those measurements in which it accurately applies.

TABLE 2.—Radiographic Assessment of Degenerative Changes and Proximal Translation of the Radius

Measure		Group I	Group II
Degenerative osteoarthritis of the elbow*	Grade 0	5 (20.8%)	15 (42.9%)
	Grade 1	10 (41.7%)	18 (51.4%)
	Grade 2	4 (16.7%)	2 (5.7%)
	Grade 3	5 (20.8%)	0
Degenerative osteoarthritis of the wrist*	Grade 0	16 (66.7%)	31 (88.6%)
	Grade 1	5 (20.8%)	4 (11.4%)
	Grade 2	3 (12.5%)	0
Periarticular ossification*		29.2%	
Increase in ulnar variance (mm)†		2.50 ± 1.50	

*The values are given as number of cases and percentage.
†The values are given as mean and standard deviation.

confirmed the results. ORIF should be our procedure for displaced radial head Mason 2 fractures.

M. F. Swiontkowski, MD

Amputation Surgery: Outcome

The Contribution of Sympathetic Mechanisms to Postamputation Phantom and Residual Limb Pain: A Pilot Study

Cohen SP, Gambel JM, Raja SN, et al (Johns Hopkins School of Medicine, Baltimore, MD; Walter Reed Army Med Ctr, Washington, DC)
J Pain 12:859-867, 2011

Postamputation pain (PAP) affects over 60% of major limb amputees. One of the main challenges in treating PAP is the difficulty involved in identifying pain mechanism(s), which pertains to both residual limb pain (RLP) and phantom limb pain (PLP). In this study, sympathetic blocks were performed on 17 major limb amputees refractory to treatment, including 2 placebo-controlled blocks done for bilateral amputations. One hour postinjection, mean RLP scores at rest declined from 5.2 (SD 2.8) to 2.8 (SD 2.6) ($P = .0002$), and PLP decreased from 5.3 (SD 3.1) to 2.3 (SD 2.1) ($P = .0009$). By 1 week, mean pain scores for RLP and PLP were 4.3 (SD 2.9) and 4.2 (SD 3.0), respectively. Overall, 8 of 16 (50%) patients experienced ≥50% reduction in RLP 1-hour postinjection, with the beneficial effects being maintained at 1 and 8 weeks in 4 and 1 patient(s), respectively. For PLP, 8 of 15 (53%) patients obtained ≥50% decrease in pain 1-hour postblock, with these numbers decreasing to 2 patients at both 1 and 8 weeks. In the 2 bilateral amputees who received controlled injections, mean PLP and RLP at rest scores went from 4.0 and 3.3 to 4.0 and 2.5 1-hour postblock, respectively, on the placebo side. On the treatment side, mean PLP and RLP scores decreased from 7.5 and 6.5, respectively, to 0.

Perspective.—The results of this study suggest that sympathetic mechanisms play a role in PLP and to a lesser extent, RLP, but that blocks confer long-term benefits in only a small percentage of patients (Figs 1 and 2, Table 1).

▶ Refractory postamputation pain is a very common clinical issue in both dysvascular and traumatic amputees. This investigation supports the continued investigation of sympathetic block techniques for both short-term and long-term benefit. This approach has benefit both for residual limb pain and for the phantom limb phenomenon in both time frames. The results of placebo-controlled injections in bilateral amputees add strength to the conclusions generated in the larger population. The technique should be evaluated in a larger population of amputees with adequate numbers of traumatic and dysvascular study participants. However, this study is enough to prompt recommendations

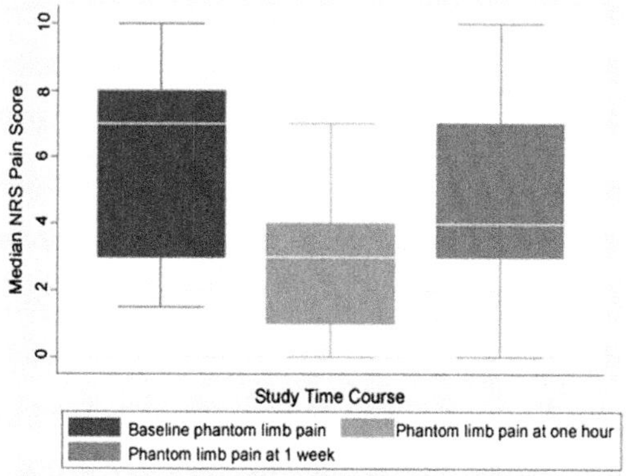

FIGURE 1.—Box plot showing the mean phantom limb pain scores with standard deviation during the study course. (Reprinted from Cohen SP, Gambel JM, Raja SN, et al. The contribution of sympathetic mechanisms to postamputation phantom and residual limb pain: a pilot study. *J Pain.* 2011;12:859-867, with permission from Elsevier.)

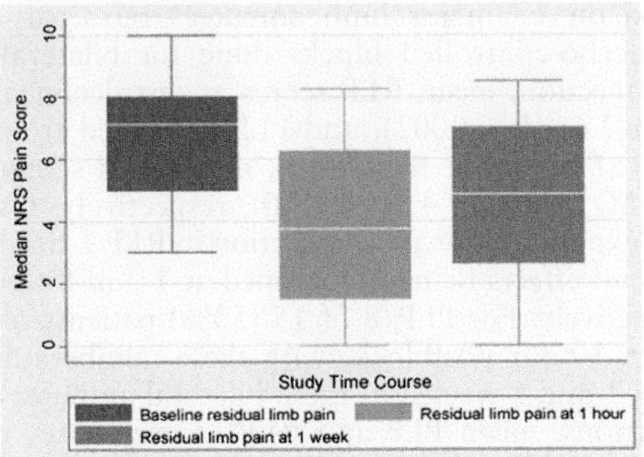

FIGURE 2.—Box plot showing the mean categorical residual limb pain scores with standard deviation during the study course. (Reprinted from Cohen SP, Gambel JM, Raja SN, et al. The contribution of sympathetic mechanisms to postamputation phantom and residual limb pain: a pilot study. *J Pain.* 2011;12:859-867, with permission from Elsevier.)

TABLE 1.—Baseline and Post-Procedure Pain Scores

Clinical Variable	Pre-Procedure Mean, SD	1-Hour Post-Procedure Mean, SD	*P* Value	1-Week Post-Procedure Mean, SD	*P* Value	2-Months Post-Procedure* Mean, SD	*P* Value
RLP- rest	5.1 (2.8)	2.8 (2.6)	.0002	4.3 (2.9)	.11	4.2 (2.4)	.29
RLP- activity	7.1 (2.9)	4.4 (3.4)	.001	4.6 (3.0)	.004	5.8 (2.9)	.02
Phantom limb pain	5.3 (3.1)	2.3 (2.1)	.0009	4.2 (3.0)	.03	3.2 (3.7)	.21
Temperature	29.4 (1.7)	31.8 (2.2)	<.00001	N.R.	N/A	N.R.	N/A

NOTE. P-values represent change from baseline.
*N = 5 followed out to 2 months (subgroup analysis).

for sympathetic block techniques for amputees with postamputation pain and phantom limb phenomenon in centers where experienced anesthesia personnel are available.

M. F. Swiontkowski, MD

A Prospective Randomized Double-blinded Pilot Study to Examine the Effect of Botulinum Toxin Type A Injection Versus Lidocaine/Depomedrol Injection on Residual and Phantom Limb Pain: Initial Report

Wu H, Sultana R, Taylor KB, et al (Med College of Wisconsin, Milwaukee)
Clin J Pain 28:108-112, 2012

Objective.—Botulinum toxin type A (Botox) injection has been used to manage pain. However, it remains to be proved whether Botox injection is effective to relieve residual limb pain (RLP) and phantom limb pain (PLP).

Design.—Randomized, double-blinded pilot study.

Setting.—Medical College and an outpatient clinic in Department of Physical Medicine and Rehabilitation.

Participants.—Amputees (n=14) with intractable RLP and/or PLP who failed in the conventional treatments.

Interventions.—Study amputees were randomized to receive 1 Botox injection versus the combination of Lidocaine and Depomedrol injection. Each patient was evaluated at baseline and every month after the injection for 6 months.

Main Outcome Measure.—The changes of RLP and PLP as recorded by VAS, and the changes of the pressure pain tolerance as determined by a pressure algometer.

Results.—All patients completed the protocol treatment without acute side effects, and monthly assessments of RLP, PLP, and pain tolerance after the treatment. The time trend in the outcomes was modeled as an immediate change owing to the treatment followed by a linear tread afterward. Repeated measures were incorporated using mixed effects modeling. We found that both Botox and Lidocaine/Depomedrol injections resulted in immediate improvements of RLP (Botox: $P=0.002$; Lidocaine/Depomedrol: $P=0.06$) and pain tolerance (Botox: $P=0.01$; Lidocaine/Depomedrol: $P=0.07$). The treatment effect lasted for 6 months in both groups. The patients who received Botox injection had higher starting pain than those who received Lidocaine/Depomedrol injection ($P=0.07$). However, there were no statistical differences in RLP and pain tolerance between these 2 groups. In addition, no improvement of PLP was observed after Botox or Lidocaine/Depomedrol injection.

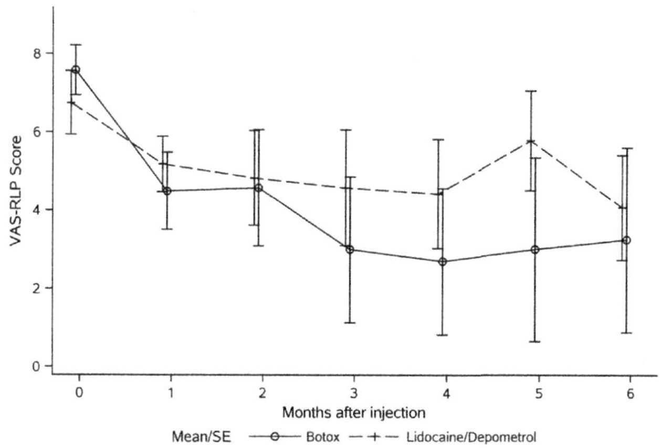

FIGURE 1.—Average VAS-RLP (VAS-R) in amputees treated with Botox injection (solid line) and Lidocaine/Depomedrol injection (dotted line). RLP indicates residual limb pain; VAS, visual analog score. (Reprinted from Wu H, Sultana R, Taylor KB, et al. A prospective randomized double-blinded pilot study to examine the effect of botulinum toxin type A injection versus lidocaine/depomedrol injection on residual and phantom limb pain: initial report. *Clin J Pain.* 2012;28:108-112, with permission from Lippincott Williams & Wilkins.)

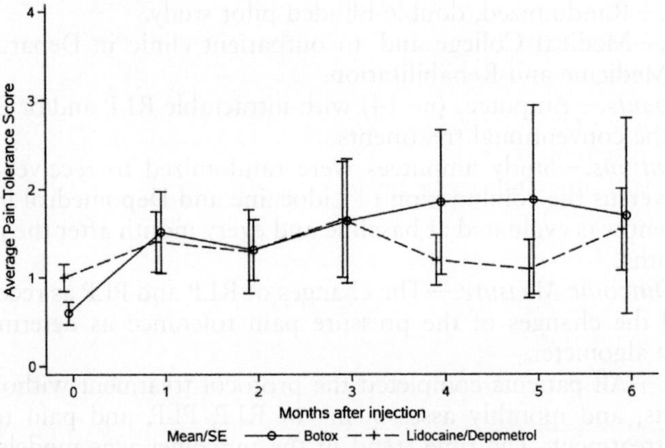

FIGURE 2.—Average pain tolerance scores in amputees treated with Botox injection (solid line) and Lidocaine/Depomedrol injection (dotted line). (Reprinted from Wu H, Sultana R, Taylor KB, et al. A prospective randomized double-blinded pilot study to examine the effect of botulinum toxin type A injection versus lidocaine/depomedrol injection on residual and phantom limb pain: initial report. *Clin J Pain.* 2012;28:108-112, with permission from Lippincott Williams & Wilkins.)

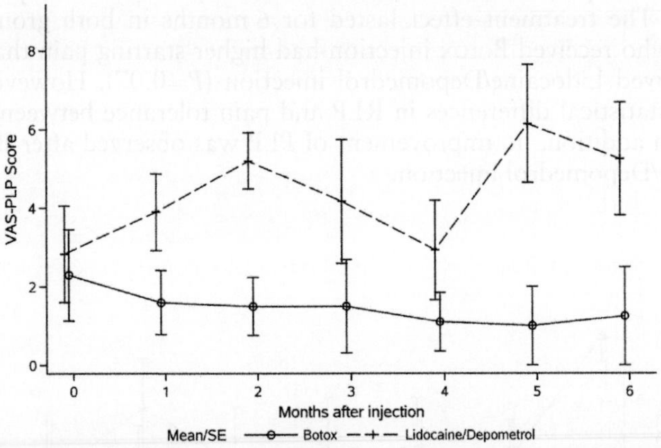

FIGURE 3.—Average VAS-PLP (VAS-P) in amputees treated with Botox injection (solid line) and Lidocaine/Depomedrol injection (dotted line). PLP indicates phantom limb pain; VAS, visual analog score. (Reprinted from Wu H, Sultana R, Taylor KB, et al. A prospective randomized double-blinded pilot study to examine the effect of botulinum toxin type A injection versus lidocaine/depomedrol injection on residual and phantom limb pain: initial report. *Clin J Pain.* 2012;28:108-112, with permission from Lippincott Williams & Wilkins.)

Conclusions.—Both Botox and Lidocaine/Depomedrol injections resulted in immediate improvement of RLP (not PLP) and pain tolerance, which lasted for 6 months in amputees who failed in conventional treatments (Figs 1-3).

▶ This very well done double-blind, randomized pilot study shows benefits for both Botox and lidocaine/depomedrol in decreasing residual limb pain but not phantom limb pain. Importantly, the cohort consisted of 14 patients who have not responded to conventional approaches to these residual symptoms. The significant impact in diminishing residual limb pain and pain tolerance persists for at least 6 months; there was no significant difference between the 2 groups. These findings will hopefully be used to power a definitive trial to determine the impact of these 2 approaches on both residual and phantom limb pain in patients with below-knee amputation. For centers and practitioners not participating in such a trial, either approach seems reasonable for patients with these symptoms who have not responded to prosthetic and standard pharmacologic approaches.

M. F. Swiontkowski, MD

A Randomized Controlled Study to Evaluate the Efficacy of Noninvasive Limb Cover for Chronic Phantom Limb Pain Among Veteran Amputees

Hsiao A-F, York R, Hsiao I, et al (VA Long Beach Healthcare System, CA; et al)

Arch Phys Med Rehabil 93:617-622, 2012

Objective.—To assess the efficacy of a noninvasive limb cover for treating chronic phantom limb pain (PLP).

Design.—Randomized, double-blind, placebo-controlled trial.

Setting.—Outpatient clinic.

Participants.—We randomly assigned 57 subjects to 2 groups: true noninvasive limb cover (n=30) and sham noninvasive limb cover (n=27). Inclusion criteria included age of 18 years or greater, upper or lower extremity amputation with healed residual limb, and 3 or more episodes of PLP during the previous 6 weeks.

Interventions.—Subjects received 2 true or sham noninvasive limb covers to be worn over the prosthesis and residual limbs 24 hours a day for 12 weeks.

Main Outcome Measures.—Primary outcome measure was the numerical pain rating scale of PLP level (0–10). Secondary outcomes included overall pain level (0–10), PLP frequency per week, and the Veterans RAND 12-Item Health Survey (VR-12). We collected data at baseline and at 6- and 12-week follow-up visits.

Results.—Demographic and clinical characteristics were not significantly different between groups. The true noninvasive limb cover group reported nonsignificant reductions in PLP from 5.9 ± 1.9 at baseline to 3.9 ± 1.7 at the 12-week follow-up. The sham noninvasive limb cover group also had nonsignificant reducations in PLP from 6.5 ± 1.8 to 4.2 ± 2.3. PLP did not differ significantly between the 2 groups at 6 weeks (mean difference, 0.8; 95% confidence interval [CI], −1.4 to 3) or at 12 weeks (mean difference, 0.2; 95% CI, −1.9 to 2.3). Similarly, overall pain level, PLP episodes per week, and VR-12 physical and mental health component scores did not differ between the 2 groups at 6 and 12 weeks.

Conclusions.—A true noninvasive limb cover did not significantly decrease PLP levels or the frequency of PLP episodes per week, overall

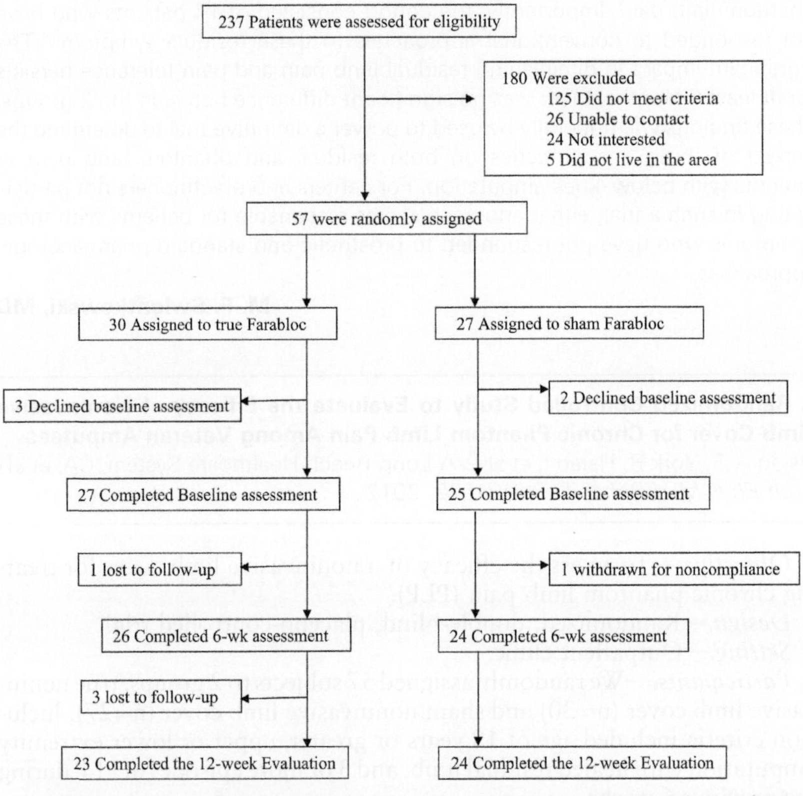

FIGURE 1.—Participant flowchart. (Reprinted from Hsiao A-F, York R, Hsiao I, et al. A randomized controlled study to evaluate the efficacy of noninvasive limb cover for chronic phantom limb pain among veteran amputees. *Arch Phys Med Rehabil.* 2012;93:617-622. Copyright 2012, with permission from the American Congress of Rehabilitation Medicine and the American Academy of Physical Medicine and Rehabilitation.)

bodily pain levels, or VR-12 physical and mental health component scores compared with a sham noninvasive limb cover in our veteran amputee sample (Figs 1 and 2, Tables 1 and 2).

► Phantom pain, particularly for dysvascular amputations, can be particularly difficult to manage effectively. This therapeutic cover had shown promise in prior studies of shorter duration and limited sample size. This well-done, placebo-controlled trial demonstrated no efficacy for this intervention. The search for effective interventions for this clinical issue continues. This trial design should serve as the model for evaluating other interventions for phantom limb pain.

M. F. Swiontkowski, MD

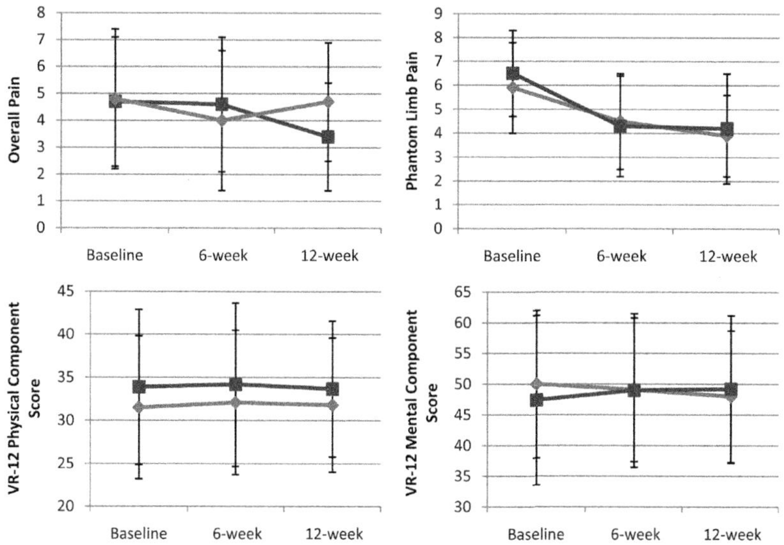

FIGURE 2.—Mean changes in 4 outcomes at 6 and 12 weeks, according to treatment groups. Outcome scores are shown for the true Farabloc group (blue diamonds) and sham Farabloc group (red squares). The values shown are unadjusted means; I bars indicate 95% CIs. Measurements were obtained at baseline, 6 weeks, and 12 weeks. Overall pain and PLP assessments were made on a visual analog scale from 0 (no pain) to 10 (excruciating pain). Summary scores on the physical and mental components of the VR-12 are scored on a T-score metric (mean ± SD: 50 ± 10), with higher scores indicating better health status. For interpretation of the references to color in this figure legend, the reader is referred to web version of this article. (Reprinted from Hsiao A-F, York R, Hsiao I, et al. A randomized controlled study to evaluate the efficacy of noninvasive limb cover for chronic phantom limb pain among veteran amputees. *Arch Phys Med Rehabil.* 2012;93:617-622. Copyright 2012, with permission from the American Congress of Rehabilitation Medicine and the American Academy of Physical Medicine and Rehabilitation.)

TABLE 1.—Study Population Demographic and Clinical Characteristics

Characteristic	True Farabloc (n=30)	Sham Farabloc (n=27)
Age (y)	61.8±12.3	65.8±13.4
Sex		
Men	97	100
Women	3	0
Cause of amputation		
Diabetes/PVD/infection/osteomyelitis	73	70
Trauma	17	26
Other	10	4
Type of amputation		
Below knee	53	59
Above knee	47	41
Time since amputation (y)	10.5±15.3	15.6±19.5
Baseline PLP level	4.7±2.4	4.7±2.6
Baseline overall pain levels	5.9±1.9	4.5±2.2

NOTE. Values are mean ± SD or percentages.
Abbreviation: PVD, peripheral vascular disease.

TABLE 2.—Comparison of True Farabloc and Sham Farabloc Groups on Pain and Health-Related Quality of Life

Variable	True Farabloc (n=30) Baseline	True Farabloc (n=30) 6wk	True Farabloc (n=30) 12wk	Sham Farabloc (n=27) Baseline	Sham Farabloc (n=27) 6wk	Sham Farabloc (n=27) 12wk
PLP level	5.9±1.9	4.5±2.0	3.9±1.7	6.5±1.8	4.3±2.1	4.2±2.3
Overall pain level	4.7±2.4	4.6±2.5	3.4±2.0	4.8±2.6	4.0±2.6	4.7±2.2
PLP frequency/wk	10.7±15.4	6.1±12.4	4.3±9.8	20.0±27.0	11.5±23.0	11.9±23.4
PLP frequency/mo	48.7±68.9	24.1±49.5	17.5±39.3	62.3±84.2	21.2±37.4	21.1±39.2
VR-12 physical component score	31.5±8.3	32.1±8.4	31.8±7.8	33.9±9.0	34.2±9.5	33.7±7.9
VR-12 mental health component score	50.0±12.0	49.1±11.7	48.0±10.7	47.4±13.8	49.0±12.5	49.2±12.0

NOTE. Values are mean ± SD.

4 Forearm, Wrist, and Hand

Evaluation and Diagnosis

Opioid Consumption Following Outpatient Upper Extremity Surgery

Rodgers J, Cunningham K, Fitzgerald K, et al (Des Moines Orthopaedic Surgeons and Des Moines Univ, IA)

J Hand Surg 37A:645-650, 2012

Purpose.—After elective outpatient upper extremity surgery, patients' need for opioid analgesic medication may be considerably less than typically dispensed. Our goal for this study was to evaluate pain control and quantify the amount of leftover pain medication.

Methods.—We recruited patients scheduled for elective outpatient upper extremity surgery, who met the inclusion criteria, to participate in a phone interview 7 to 14 days after surgery. Information collected included age, gender, procedure performed, analgesic medication and regimen prescribed, satisfaction with pain control, number of tablets remaining, reasons for not taking medication, other analgesic medications used, payer classification, and any adverse drug reactions.

Results.—A total of 287 eligible subjects consented to participate. Of these, 36 patients failed phone contact and 1 patient canceled surgery, which left 250 patients who completed the study. Oxycodone, hydrocodone, and propoxyphene accounted for over 95% of the prescription medications, with adequate pain control reported by 230 (92%) patients. Patients most frequently received 30 pills. Patients undergoing bone procedures reported the highest medication use (14 pills), whereas patients undergoing soft tissue procedures reported the lowest use (9 pills). Over half of the subjects reported taking the opioid medication for 2 days or less. Medicare patients consumed significantly less medication (7 pills, $P < .05$) than patients covered by all other types of insurance. Overall, patients consumed a mean of 10 opioid pills, whereas 19 pills per subject were reported unused, which resulted in 4,639 leftover tablets for the entire cohort.

Conclusions.—Our data show that excess opioid analgesics are made available after elective upper extremity surgery and could potentially become a source for diversion. A prescription of 30 opioid pills for outpatient surgery

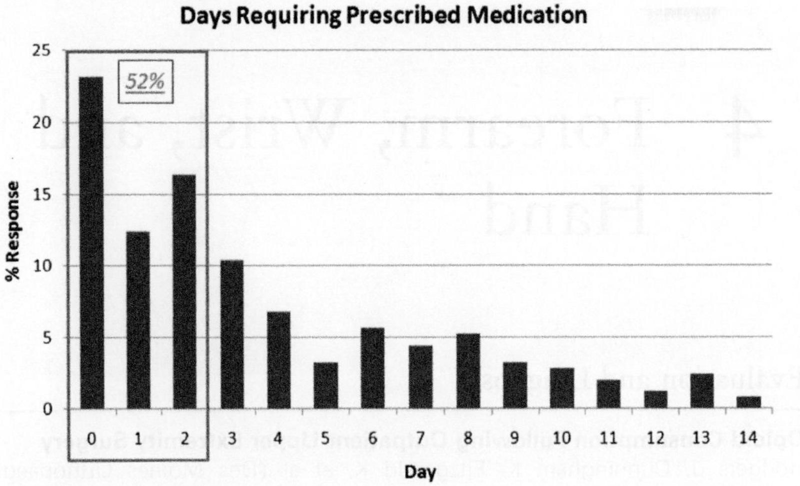

FIGURE 2.—Patient-reported number of days prescribed opioid pain medication was taken. (Reprinted from Rodgers J, Cunningham K, Fitzgerald K, et al. Opioid consumption following outpatient upper extremity surgery. *J Hand Surg*. 2012;37A:645-650, Copyright 2012, with permission from the American Society for Surgery of the Hand.)

TABLE 1.—Summary Description of Study Group

Age (mean ± SD [range])	54 ± 12.8 (19–88)
Gender	167 (66.8%) female, 83 (33.2%) male
Surgery type	
Hard tissue	58 (23.3%)
Hand and wrist (ORIF, arthroplasty)	46
Elbow (ORIF, tennis elbow release, reinsert bicep tendon)	9
Shoulder rotator cuff repair	3
Soft issue	191 (76.7%)
Hand and wrist (carpal tunnel release, ganglion excision, trigger finger release, tendon or nerve repair, excision mass)	156
Elbow (cubital tunnel release, ulnar nerve transposition, elbow arthroscopy)	29
Shoulder (shoulder manipulation, shoulder arthroscopy, not rotator cuff repair)	6
Payer type	
Workers' compensation	41 (16%)
Private	155 (62%)
Medicaid	5 (2%)
Medicare	49 (20%)

ORIF, open reduction internal fixation.

appears excessive and unnecessary, especially for soft tissue procedures of the hand and wrist.

Type of Study/Level of Evidence.—Prognostic I (Fig 2, Table 1).

▶ It is not far-fetched to imagine that we as orthopedic surgeons are being squeezed in a vice with respect to prescribing of postoperative opioid narcotics.

On one side of the vice we have a group of government agencies that mandate we adhere to an arduous documentation of patient-reported pain assessments and alleviate pain accordingly. On the other side we are faced with the recognition that opioid dependence and misuse is an exploding socioeconomic problem and that many abused narcotics are obtained from legitimate prescriptions that are unused by patients and are stolen. In addition, we know from experience that postoperative pain after bone and joint surgery hurts quite a bit in the early postoperative period compared with other procedures. The findings of this study are elucidating and important and should cause readers to reflect on their current opioid prescribing practices.

S. D. Trigg, MD

Subluxation of the Distal Radioulnar Joint as a Predictor of Foveal Triangular Fibrocartilage Complex Tears

Ehman EC, Hayes ML, Berger RA, et al (Mayo Clinic, Rochester, MN)
J Hand Surg 36A:1780-1784, 2011

Purpose.—The triangular fibrocartilage complex (TFCC) with its ulnar foveal attachment is the primary stabilizer of the distal radioulnar joint (DRUJ). The purpose of this study was to describe a technique for measuring the degree of subluxation of the DRUJ in wrist magnetic resonance imaging (MRI) examinations to predict tears involving the foveal attachment of the TFCC.

Methods.—We measured DRUJ geometry in wrist MRI examinations of 34 patients who were found to have foveal TFCC tears at surgery. We compared the results with DRUJ geometry in 11 asymptomatic controls. Subluxation of the ulnar head was assessed using transaxial MRI images obtained at the level of the DRUJ with the wrist in pronation. We quantified subluxation with a line spanning the sigmoid notch of the radius and a perpendicular line through the center of curvature of the articulating surface of the ulna. We calculated the ratio of the lengths of the dorsal and volar segments and normalized it to the center of the sigmoid notch.

Results.—A total of 34 patients with intraoperatively confirmed tears of the foveal attachment of the TFCC had a mean dorsal ulnar subluxation measurement of 16% ± 4%, whereas the 11 controls had a mean subluxation measurement of 5% ± 4%.

Conclusions.—The results confirm the hypothesis that subluxation of the ulnar head relative to the sigmoid notch of the radius, as assessed by MRI with the wrist in pronation, is a predictor of tears of the foveal attachment of the TFCC.

Type of Study/Level of Evidence.—Diagnostic II (Fig 1).

▶ The physical examination of a patient with a suspected triangular fibrocartilage complex (TFCC) tear can be challenging, particularly in the acute setting in which the examiner's attempts to establish distal radioulnar joint (DRUJ) instability can be painful and thus limit a complete examination. Moreover,

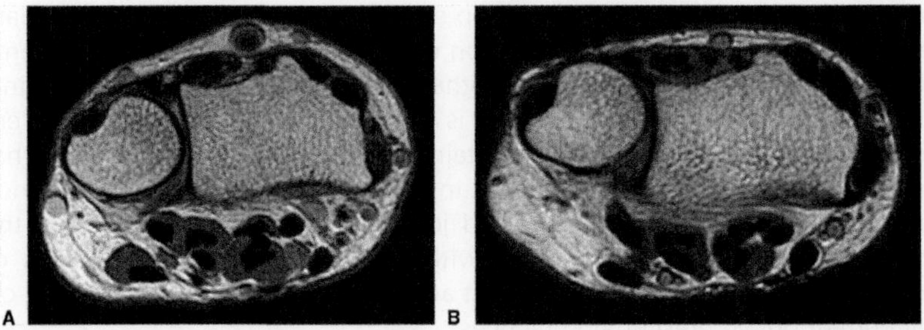

FIGURE 1.—A Axial T1-weighted fast spin echo MR image (TR/TE of 500/12 at 1.5 T) of the left wrist from a subject with no known wrist pathology. B Axial MR image of the left wrist from a patient with a tear of the foveal attachment of the TFCC using the same imaging parameters. We selected the image with the greatest cross-sectional profile of the radius and the ulna from axial datasets and measured it to assess DRUJ geometry. (Reprinted from Ehman EC, Hayes ML, Berger RA, et al. Subluxation of the distal radioulnar joint as a predictor of foveal triangular fibrocartilage complex tears. *J Hand Surg*. 2011;36A:1780-1784, Copyright 2011, with permission from the American Society for Surgery of the Hand.)

confidence in distinguishing a stable from an unstable DRUJ in patients with increased ligamentous laxity can be especially difficult. MRI of the wrist is generally accepted as an important diagnostic imaging tool to image the soft tissues about the wrist, including disruptions of the foveal attachment of the TFCC. This study is important because it furthers our understanding of the anatomic geometry of the unstable DRUJ in patients with arthroscopically proven foveal disruptions of the dorsal and palmar radioulnar ligaments. Their method establishes important technical guidelines for how we should order an MRI study, showing the importance of the axial views with forearm pronation in patients suspected of having DRUJ instability.

S. D. Trigg, MD

Forearm and Wrist

The Effects of Screw Length on Stability of Simulated Osteoporotic Distal Radius Fractures Fixed With Volar Locking Plates

Wall LB, Brodt MD, Silva MJ, et al (Washington Univ School of Medicine, St Louis, MO)
J Hand Surg 37A:446-453, 2012

Purpose.—Volar plating for distal radius fractures has caused extensor tendon ruptures resulting from dorsal screw prominence. This study was designed to determine the biomechanical impact of placing unicortical distal locking screws and pegs in an extra-articular fracture model.

Methods.—We applied volar-locking distal radius plates to 30 osteoporotic distal radius models. We divided radiuses into 5 groups based on distal locking fixation: bicortical locked screws, 3 lengths of unicortical locked screws (abutting the dorsal cortex [full length], 75% length, and 50% length to dorsal cortex), and unicortical locked pegs. Distal radius osteotomy simulated a dorsally comminuted, extra-articular fracture. We determined each construct's stiffness under physiologic loads (axial compression, dorsal bending, and volar bending) before and after 1,000 cycles of axial conditioning and before axial loading to failure (2 mm of displacement) and subsequent catastrophic failure.

Results.—Cyclic conditioning did not alter the constructs' stiffness. Stiffness to volar bending and dorsal bending forces were similar between groups. Final stiffness under axial load was statistically equivalent for all groups: bicortical screws (230 N/mm), full-length unicortical screws (227 N/mm), 75% length unicortical screws (226 N/mm), 50% length unicortical screws (187 N/mm), and unicortical pegs (226 N/mm). Force at 2-mm displacement was significantly less for 50% length unicortical screws (311 N) compared with bicortical screws (460 N), full-length unicortical screws (464 N), 75% length unicortical screws (400 N), and unicortical pegs (356 N). Force to catastrophic fracture was statistically equivalent between groups, but mean values for pegs (749 N) and 50% length unicortical (702 N) screws were 16% to 21% less than means for bicortical (892 N), full-length unicortical (860 N), and 75% length (894 N) unicortical constructs.

Conclusions.—Locked unicortical distal screws of at least 75% length produce construct stiffness similar to bicortical fixation. Unicortical distal fixation for extra-articular distal radius fractures should be entertained to avoid extensor tendon injury because this technique does not appear to compromise initial fixation.

Clinical Relevance.—Using unicortical fixation during volar distal radius plating may protect extensor tendons without compromising fixation.

▶ The acceleration in the use of volar locking plates for the treatment of unstable adult distal radius fractures remains unabated. Volar locking plates have largely relegated dorsal plating to "specialty" plate status, with the latter used in more unusual or complex fractures and malunions. The reasoning behind the increased popularity of volar locking plates over dorsal locking plates includes evidence of increased stiffness and strength and superior functional outcomes, along with the recognition of potential hardware-related complications associated with some dorsal plate designs. However, the hazards of intra-articular and dorsal screw penetration with volar locking plates are a consideration if meticulous intraoperative fluoroscopic inspection of screw length and positioning are not adhered to. This in vitro study is important because it furthers our knowledge of the strength of volar plating using unicortical locking screws, which should reduce the potential for dorsal cortex screw protrusion—related tendon injury while maintaining sufficient stiffness and strength to allow an appropriate early range-of-motion program.

S. D. Trigg, MD

A Prospective Randomized Controlled Trial Comparing Occupational Therapy with Independent Exercises After Volar Plate Fixation of a Fracture of the Distal Part of the Radius

Souer JS, Buijze G, Ring D (Massachusetts General Hosp, Boston)

J Bone Joint Surg Am 93:1761-1766, 2011

Background.—The effect of formal occupational therapy on recovery after open reduction and volar plate fixation of a fracture of the distal part of the radius is uncertain. We hypothesized that there would be no difference in wrist function and arm-specific disability six months after open reduction and volar plate fixation of a distal radial fracture between patients who receive formal occupational therapy and those with instructions for independent exercises.

Methods.—Ninety-four patients with an unstable distal radial fracture treated with open reduction and volar locking plate fixation were enrolled in a prospective randomized controlled trial comparing exercises done under the supervision of an occupational therapist with surgeon-directed independent exercises. The primary study question addressed combined wrist flexion and extension six months after surgery. Secondary study questions addressed wrist motion, grip strength, Gartland and Werley scores, Mayo wrist scores, and DASH (Disabilities of the Arm, Shoulder and Hand) scores at three months and six months after surgery.

Results.—There was a significant difference in the mean arc of wrist flexion and extension six months after surgery (118° versus 129°), favoring patients prescribed independent exercises. Three months after surgery, there was a significant difference in mean pinch strength (80% versus 90%), mean grip strength (66% versus 81%), and mean Gartland and Werley scores, favoring patients prescribed independent exercises. At six months, there was a significant difference in mean wrist extension (55° versus 62°), ulnar deviation (82% versus 93%), mean supination (84° versus 90°), mean grip strength (81% versus 92%), and mean Mayo score, favoring patients prescribed independent exercises. There were no differences in arm-specific disability (DASH score) at any time point.

Conclusions.—Prescription of formal occupational therapy does not improve the average motion or disability score after volar locking plate fixation of a fracture of the distal part of the radius.

▶ This is an important study on several fronts. First, and most obvious, is that the authors' conclusions that formal postsurgical supervised hand therapy does not improve either disability scores or functional range of motion and grip strength compared with a physician-instructed exercise program following open reduction and volar plating of distal radius fractures has far-reaching economic considerations. Supervised hand therapy can add significantly to the total cost of treatment of this commonly performed procedure even when the time-value costs that patients incur when attending a scheduled supervised hand therapy program are not factored in. The second reason for recommending this article is that it is clear from a careful reading of how the treating physicians implement their instructions for the patient independent exercise program, which addresses a healthy dose of patient education of the psychologic and physiologic experience of pain as part of their rehab program, is no small matter in the reported outcomes. The exercises are straightforward; the key here is in the message of patient education in instructing how one should transition from a nociceptive protective response of pain with exercise to experience the pain associated with a therapeutic "healthy stretch."

S. D. Trigg, MD

The Role of Bone Allografts in the Treatment of Angular Malunions of the Distal Radius

Ozer K, Kiliç A, Sabel A, et al (Univ of Colorado, Denver; Colorado School of Public Health, Denver)
J Hand Surg 36A:1804-1809, 2011

Purpose.—Two cohorts of patients who had corrective osteotomies and volar platings for malunited fractures of the distal radius were compared retrospectively to determine whether the time to union and the outcome were affected by bone allograft.

Methods.—Patients in the first group (n = 14) did not receive any bone graft; patients in the second group (n = 14) had allograft bone chips following volar plating. Indications for surgery, surgical technique, and postoperative rehabilitation were the same in both groups. Volar cortical contact was maintained using a volar locking plate in all patients. Radiographic parameters of deformity correction, time to union, wrist and forearm range of motion, grip strength, patient-rated wrist evaluation and Disabilities of the Arm, Shoulder, and Hand questionnaire were used to evaluate the outcome before and after the surgery. Average follow-up time was 36 weeks. Patients who had diabetes, who smoked, who had a body mass index of more than 35, and who required lengthening for deformity correction were excluded from the study.

Results.—Osteotomies in both groups healed without loss of surgical correction. Final outcome and time to union revealed no significant differences, clinically or statistically, between the 2 groups. The Disabilities of the Arm, Shoulder, and Hand score was improved in both groups.

Conclusions.—When volar cortical contact was maintained using a volar locked plate, bone allograft at the osteotomy site did not improve the final outcome.

Type of Study/Level of Evidence.—Therapeutic III.

► In the early days of our experience with open reduction and internal fixation of unstable displaced distal radius fractures with dorsal and volar locked plating, many investigators recommended autologous bone grafting, which for a time was considered the standard of care. With improved strength and rigidity of later plate designs coupled with experience of comparative time to union, allografting supplanted autologous bone grafting. Currently, allografting is not considered necessary when using volar locked plating for the majority of fractures because nonunions are rare when proper techniques are followed. Following a similar historical line has been the experience of the need for autologous structural bone grafting with less rigid plate fixation for opening wedge corrective osteotomy for distal radius fracture malunions; with advances in implant design, nonstructural allografts produced similar outcomes compared with autologous grafting. The authors of this study present their early experience of the outcomes of volar plating of simple opening wedge corrective osteotomies with and without nonstructural allograft. Because cost analysis will no doubt continue to be a major driver in evidence-based medicine going forward, the authors' experience and techniques are worthy of your review.

S. D. Trigg, MD

A Prospective Randomized Trial Comparing Nonoperative Treatment with Volar Locking Plate Fixation for Displaced and Unstable Distal Radial Fractures in Patients Sixty-Five Years of Age and Older

Arora R, Lutz M, Deml C, et al (Med Univ Innsbruck (MUI), Anichstrasse, Austria)

J Bone Joint Surg Am 93:2146-2153, 2011

Background.—Despite the recent trend toward the internal fixation of distal radial fractures in older patients, the currently available literature lacks adequate randomized trials examining whether open reduction and internal fixation (ORIF) with a volar locking plate is superior to nonoperative (cast) treatment. The purpose of the present randomized clinical trial was to compare the outcomes of two methods that were used for the treatment of displaced and unstable distal radial fractures in patients sixty-five years of age or older: (1) ORIF with use of a volar locking plate and (2) closed reduction and plaster immobilization (casting).

Methods.—A prospective randomized study was performed. Seventy-three patients with a displaced and unstable distal radial fracture were randomized to ORIF with a volar locking plate ($n = 36$) or closed reduction and cast immobilization ($n = 37$). The outcome was measured on the basis of the Patient-Rated Wrist Evaluation (PRWE) score; the Disabilities of the Arm, Shoulder and Hand (DASH) score; the pain level; the range of wrist motion; the rate of complications; and radiographic measurements including dorsal radial tilt, radial inclination, and ulnar variance.

Results.—There were no significant differences between the groups in terms of the range of motion or the level of pain during the entire follow-up period ($p > 0.05$). Patients in the operative treatment group had lower DASH and PRWE scores, indicating better wrist function, in the early postoperative time period ($p < 0.05$), but there were no significant differences between the groups at six and twelve months. Grip strength was significantly better at all times in the operative treatment group ($p < 0.05$). Dorsal radial tilt, radial inclination, and radial shortening were significantly better in the operative treatment group than in the nonoperative treatment group at the time of the latest follow-up ($p < 0.05$). The number of complications was significantly higher in the operative treatment group (thirteen compared with five, $p < 0.05$).

Conclusions.—At the twelve-month follow-up examination, the range of motion, the level of pain, and the PRWE and DASH scores were not different between the operative and nonoperative treatment groups. Patients in the operative treatment group had better grip strength through the entire time period. Achieving anatomical reconstruction did not convey any improvement in terms of the range of motion or the ability to perform daily living activities in our cohorts.

▶ The correlation between anatomic restoration of articular congruity and alignment of distal radius fractures and improved functional outcomes in younger and higher-demand patients is well known. The optimum treatment for older and lower-demand patients with similar fractures is less clear. The use of volar locking plates for the treatment of unstable and complex distal radius fractures is ever increasing and has been advocated for use in older patients as well. This study breaks new ground, as it is one of the only prospective, randomized, clinical trials to directly compare the outcomes of operative treatment using volar locking plates with nonoperative cast immobilization in older patients at 1-year follow-up. Their results are surprising in many respects and warrant your review.

S. D. Trigg, MD

Hand

Five- to 18-Year Follow-Up for Treatment of Trapeziometacarpal Osteoarthritis: A Prospective Comparison of Excision, Tendon Interposition, and Ligament Reconstruction and Tendon Interposition

Gangopadhyay S, McKenna H, Burke FD, et al (Nottingham Univ Hosps, UK; Royal Derby Hosp, UK)
J Hand Surg 37A:411-417, 2012

Purpose.—To investigate whether palmaris longus interposition or flexor carpi radialis ligament reconstruction and tendon interposition improve the outcome of trapezial excision for the treatment of basal joint arthritis after a minimum follow-up of 5 years.

Methods.—We randomized 174 thumbs with trapeziometacarpal osteoarthritis into 3 groups to undergo simple trapeziectomy, trapeziectomy with palmaris longus interposition, or trapeziectomy with ligament reconstruction and tendon interposition using 50% of the flexor carpi radialis tendon. A K-wire was passed across the trapezial void and retained for 4 weeks, and a thumb spica was used for 6 weeks in all 3 groups. We reviewed 153 thumbs after a minimum of 5 years (median, 6 y; range, 5–18 y) after surgery with subjective and objective assessments of thumb pain, function, and strength.

Results.—There was no difference in the pain relief achieved in the 3 treatment groups, with good results in 120 (78%) patients. Grip strength and key and tip pinch strengths did not differ among the 3 groups and range of movement of the thumb was similar. Few complications persisted after 5 years, and these were distributed evenly among the 3 groups. Compared with the results at 1 year in the same group of patients, the good pain relief achieved was maintained in the longer term, irrespective of the type of surgery. While improvements in grip strength achieved at 1 year after surgery were preserved, the key and tip pinch strengths deteriorated with time, but the type of surgery did not influence this.

Conclusions.—The outcomes of these 3 variations of trapeziectomy were similar after a minimum follow-up of 5 years. There appears to be no benefit to tendon interposition or ligament reconstruction in the longer term.

▶ Trapeziometacarpal osteoarthritis is one of the most frequently presenting arthritic conditions for most hand surgical practices. In the United States, trapeziectomy with ligament reconstruction and tendon interposition (LRTI) is the most frequently performed reconstructive surgical procedure performed for recalcitrant pain and dysfunction.[1] Elsewhere, trapeziectomy with or without tendon interposition remains popular. Bias toward one procedure over another may be based on surgeon training as much as anything else. Despite the commonality of the condition and the frequency of procedures performed, no single method has proven optimal. This is one of the longest-term prospective randomized studies to compare outcomes from the 3 most frequently performed reconstructive procedures for trapeziometacarpal osteoarthritis and as such warrants our review. Longitudinal metacarpal subsidence and/or convergence resulting in later bone-to-bone contact is among the major perceived reasons for selecting interposition or LRTI. One major weakness of this study is that no long-term radiographic data are included, which would add important information to the clinical outcome data.

S. D. Trigg, MD

Reference

1. Wolf JM, Delaronde S. Current trends in nonoperative and operative treatment of trapeziometacarpal osteoarthritis: a survey of US hand surgeons. *J Hand Surg Am.* 2012;37:77-82.

Assessing the Impact of Antibiotic Prophylaxis in Outpatient Elective Hand Surgery: A Single-Center, Retrospective Review of 8,850 Cases

Bykowski MR, Sivak WN, Cray J, et al (Dept of Plastic and Reconstructive Surgery, Pittsburgh, PA; Hand and Upper Extremity Ctr, Wexford, PA; Johns Hopkins Univ School of Medicine, Baltimore, MD)

J Hand Surg 36A:1741-1747, 2011

Purpose.—Prophylactic antibiotics have been shown to prevent surgical site infection (SSI) after some gastrointestinal, orthopedic, and plastic surgical procedures, but their efficacy in clean, elective hand surgery is unclear. Our aims were to assess the efficacy of preoperative antibiotics in preventing SSI after clean, elective hand surgery, and to identify potential risk factors for SSI.

Methods.—We queried the database from an outpatient surgical center by Current Procedural Terminology code to identify patients who underwent elective hand surgery. For each medical record, we collected patient demographics and characteristics along with preoperative, intraoperative, and postoperative management details. The primary outcome of this study was SSI, and secondary outcomes were wound dehiscence and suture granuloma.

Results.—From October 2000 through October 2008, 8,850 patient records met our inclusion criteria. The overall SSI rate was 0.35%, with an average patient follow-up duration of 79 days. The SSI rates did not significantly differ between patients receiving antibiotics (0.54%; 2,755 patients) and those who did not (0.26%; 6,095 patients). Surgical site infection was associated with smoking status, diabetes mellitus, and longer procedure length irrespective of antibiotic use. Subgroup analysis revealed that prophylactic antibiotics did not prevent SSI in male patients, smokers, or diabetics, or for procedure length less than 30 minutes, 30 to 60 minutes, and greater than 60 minutes.

Conclusions.—Prophylactic antibiotic administration does not reduce the incidence of SSI after clean, elective hand surgery in an outpatient population. Moreover, subgroup analysis revealed that prophylactic antibiotics did not reduce the frequency of SSI among patients who were found to be at higher risk in this study. We identified 3 factors associated with the development of SSI in our study: diabetes mellitus status, procedure length, and smoking status. Given the potential harmful complications associated with antibiotic use and the lack of evidence that prophylactic antibiotics prevent SSIs, we conclude that antibiotics should not be routinely administered to patients who undergo clean, elective hand surgery.

Type of Study/Level of Evidence.—Therapeutic III.

▶ Chasing zero. We are practicing in an era of ever-increasing scrutiny by governmental and third-party payers targeting improvement of patient safety and quality of health care. Reducing the rate of surgical site infections is currently among the key quality metrics that are studied to assess ratings for hospitals and medical institutions. This is no small matter when reimbursement will likely be increasingly tied to an institution's ratings going forward. Prophylactic antibiotics have been shown to reduce the rate of surgical site infections in some hip procedures, but their role for routine elective outpatient soft tissue hand surgery cases is less clear. This is one of the largest studies to date to assess the efficacy of prophylactic antibiotics in such cases.

S. D. Trigg, MD

A Percutaneous Technique to Treat Unstable Dorsal Fracture–Dislocations of the Proximal Interphalangeal Joint

Vitale MA, White NJ, Strauch RJ (Columbia Univ, NY)
J Hand Surg 36A:1453-1459, 2011

Purpose.—Unstable dorsal fracture–dislocations of the proximal interphalangeal (PIP) joint are complex injuries that are difficult to treat and usually require operative fixation. There are a number of surgical techniques for treating these injuries but none has emerged as superior. The purposes of this study were to describe a simple percutaneous technique to treat unstable dorsal fracture–dislocations of the PIP joint and to report short-term postoperative results.

Methods.—We treated 6 patients with unstable dorsal fracture–dislocations of the PIP joint with the technique of closed reduction, percutaneous fracture reduction, and pinning via a volar approach and also with dorsal block pinning. We collected information on postoperative stability, range of motion at the PIP and distal interphalangeal joints, and radiographic outcomes. We also administered the Disabilities of the Arm, Shoulder, and Hand and visual analog pain scale questionnaires.

Results.—At a mean follow-up of 18 months (range, 6–57 mo), there were no subluxation or dislocation events. The mean range of motion was from 4° of extension to 93° of flexion at the PIP joint and from 1° of extension to 73° of flexion at the distal interphalangeal joint. Radiographic

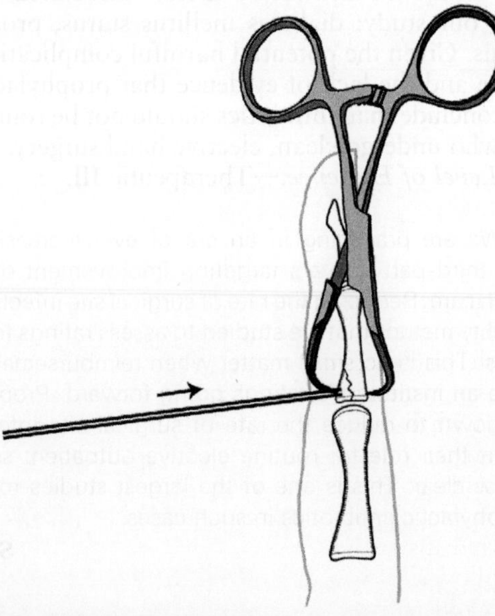

FIGURE 4.—Fixation with 2 K-wires through base of middle phalanx, volar to dorsal. (Reprinted from Vitale MA, White NJ, Strauch RJ. A percutaneous technique to treat unstable dorsal fracture–dislocations of the proximal interphalangeal joint. *J Hand Surg*. 2011;36A:1453-1459, with permission from the American Society for Surgery of the Hand.)

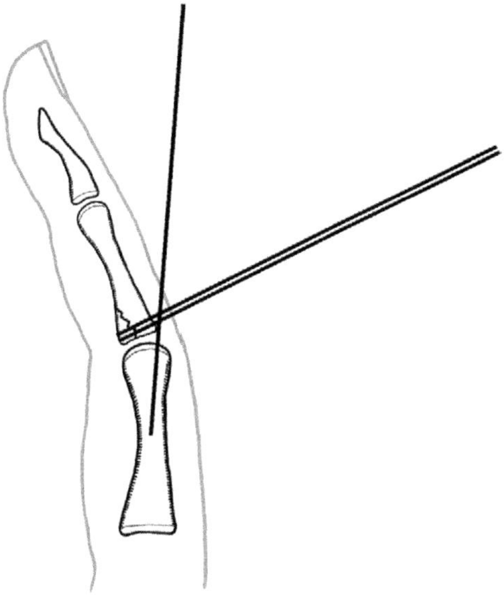

FIGURE 6.—Insertion of dorsal blocking K-wire through the head of the proximal phalanx. (Reprinted from Vitale MA, White NJ, Strauch RJ. A percutaneous technique to treat unstable dorsal fracture—dislocations of the proximal interphalangeal joint. *J Hand Surg.* 2011;36A:1453-1459, Copyright 2011, with permission from the American Society for Surgery of the Hand.)

analysis revealed a concentric reduction and union in all cases. The mean Disabilities of the Arm, Shoulder, and Hand score was 8 and the mean visual analog pain score was 1.4 out of 10. There were no minor or major complications.

Conclusions.—This percutaneous technique reliably restored stability to the PIP joint, allowed for concentric reduction of the joint, and produced excellent radiographic and clinical outcomes. The postoperative management course with this technique is critical to the outcome (Figs 4 and 6).

► Dorsal fracture dislocation injuries of the proximal interphalangeal joints (pilon fractures) are relatively common and unfortunately all too commonly result in posttreatment complications, including joint stiffness, pain, and instability no matter what treatment method is used. Establishing and maintaining a congruent joint reduction is a critical factor. Although numerous operative methods have been reported, no technique has been proven superior, and there are few comparative studies. Moreover, many reports are retrospective small case studies, and this one is no different in this regard. However, this study proposes a novel approach, which, at first glance would seem somewhat crude, as it initially violates the flexor tendons with a towel clip tine and 2 K-wires. That said, their reported outcomes are nothing to sneer at and I think are deserving of your consideration.

S. D. Trigg, MD

Surgical Repair of Multiple Pulley Injuries—Evaluation of a New Combined Pulley Repair

Schöffl V, Küpper T, Hartmann J, et al (Friedrich Alexander Univ Erlangen-Nuremberg; Aachen Technical Univ, Germany; Dept of Pediatrics, Klinikum Bamberg, Germany)

J Hand Surg 37A:224-230, 2012

Purpose.—We report on a combined repair of multiple annular pulley tears using 1 continuous palmaris longus tendon graft to restore strength and function.

Methods.—We treated 6 rock climbers with grade 4 pulley injuries (multiple pulley injuries) using the combined repair technique and re-evaluated them after a mean of 28 months.

Results.—All patients had excellent Buck-Gramcko scores; the functional outcome was good in 4, satisfactory in 1, and fair in 1. The sport-specific outcome was excellent in 5 and satisfactory in 1. Proximal interphalangeal joint flexion deficit slightly increased in 1 patient and remained the same in the other 5. Climbing level after the injury was the same as before in 4 and decreased slightly in 2 climbers.

Conclusions.—The technique is effective with good results and has since become our standard treatment. Nevertheless, it is limited in patients with flexion contracture of the proximal interphalangeal joint.

Type of Study/Level of Evidence.—Therapeutic III (Fig 1).

▶ Flexor tendon annular pulley ruptures have frequently been reported in rock climbers. However, multiple annular pulley ruptures are considered rare even for this sport. In my experience, these injuries also occur in other sports, including water skiing, wake boarding, and kite surfing. Most reports on the repair and reconstruction on ruptured annular pulleys have focused on single pulley or A2/A3 repairs. The authors of this study have proposed a novel method of a combined repair of multiple pulley ruptures using a continuous palmaris longus tendon graft. Their method is based on sound known biomechanical and cadaveric studies.

S. D. Trigg, MD

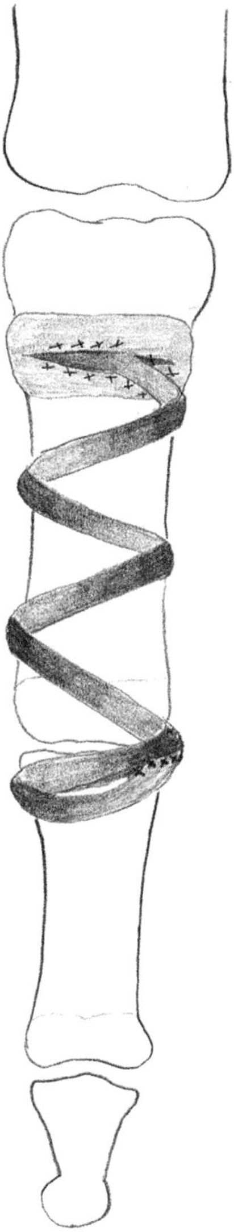

FIGURE 1.—Our continuous repair technique. (Reprinted from Schöffl V, Küpper T, Hartmann J, et al. Surgical repair of multiple pulley injuries—evaluation of a new combined pulley repair. *J Hand Surg*. 2012;37A:224-230, Copyright 2012, with permission from the American Society for Surgery of the Hand.)

An Analysis of the Pull-Out Strength of 6 Suture Loop Configurations in Flexor Tendons

Karjalainen T, He M, Chong AKS, et al (Oulu Univ Hosp, Finland; Natl Univ Hosp of Republic of Singapore)
J Hand Surg 37A:217-223, 2012

Purpose.—New, stronger suture materials have been introduced for flexor tendon surgery. The advantage of these materials can be lost if the suture loop pulls out from the tendon. The aim of this study was to compare the ability of various locking loops to grip the tendon.

Methods.—We inserted 4 different standard and 2 experimental locking loops with 200-μm nitinol wire into human cadaveric flexor digitorum profundus tendons. The standard loops were: group 1, cruciate; group 2, Pennington modified Kessler; group 3, cross-stitch; and group 4, Lim-Tsai. The experimental loops were: group 5, a composition of Pennington modified Kessler with a cross-stitch loop; and group 6, a locking Kessler type of loop with a superficial transverse component. We loaded the loops until failure. We recorded the pull-out strength and stiffness and documented failure mechanisms during the pull-out test.

Results.—The cruciate loop had the weakest holding capacity, 20 N, which was significantly less than in groups 2 to 6. The cross-stitch loop, Lim-Tsai loop, and modified Kessler loop performed similarly (36 N, 37 N, and 39 N, respectively). The experimental loops had the highest pull-out strength (group 5, 59 N; and group 6, 60 N, both significantly greater than groups 1 to 4). The mode of failure was pull-out for all of the standard loops and 7 of the experimental loops. Of 20 experimental loops, 13 failed by suture rupture.

Conclusions.—The 2 experimental loop configurations demonstrated higher pull-out strength and may have advantages when used with newer and stronger suture materials. The number of the locking components in the loops and the way the tension is transmitted to the tendon fibrils explain the results.

Clinical Relevance.—The loops presented in this study and that grip the tendon better may be useful with new materials that have high tensile strength.

▶ Research activity in flexor tendon repair has increased significantly in the last decade. We have established the benefits of early motion on tendon healing and resultant clinical outcomes. Early motion/gliding requires a strong, low-profile repair, and numerous multistrand locking and grasping suture repair techniques using conventional materials have been proposed and comparatively studied. Despite the current trend for the use of multistrand suture repairs, material failure remains a concern. The newer so-called "super braid" and stronger high-tensile-strength monofilament suture materials are sufficiently strong that repair failure by suture pull-out (through) and not material rupture has become a reality.

This then requires a new look at loop configuration and suturing patterns using these materials, and this study is one of the best to date.

S. D. Trigg, MD

Nerve

A Method to Localize The Radial Nerve Using the 'Apex Of Triceps Aponeurosis' as a Landmark

Arora S, Goel N, Cheema GS, et al (The Maulana Azad Med College & Associated Lok Nayak Hosp, New Delhi, India; Sushruta Trauma Centre, Delhi, India; et al)

Clin Orthop Relat Res 469:2638-2644, 2011

Background.—The relationship of the radial nerve is described with various osseous landmarks, but such relationships may be disturbed in the setting of humerus shaft fractures. Alternative landmarks would be helpful to more consistently and reliably allow the surgeon to locate the radial nerve during the posterior approach to the arm.

Questions/Purposes.—We investigated the relationship of the radial nerve with the apex of triceps aponeurosis, and describe a technique to locate the nerve.

Materials and Methods.—We performed dissections of 10 cadavers and gathered surgical details of 60 patients (30 patients and 30 control patients) during the posterior approach of the humerus. We measured the distance of the radial nerve from the apex of the triceps aponeurosis along the long axis of the humerus in cadaveric dissections and patients. This distance was correlated with the height and arm length. For all patients, we recorded time until first observation of the radial nerve, blood loss, and postoperative radial nerve function.

Results.—The mean distance of the radial nerve from the apex of the triceps aponeurosis was 2.5 cm, which correlated with the patients' height and arm length. The mean time until the first observation of the radial nerve from beginning the skin incision was 6 minutes, as compared with 16 minutes in the control group. Mean blood loss was 188 mL and 237 mL, respectively. With the numbers available, we observed no difference in the incidence of patients with postoperative nerve palsy: none in the study group and three in the control group.

Conclusion.—The apex of the triceps aponeurosis appears to be a useful anatomic landmark for localization of the radial nerve during the posterior approach to the humerus (Fig 2, Table 1).

▶ One of the more satisfying outcomes from the practice of orthopedic surgery is that we remain students of anatomy throughout our careers. We are all aware of both the perilous potential for iatrogenic injury to the radial nerve during operative treatment of the humerus as well as the frequent necessity to explore the radial nerve associated with fracture treatment. The posterior approach to the humerus is a workhorse approach for exposure of the middle and distal thirds of the humerus. Classically, the location and course of the radial nerve have

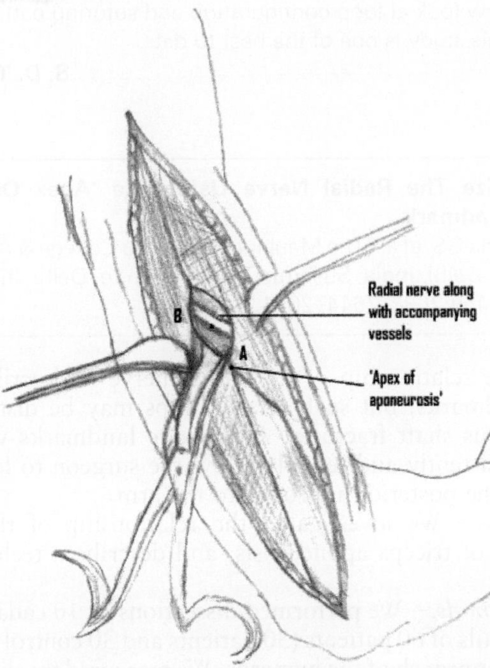

FIGURE 2.—A diagram shows how, during the posterior approach to the humerus, the radial nerve and accompanying vessels can be seen in the tunnel made approximately 2.5 cm proximal to the apex of the triceps aponeurosis. Point "A" denotes the apex of the aponeurosis, whereas point "B" denotes the most distal extent of the radial nerve along the long axis of the humerus in the plane between the long and lateral heads of the triceps. (Reprinted from Arora S, Goel N, Cheema GS, et al. A method to localize the radial nerve using the 'apex of triceps aponeurosis' as a landmark. *Clin Orthop Relat Res.* 2011;469:2638-2644, with kind permission from Springer Science+Business Media.)

TABLE 1.—Mean Distance of Radial Nerve From the Apex of Triceps Aponeurosis

Number of Patients (N = 30)	Body Height (cm)	Arm Length (cm)	Mean Distance of the Radial Nerve From the Apex of the Triceps Aponeurosis (cm)
3	≤150	<26	2.27
9	151–165	26–32.5	2.48
15	166–180	32.6–36	2.57
3	>180	>36	2.73
			p <0.001

been referenced from distances from osseous landmarks, including the humeral epicondyles and acromion. The anatomic relationship of the radial nerve in the spiral groove to these osseous landmarks is variable according to the stature of the patient and, of course, is changed with fracture displacement. This article provides us with important information on another method to reliably locate the radial nerve when utilizing the posterior approach to the humerus.

S. D. Trigg, MD

Comparisons of Outcomes from Repair of Median Nerve and Ulnar Nerve Defect with Nerve Graft and Tubulization: A Meta-Analysis

Yang M, Rawson JL, Zhang EW, et al (Univ of Mississippi Med Ctr, Jackson; et al)

J Reconstr Microsurg 27:451-460, 2011

In this study, an updated meta-analysis of all published human studies was presented to evaluate the recovery of the median and the ulnar nerves in the forearm after defect repair by nerve conduit and autologous nerve graft. Up to June of 2010, search for English language articles was conducted to collect publications on the outcome of median or ulnar nerve defect repair. A total of 33 studies and 1531 cases were included in this study. Patient information was extracted from these publications and the postoperative outcome was analyzed using meta-analysis. There was no significant difference in the postoperative recovery between the median and the ulnar nerves (odds ratio = 0.98). Sensory nerves were found to achieve a more satisfactory recovery after nerve defect repair than motor nerves ($p < 0.05$). Median nerve can also achieve more satisfactory recovery in both sensory and motor function than ulnar nerve ($p < 0.05$). There was no statistical difference between tubulization and autologous nerve graft in repairing defects less than 5 cm. Based on the results of this study, a median nerve with sensory impairment was associated with improved postoperative prognosis, while an ulnar nerve with motor nerve damage was prone to a worse prognosis. Tubulization can be a good alternative in the reconstruction of small defects.

▶ Among reports on repair and reconstruction of peripheral nerve injuries of the upper extremity, injuries to the median and ulnar nerves are second in reported frequency to digital nerve injuries. Research continues to investigate alternatives to conventional autologous nerve grafts, which includes the use and outcomes of nerve conduits. The authors of this meta-analysis study correctly point out that there is a paucity of data that compare the outcomes of nerve conduits with autologous nerve grafting for injuries to the median and ulnar nerve in the forearm. Only with future prospective controlled comparative research studies on nerve conduits compared directly with autologous nerve grafting will the limitations of heterogenicity inherent in a meta-analysis be better controlled. That said, this study was well done, and the authors' derived conclusions add to our knowledge base on the treatment of these devastating injuries.

S. D. Trigg, MD

Processed nerve allografts for peripheral nerve reconstruction: a multicenter study of utilization and outcomes in sensory, mixed, and motor nerve reconstructions

Brooks DN, Weber RV, Chao JD, et al (The Buncke Clinic, San Francisco, CA; Albert Einstein College of Medicine, Bronx, NY; Albany Med College, NY; et al)

Microsurgery 32:1-14, 2012

Purpose.—As alternatives to autograft become more conventional, clinical outcomes data on their effectiveness in restoring meaningful function is essential. In this study we report on the outcomes from a multicenter study on processed nerve allografts (Avance® Nerve Graft, AxoGen, Inc).

Patients and Methods.—Twelve sites with 25 surgeons contributed data from 132 individual nerve injuries. Data was analyzed to determine the safety and efficacy of the nerve allograft. Sufficient data for efficacy analysis were reported in 76 injuries (49 sensory, 18 mixed, and 9 motor nerves). The mean age was 41 ± 17 (18–86) years. The mean graft length was 22 ± 11 (5–50) mm. Subgroup analysis was performed to determine the relationship to factors known to influence outcomes of nerve repair such as nerve type, gap length, patient age, time to repair, age of injury, and mechanism of injury.

Results.—Meaningful recovery was reported in 87% of the repairs reporting quantitative data. Subgroup analysis demonstrated consistency, showing no significant differences with regard to recovery outcomes between the groups ($P > 0.05$ Fisher's Exact Test). No graft related adverse experiences were reported and a 5% revision rate was observed.

Conclusion.—Processed nerve allografts performed well and were found to be safe and effective in sensory, mixed and motor nerve defects between 5 and 50 mm. The outcomes for safety and meaningful recovery observed in this study compare favorably to those reported in the literature for nerve autograft and are higher than those reported for nerve conduits.

▶ Over the past several years, research has intensified to find alternatives to autologous nerve grafts for peripheral nerve injuries. This research has largely proceeded down 2 investigative lines: processed nerve allografts and nerve conduits. This is the largest study to date reporting on the use and outcomes of processed nerve allografts. This study suffers from many of the same limitations inherent to most retrospective multicenter observational studies, but the authors' data are worthy of your review because they add to our foundational knowledge and expectation of outcomes from the use of nerve allografts.

S. D. Trigg, MD

Reconstruction of Digital Nerves With Collagen Conduits

Taras JS, Jacoby SM, Lincoski CJ (Thomas Jefferson Univ, Philadelphia, PA; Drexel Univ College of Medicine, Philadelphia, PA; Univ Orthopedics Ctr, State College, PA)

J Hand Surg 36A:1441-1446, 2011

Purpose.—Digital nerve reconstruction with a biodegradable conduit offers the advantage of providing nerve reconstruction while providing a desirable environment for nerve regeneration. Many conduit materials have been investigated, but there have been few reports of human clinical trials of purified type I bovine collagen conduits.

Methods.—We report a prospective study of 22 isolated digital nerve lacerations in 19 patients reconstructed with a bioabsorbable collagen conduit. The average nerve gap measured 12 mm. An independent observer performed the postoperative evaluation, noting the return of protective sensation, static 2-point discrimination, and moving 2-point discrimination, and recording the patient's pain level using a visual analog scale. Minimal follow-up was 12 months and mean follow-up was 20 months after surgery.

Results.—All patients recovered protective sensation. The mean moving 2-point discrimination and static 2-point discrimination measured 5.0 and 5.2 mm, respectively, for those with measurable recovery at final follow-up visit. Excellent results were achieved in 13 of 22 digits, good results in 3 of 22 digits, and fair results in 6 of 22 digits, and there were no poor results. Reported pain scores at the last postoperative visit were measured universally as 0 on the visual analog scale.

Conclusions.—Our data suggest that collagen conduits offer an effective method of reconstruction for digital nerve lacerations. This study confirms that collagen conduits reliably provide a repair that restores nerve function for nerve gaps measuring less than 2 cm.

▶ The use of nerve conduits as an alternative to autologous nerve grafts is an evolving science. To date, synthetic bioabsorbable polyglycolic (PGA) tubes have been the most frequently studied nerve conduit material. More recently, type I collagen conduits have compared favorably to PGA tubes in animal studies. Pliability of collagen conduits is often listed as a usage selection factor but the optimum nerve conduit material is unknown. This prospective study is one of the largest to date to further our clinical knowledge on the surgical techniques and outcomes of collagen nerve conduits in shorter nerve-gap (5–15 mm) digital nerve injuries.

S. D. Trigg, MD

5 Shoulder and Elbow

Introduction

Over the last decade, shoulder and elbow has been one of the fastest growing areas of specialty interest, particularly the shoulder. Over the last 10 years the emergence of the reverse total shoulder replacement is probably the most significant event along with the ever-evolving and more sophisticated arthroscopic intervention. Today we find that arthroscopic techniques are becoming the standard, not just for diagnosis and debridement but also for instability, rotator cuff disease, and the like. Unless arthroscopic procedures are part of the armamentarium, it is difficult to consider how one might be relevant and on the cutting edge of shoulder surgery going forward. An exception, of course, is offered to those who focus on joint replacement arthroplasty, which are relatively few. My major focus in this volume with regard to the elbow continues to be that of trauma. Although there are some interesting developments occurring in joint replacement, particularly partial replacement, the literature has lagged behind the clinical practice. Hence, we have tended to focus more on the common elbow problems, those that are most typically seen in the orthopedic surgeon's office, including traumatic conditions that continue to be problematic for many of us.

Bernard F. Morrey, MD

Platelet-Rich Plasma Versus Autologous Whole Blood for the Treatment of Chronic Lateral Elbow Epicondylitis: A Randomized Controlled Clinical Trial

Thanasas C, Papadimitriou G, Charalambidis C, et al (Red Cross Hosp, Athens, Greece)
Am J Sports Med 39:2130-2134, 2011

Background.—Chronic lateral elbow epicondylitis is a tendinosis with angiofibrolastic degeneration of the wrist extensors' origin. Healing of this lesion is reported with the use of autologous blood as well as with platelet-rich plasma (PRP).

Purpose.—A comparative study of these 2 treatments was conducted in an effort to investigate the possible advantages of PRP.

Study Design.—Randomized controlled trial; Level of evidence, 1.

Methods.—Twenty-eight patients were divided equally into 2 groups, after blocked randomization. Group A was treated with a single injection of 3 mL of autologous blood and group B with 3 mL of PRP under ultrasound guidance. A standardized program of eccentric muscle strengthening was followed by all patients in both groups. Evaluation using a pain visual analog scale (VAS) and Liverpool elbow score was performed at 6 weeks, 3 months, and 6 months.

Results.—The VAS score improvement was larger in group B at every follow-up interval but the difference was statistically significant only at 6 weeks, when mean improvement was 3.8 points (95% confidence interval [CI], 3.1-4.5) in group B (61.47% improvement) and 2.5 points (95% CI, 1.9-3.1) in group A (41.6% improvement) ($P < .05$). No statistically significant difference was noted between groups regarding Liverpool elbow score.

Conclusion.—Regarding pain reduction, PRP treatment seems to be an effective treatment for chronic lateral elbow epicondylitis and superior to autologous blood in the short term. Defining details of indications, best PRP concentration, number and time of injections, as well as rehabilitation protocol might increase the method's effectiveness. Additionally, the possibility of cost reduction of the method might justify the use of PRP over autologous whole blood for chronic or refractory tennis elbow (Fig 1).

► There are few prospective, randomized studies in orthopedics. Treatment of epicondylitis does lend itself to such studies. The abstract accurately summarizes the findings that platelet-rich plasma (PRP) is superior to whole blood; the reader should note the residual pain for both groups still is around or exceeds 2 on the visual analogue scale (Fig 1). This, coupled with problems

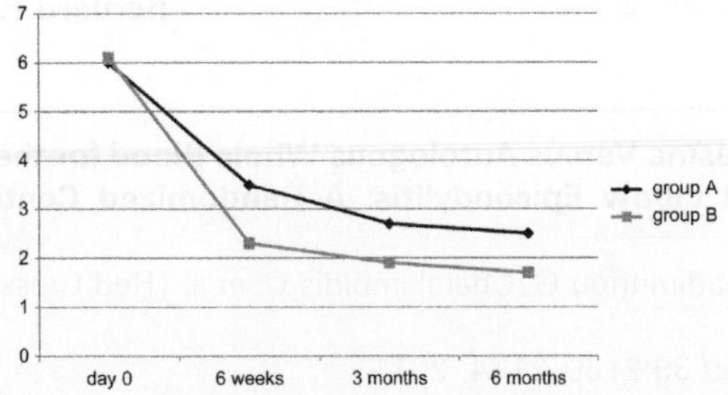

group	day 0	6 weeks*	3 months	6 months
A	6.0 (5.32-6.68)	3.5 (2.82-4.18)	2.78 (2.28-3.28)	2.53 (1.89-3.17)
B	6.1 (5.43-6.77)	2.35 (1.83-2.87)	1.92 (1.41-2.43)	1.78 (1.14-2.42)

FIGURE 1.—Pain visual analog scale score distribution (95% confidence interval). 0, no pain; 10, max pain. *Indicates significant difference between groups. (Reprinted from Thanasas C, Papadimitriou G, Charalambidis C, et al. Platelet-rich plasma versus autologous whole blood for the treatment of chronic lateral elbow epicondylitis: a randomized controlled clinical trial. *Am J Sports Med.* 2011;39:2130-2134, with permission from The Author(s).)

of cost and procedural discomfort, continues to prompt one to feel PRP may not be the ultimate solution for this problem.

B. F. Morrey, MD

Comparison of Autologous Blood, Corticosteroid, and Saline Injection in the Treatment of Lateral Epicondylitis: A Prospective, Randomized, Controlled Multicenter Study

Wolf JM, Ozer K, Scott F, et al (Univ of Colorado—Denver; Denver Health Med Ctr, CO; Denver Veterans Administration Med Ctr, CO)

J Hand Surg 36A:1269-1272, 2011

Purpose.—We compared saline, corticosteroid, and autologous blood injections for lateral epicondylitis in a prospective, blinded, randomized, controlled trial. The null hypothesis was that patient-rated outcomes after autologous blood injection would not be superior to corticosteroid and saline injections.

Methods.—Patients with clinically diagnosed lateral epicondylitis of less than 6 months' duration were randomized into 1 of 3 groups to receive a 3-mL injection of saline and lidocaine, corticosteroid and lidocaine, or autologous blood and lidocaine. Of 34 subjects who enrolled, 28 completed follow-up. A total of 10 were randomized to the saline group, 9 to the autologous blood group, and 9 to the steroid group. Every participant had 3 mL blood drawn, and the injection syringe was foil-covered to prevent the subject from knowing the contents. The primary outcome measure was the Disabilities of the Arm, Shoulder, and Hand (DASH) score. Patients completed a pain visual analog scale, DASH, and the Patient-Rated Forearm Evaluation before injection and at 2 weeks, 2 months, and 6 months after injection. We performed statistical analysis using repeated measures of analyses of variance.

Results.—There were no significant differences in DASH scores among the 3 groups at 2- and 6-month follow-up points, with the mean scores for saline at 20 and 10, respectively, compared with 28 and 20 for autologous blood and 28 and 13 for steroid injections. Secondary measures showed similar findings, with outcomes scores showing improvement in all 3 groups.

Conclusions.—In this prospective, randomized, controlled trial, autologous blood, corticosteroid, and saline injection provide no advantage over placebo saline injections in the treatment of lateral epicondylitis. Patients within each injection group demonstrated improved outcome scores over a 6-month period.

▶ The patient and surgeon alike continue to grope for a solution to tennis elbow. The major advantage of this study is the authors' effort to perform a randomized study. Unfortunately, it is difficult to consider it definitive. As the authors point out, many patients refused to participate, and the dropout rate was considerable. The surgeons were not blinded, and this adds an additional variable. The resulting small sample size further complicates the ability to feel strongly about the conclusions. What can be said is that there is no obvious advantage to any of the treatments offered here, in the short or intermediate term, with the obvious limitations of the study.

B. F. Morrey, MD

A Fragment-Specific Approach to Type IID Monteggia Elbow Fracture–Dislocations

Beingessner DM, Nork SE, Agel J, et al (Harborview Med Ctr, Seattle, WA; et al)

J Orthop Trauma 25:414-419, 2011

Objectives.—To describe the pattern of injury, surgical technique, and outcomes of Monteggia Type IID fracture dislocations.

Design.—Retrospective review of prospectively collected clinical and radiographic patient data in an orthopaedic trauma database.

Setting.—Level I university-based trauma center.

Patients/Participants.—All patients with Monteggia Type IID fracture–dislocations admitted from January 2000 to July 2005.

Intervention.—Review of patient demographics, fracture pattern, method of fixation, complications, additional surgical procedures, and clinical and radiographic outcome measures. Main Outcome Measurements: Clinical outcomes: elbow range of motion, complications. Radiographic outcomes: characteristic fracture fragments, quality of fracture reduction, healing time, degenerative changes, and heterotopic ossification.

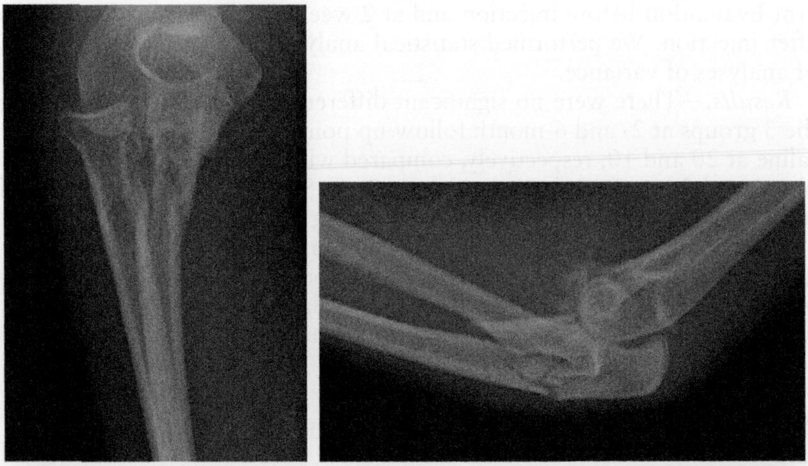

FIGURE 2.—Anteroposterior (A) and traction (C) radiographs of a typical Monteggia IID injury. Note the multifragmentary coronoid fracture with displacement posterior to the olecranon, the anterior oblique fragment, and a comminuted radial head fracture. (Reprinted from Beingessner DM, Nork SE, Agel J, et al. A fragment-specific approach to type IID monteggia elbow fracture–dislocations. *J Orthop Trauma.* 2011;25:414-419, with permission from Lippincott Williams & Wilkins.)

Results.—Sixteen patients were included in the study. All fractures united. There were six complications in six patients, including three contractures with associated heterotopic ossification, one pronator syndrome and late radial nerve palsy, one radial head collapse, and one with prominent hardware.

Conclusions.—Monteggia IID fracture–dislocations are complex injuries with typical specific fracture fragments. Anatomic fixation of all injury components and avoidance of complications where possible can lead to a good outcome in these challenging injuries (Figs 2A, C and 5B, C).

▶ The authors correctly point out that the so called Monteggia IID fracture is both uncommon (hence only 16 cases reported) and difficult to treat. I personally tend to think of this less as a Monteggia variant and more as a transolecranon fracture dislocation (Fig 2A and C). The value of offering a step-by-step approach is confirmed by the good results reported here. Although the authors report 6 steps, which I think is appropriate, we have typically collapsed the treatment into 4 surgical considerations, but in the same order as the authors': radial head, coronoid/distal shaft, proximal ulna, and lateral ulnar collateral ligament. That 9 of 16 had a functional arc of flexion (30–130°) is quite good given the nature of the injury. In my experience, the most difficult and significant

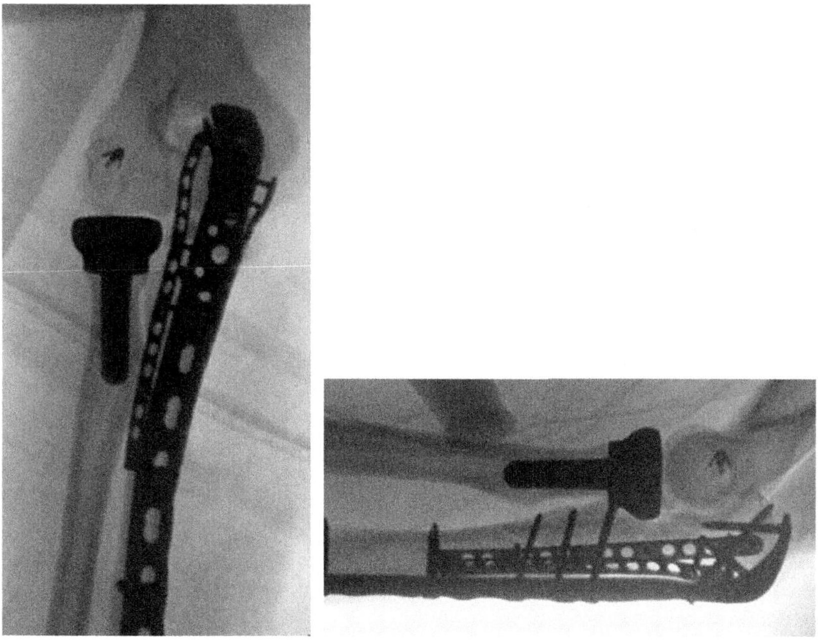

FIGURE 5.—Radiocapitellar (B), and lateral (C) radiographs of elbow after repair of olecranon and shaft components. A periarticular proximal ulna plate (3.5-mm thickness) spans both components of the injury and the proximal radioulnar joint is imaged to verify that it is clear of hardware (B). (Reprinted from Beingessner DM, Nork SE, Agel J, et al. A fragment-specific approach to type IID monteggia elbow fracture–dislocations. *J Orthop Trauma.* 2011;25:414-419, with permission from Lippincott Williams & Wilkins.)

complication is that of ectopic bone, reported in 3 of 16 cases in this series. It is difficult to know how much should be attributed to the injury or to the treatment. Regardless, this is a useful contribution to assist in the management of this type of injury (Fig 5B and C).

B. F. Morrey, MD

Outcomes of open arthrolysis of the elbow without post-operative passive stretching

Higgs ZCJ, Danks BA, Sibinski M, et al (Glasgow Royal Infirmary, UK)
J Bone Joint Surg Br 94-B:348-352, 2012

The use of passive stretching of the elbow after arthrolysis is controversial. We report the results of open arthrolysis in 81 patients. Prospectively collected outcome data with a minimum follow-up of one year were analysed. All patients had sustained an intra-articular fracture initially and all procedures were performed by the same surgeon under continuous brachial plexus block anaesthesia and with continuous passive movement (CPM) used postoperatively for two to three days. CPM was used to maintain the movement achieved during surgery and passive stretching was not used at any time. A senior physiotherapist assessed all the patients at regular intervals. The mean range of movement (ROM) improved from 69° to 109° and the function and pain of the upper limb improved from 32 to 16 and from 20 to 10, as assessed by the Disabilities of the Arm Shoulder and Hand score and a visual analogue scale, respectively. The greatest improvement was obtained in the stiffest elbows: nine patients with a pre-operative ROM <30° achieved a mean post-operative ROM of 92° (55° to 125°). This study demonstrates that in patients with a stiff elbow after injury, good results may be obtained after open elbow arthrolysis without using passive stretching during rehabilitation.

▶ This is an important contribution for several reasons. The authors offer a very careful and thoughtful analysis of management of the number 1 complication of elbow pathology—stiffness. The central conclusion is that manipulation is not necessary, as motion will gradually be regained over time after the initial treatment (Fig 3 in the original article). In general, I completely agree that does occur. However, notice the trends in Fig 3 in the original article. The rather dramatic motion gained at surgery is, in fact, lost after the procedure. It recovers, somewhat, but not dramatically. Hence, I do selectively examine the elbow after stiffness surgery, that is, stretch it out. This has been documented as being effective. The key issue, to be honest, is that we do not understand this process very well—but we are working on it.

B. F. Morrey, MD

Distal Humerus Hemiarthroplasty of the Elbow for Comminuted Distal Humeral Fractures in the Elderly Patient

Burkhart KJ, Nijs S, Mattyasovszky SG, et al (Univ Med Ctr, Cologne, Germany; Univ Hosp of the Catholic Univ of Leuven, Belgium; Univ Med Ctr of the Johannes Gutenberg-Univ Mainz, Germany)

J Trauma 71:635-642, 2011

Background.—The purpose of our study was to evaluate the objective and subjective outcomes, as well as the radiographic results after elbow hemiarthroplasty (HA) for comminuted distal humerus fractures in elderly patients.

Methods.—Ten female patients with a mean age of 75.2 years were treated with elbow HA either for osteoporotic, comminuted distal humerus fractures (n = 8) or for early failed osteosynthesis of distal humerus fractures (n = 2). The mean follow-up period was 12.1 months. All patients were examined and evaluated using the Mayo Elbow Performance Score and the Disabilities of the Arm, Shoulder, and Hand score. Radiographic postoperative outcomes were assessed performing anteroposterior and lateral radiographs of the injured elbow.

Results.—According to the Mayo Elbow Performance Score, nine patients achieved "good" to "excellent results" and only one patient revealed a "fair" clinical outcome. The mean Disabilities of the Arm, Shoulder, and Hand score was 11.5 (range, 0–30). The flexion of the affected elbow was 124.5° (range, 95–140°), the extension deficit was 17.5° (range, 5–30°), the pronation was 80.5° (range, 60–90°), and the supination was 79.5° (range, 50–90°). The following postoperative complications were seen: one triceps weakness, one transient ulnar nerve irritation, one superficial wound infection, and two heterotopic ossifications. None of the patients required explantation of the prosthesis. There was no evidence of loosening, radiolucency, or proximal bone resorption, whereas one patient developed progressive osteoarthritis of the proximal ulnar and radial articulation.

Conclusions.—Elderly patients treated with elbow HA revealed good to excellent short-term clinical outcomes. A high rate of complications occurred but most complications found were minor and reoperation rate was low. Our results must be regarded as a report on our first experience with HA. As cartilage wear is just a question of time especially in active patients, we cautiously recommend HA only for elderly and multimorbid low-demand patients (Fig 4).

► Selecting this article bumps up against one of my basic rules in article selection—keep it in the mainstream. But I also try to introduce emerging thoughts and treatments, especially when I feel there will be long-term acceptance. The use of a hemi-replacement at the elbow has of course been around for years in the form of a radial head implant. However, a distal humeral replacement was also described as early as the 1950s. The indication today is just as is described here: the fracture is not amenable to osteosynthesis, and the ulnar and radial articulations are essentially intact and the collateral ligaments are

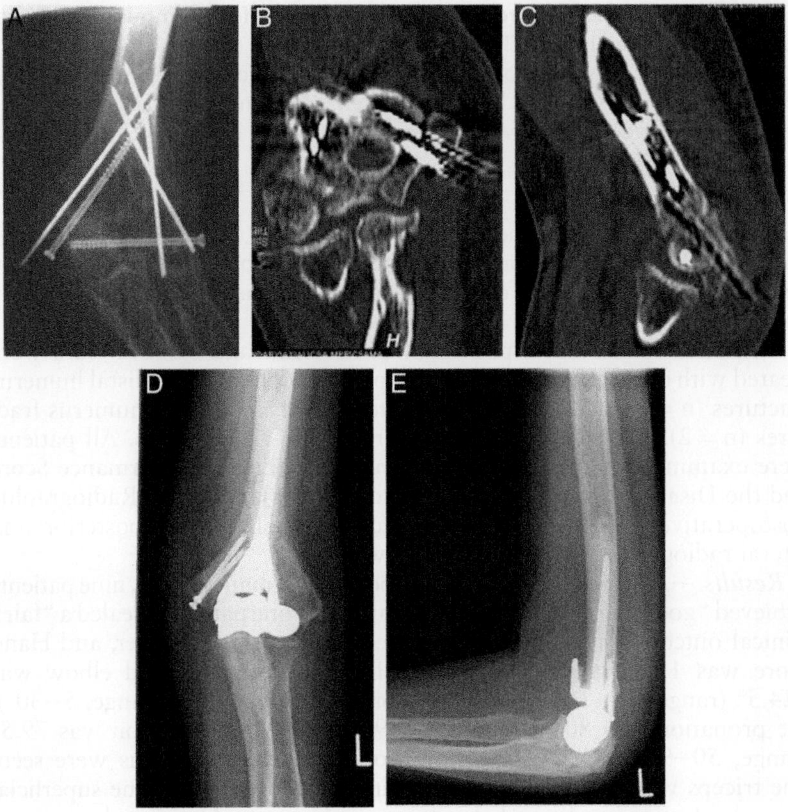

FIGURE 4.—Seventy-one-year-old woman presented to us with a painful unhealed fracture (*A–C*) of the distal humerus after unstable osteosynthesis of an AO-C3 fracture in an external hospital. HA was performed 85 days after trauma with reconstruction of the medial epicondyle (*D, E*). After 23 months, she reached an excellent result according to the MEPS. DASH was 0. (Reprinted from Burkhart KJ, Nijs S, Mattyasovszky SG, et al. Distal humerus hemiarthroplasty of the elbow for comminuted distal humeral fractures in the elderly patient. *J Trauma*. 2011;71:635-642, with permission from Lippincott Williams & Wilkins.)

competent, or can be rendered as such. In these selective instances, a hemi-replacement can be quite effective (Fig 4). Unlike the current authors, I reserve the hemi for the younger patient, still preferring a total for the older individual. The most important information to share, however, is that there is no US Food and Drug Administration—approved device in this country that can be used in this manner. So, if done, it will be an off-label application. Stay tuned.

B. F. Morrey, MD

Incidence, prevalence, and consultation rates of shoulder complaints in general practice

Greving K, Dorrestijn O, Winters JC, et al (Univ of Groningen, The Netherlands)
Scand J Rheumatol 41:150-155, 2012

Objective.—To study the incidence, prevalence, and consultation rates of patients with shoulder complaints in general practice in the Netherlands during 10 years following initial presentation.

Methods.—A primary care database with an average population of 30 000 patients per year aged 18 years or older was used to select patients who consulted their general practitioner (GP) with shoulder complaints in the northern part of the Netherlands in the year 1998. Information about consultations for shoulder complaints was extracted. Incidence and prevalence for men, women, and different age groups were calculated for 9 and 10 years.

Results.—A total of 526 patients consulted their GP with a new shoulder complaint. During an average follow-up of 7.6 years, these patients consulted their GP 1331 times because of their shoulder complaints (average of 0.33 consultations per year). Almost half of the patients consulted their GP only once. Patients in the 45–64 age category had the highest probability of repeated GP consultations during follow-up. Average incidence was 29.3 per 1000 person-years. Women and patients in the 45–64 age category have the highest incidence. The annual prevalence of shoulder complaints ranged from 41.2 to 48.4 per 1000 person-years, calculated for the period 1998 to 2007, and was higher among women than among men.

Conclusion.—Although the incidence of shoulder complaints in general practice is as high as 29.3 per 1000 person-years, GPs' workload is generally low, as nearly half of these patients consult their GP only once for their complaint.

▶ This article is included because I was very interested in a question that was not answered. Because it originates from the Netherlands, it is not surprising that the findings reported here might not be relevant to the United States. That said, the one central and interesting finding is that, while shoulder complaints account for a reasonable number of patients seeking the care of a general practitioner, they do not account for a high burden of work for the general practitioner. The reason is simple: more than half are single-visit appointments! What I was looking for, and did not find, is the frequency of referral to an orthopedic surgeon. The frequency of referral to physical therapy is 15%. My honest impression from reading this article is that we probably overtreat our patients with shoulder conditions in this country. That said, right or wrong, this probably will not change.

B. F. Morrey, MD

Correlation of MR Arthrographic Findings and Range of Shoulder Motions in Patients With Frozen Shoulder

Lee S-Y, Park J, Song S-W (The Catholic Univ of Korea, Seoul, Republic of Korea)

AJR Am J Roentgenol 198:173-179, 2012

Objective.—The purpose of this article is to correlate MRI arthrographic findings with range of shoulder motions in patients with frozen shoulder.

Materials and Methods.—Shoulder MRI studies of 40 patients (22 women and 18 men; mean age, 52.8 years) with frozen shoulder were retrospectively compared with MRI studies of 40 age- and sex-matched control subjects without frozen shoulder. The thickness of the coracohumeral ligament and the capsule in axillary recess were measured retrospectively. The range of shoulder motions, including external rotation (ER), internal rotation (IR), lateral abduction, and forward flexion (FF), were prospectively evaluated by one experienced orthopedic surgeon.

Results.—The mean (± SD) thickness of the coracohumeral ligament (4.13 ± 1.04 vs 2.51 ± 0.59 mm; $p = 0.000$) and the capsule in axillary recess (3.97 ± 1.45 vs 2.33 ± 0.87 mm; $p = 0.000$) were significantly greater in the patient group than in the control group. Multiple linear regression showed that only coracohumeral ligament thickness was significantly associated with ER ($R^2 = 0.418$; $p = 0.000$) and IR ($R^2 = 0.346$; $p = 0.001$), but not with lateral abduction and FF. Capsular thickness in axillary recess was not significantly correlated with any shoulder motion.

Conclusion.—Coracohumeral ligament thickness on MR arthrography correlates with the range limitation of ER and IR in patients with frozen shoulder.

▶ Frozen shoulder continues to be seen by many orthopedic surgeons and continues to pose treatment problems. Because this may present to a general orthopedic surgeon's office, information such as this may be of value. The authors clearly document the expected correlation between the thickening of the capsule, in its various components (Fig 4 in the original article), and loss of motion (Fig 3 in the original article). What would be of particular interest is to know whether such imaging can provide insight regarding prognosis or serve as a measure of treatment success. Logic would suggest the imaging is not necessary, and simple clinical examination is all that is required to follow the resolution of the process.

B. F. Morrey, MD

Acromioclavicular Joint Pain in Patients With Adhesive Capsulitis: A Prospective Outcome Study

Anakwenze OA, Hsu JE, Kim JS, et al (Univ of Pennsylvania, Philadelphia; Pennsylvania Hosp, Philadelphia)

Orthopedics 34:e556-e560, 2011

Diagnosis of adhesive capsulitis is a clinical diagnosis based on history and physical examination. Afflicted patients exhibit active and passive loss of motion in all planes and a positive capsular stretch sign. The effect of adhesive capsulitis on acromioclavicular biomechanics leading to tenderness has not been documented in the literature. This study reports on the incidence of acromioclavicular tenderness in the presence of adhesive capsulitis. Furthermore, we note the natural history of such acromioclavicular joint pain in relation to that of adhesive capsulitis.

Over a 2-year period (2005-2007), 84 patients undergoing initial evaluation for adhesive capsulitis were prospectively examined with the use of validated outcome measures and physical examination. Acromioclavicular joint tenderness results were compared and analyzed on initial evaluation and final follow-up of at least 1 year. Forty-eight patients (57%) with adhesive capsulitis had acromioclavicular joint pain on examination. At final follow-up, as range of motion improved, a significant increase in American Shoulder and Elbow Surgeons/Penn shoulder score and decrease in number of patients with acromioclavicular pain was noted with only 6 patients with residual pain ($P<.05$).

In the presence of adhesive capsulitis, there is not only compensatory scapulothoracic motion but also acromioclavicular motion. This often results in transient symptoms at the acromioclavicular joint, which abate as the frozen shoulder resolves and glenohumeral motion improves. This is important to recognize to avoid unnecessary invasive treatment of the acromioclavicular joint when the patient presents with adhesive capsulitis.

▶ Contrary to the ever-increasing tendency to rely on hi-tech diagnostic tools, this nice study provides valuable insight based on careful clinical assessment. The authors have carefully studied a large number of patients with adhesive capsulitis, noting more than 50% have associated pain at the acromioclavicular joint. The real value, however, is to note that this seems to be associated with the glenohumeral pathology and resolves with resolution of the underlying process. The take-home message is that the symptom need not be addressed procedurally—reassurance is all that is necessary.

B. F. Morrey, MD

Diagnostic Accuracy of Clinical Tests for Subacromial Impingement Syndrome: A Systematic Review and Meta-Analysis

Alqunaee M, Galvin R, Fahey T (Royal College of Surgeons in Ireland, Dublin, Republic of Ireland)

Arch Phys Med Rehabil 93:229-236, 2012

Objective.—To examine the accuracy of clinical tests for diagnosing subacromial impingement syndrome (SIS).

Data Sources.—A systematic literature search was conducted in January 2011 to identify all studies that examined the diagnostic accuracy of clinical tests for SIS. The following search engines were used: Cochrane Library, EMBASE, Science Direct, and PubMed.

Study Selection.—Two reviewers screened all articles. We included prospective or retrospective cohort studies that examined individuals with a painful shoulder, reported any clinical test for SIS, and used arthroscopy or open surgery as the reference standard. The search strategy yielded 1338 articles of which 1307 publications were excluded based on title/abstract. Sixteen of the remaining 31 articles were included. The PRISMA (preferred reporting items for systematic reviews and meta-analyses) guidelines were followed to conduct this review.

Data Extraction.—The number of true positives, false positives, true negatives, and false negatives for each clinical test were extracted from relevant studies, and a 2×2 table was constructed. Studies were combined using a bivariate random-effects model. Heterogeneity was assessed using the variance of logit-transformed sensitivity and specificity.

Data Synthesis.—Ten studies with 1684 patients are included in the meta-analysis. The Hawkins-Kennedy test, Neer's sign, and empty can test are shown to be more useful for ruling out rather than ruling in SIS, with greater pooled sensitivity estimates (range, .69−.78) than specificity (range, .57−.62). A negative Neer's sign reduces the probability of SIS from 45% to 14%. The drop arm test and lift-off test have higher pooled specificities (range, .92−.97) than sensitivities (range, .21−.42), indicating that they are more useful for ruling in SIS if the test is positive.

Conclusions.—This systematic review quantifies the diagnostic accuracy of 5 clinical tests for SIS, in particular the lift-off test. Accurate diagnosis of SIS in clinical practice may serve to improve appropriate treatment and management of individuals with shoulder complaints (Table 5).

▶ This is an important literature review and analysis for 2 reasons. First, a very common and controversial topic is studied—subacromial impingement. Second, emphasis is placed on clinical finding. I cannot overemphasize the necessity to accurately understand the symptom complex as well as the ubiquitous magnetic resonance imaging findings. One should have it clear that some tests are more useful to rule out the condition, such as a negative Neer test, and others are more useful to suggest the presence of a clinically relevant process if positive, such as the drop arm or lift-off tests (Table 5). If the clinician can keep the

TABLE 5.—Summary Estimates of Positive and Negative LRs Using a Bivariate Random-Effects Model

Clinical Test	LR+	95% CI	−LR	95% CI
Hawkins-Kennedy test	1.70	1.29–2.26	.46	.27–.78
Neer's sign	1.86	1.49–2.31	.37	.25–.55
Empty can test	1.81	1.16–2.83	.50	.40–.63
Drop arm test	2.62	1.60–4.30	.86	.79–.94
Lift-off test	16.47	1.46–185.61	.59	.37–.97

findings of this very credible review in mind, it will allow much better selection of appropriate candidates for surgical decompression.

B. F. Morrey, MD

Effectiveness of Surgical and Postsurgical Interventions for the Subacromial Impingement Syndrome: A Systematic Review

Gebremariam L, Hay EM, Koes BW, et al (Erasmus MC – Univ Med Ctr Rotterdam, The Netherlands; Keele Univ, UK)
Arch Phys Med Rehabil 92:1900-1913, 2011

Objective.—To provide an evidence-based overview of the effectiveness of surgical and postsurgical interventions for the subacromial impingement syndrome.

Data Sources.—The Cochrane Library, PubMed, Embase, PEDro, and CINAHL were searched.

Study Selection.—Two reviewers independently selected relevant systematic reviews and randomized controlled trials (RCTs).

Data Extraction.—Two reviewers independently extracted data and assessed the methodologic quality.

Data Synthesis.—If pooling of data was not possible, a best-evidence synthesis was used to summarize the results.

TABLE 1.—Methodologic Quality Assessment: Sources of Risk Bias

Items Risk of Bias
1. Was the method of randomization adequate?
2. Was the treatment allocation concealed?
3. Was the patient blinded to the intervention?
4. Was the care provider blinded to the intervention?
5. Was the outcome assessor blinded to the intervention?
6. Was the dropout rate described and acceptable?
7. Were all randomized participants analyzed in the group to which they were allocated?
8. Are reports of the study free of suggestion of selective outcome reporting?
9. Were the groups similar at baseline regarding the most important prognostic indicators?
10. Were cointerventions avoided or similar?
11. Was the compliance acceptable in all groups?
12. Was the timing of the outcome assessment similar in all groups?

TABLE 4.—Methodologic Quality Scores of the Included Cochrane Review of Coghlan et al[11]

Reference	Randomization?	Allocation Concealment?	Blinding Patients?	Blinding? Outcome Assessors?	Acceptable? No. Lost to Follow-up?	Intention-to-Treat Analysis?	Score Maximum	Score Study	%	Overall Validity	Quality of the Study
Brox et al[15]	+	?	—	+	+	+	6	4	66	C	Low
Haahr et al[16]	+	+	—	—	+	+	6	4	66	B–C	Low
Husby et al[17]	+	?	—	+	+	NS	6	4	66	C	Low
Murphy et al[24]	+	—	+	?	?	NS	6	2	33	C	Low
Iversen et al[20]	?	?	—	—	+	+	6	2	33	C	Low
Rahme et al[14]	+	?	—	—	+	—	6	2	33	C	Low
Spangehl et al[21]	?	?	—	+	+	NS	6	2	33	C	Low
T'Jonck et al[18]	?	?	?	?	+	+	6	2	33	C	Low
Ingvarrson et al[22]	?	?	?	?	+	NS	6	1	17	C	Low
Rubenthaler[23]	?	?	?	?	+	?	6	1	17	C	Low
Sachs et al[19]	?	?	—	—	+	NS	6	1	17	C	Low

Abbreviations: +, yes; -, no; ?, unclear; No. lost to follow-up, we defined this item positive if the percentage of lost to follow-up is <20% for the short-term follow-up and <30% for the long-term follow-up; NS, not stated but participants completed within their surgical allocation; Overall validity, A (low risk of bias), all criteria met; B (moderate risk of bias), 1 or more criteria partly met; C (high risk of bias), 1 or more criteria not met.

Editor's Note: Please refer to original journal article for full references.

Results.—One review and 5 RCTs reporting on various surgical techniques, and postsurgical interventions were included. Moderate evidence was found in favor of adding platelet-leukocyte gel versus open subacromial decompression. No evidence was found for the superiority of subacromial decompression versus conservative treatment in the short, mid, and long term or in favor of 1 surgical technique when compared with another. Limited evidence was found in favor of early activation after arthroscopic decompression in the short and long term.

Conclusions.—This review shows that there is no evidence that surgical treatment is superior to conservative treatment or that 1 particular surgical technique is superior to another. Because of possibly lower risks for complications, conservative treatment may be preferred. When choosing for surgery, arthroscopic decompression may be preferred because of the less invasive character of the procedure (Tables 1 and 4).

▶ There are a number of interesting features to this report. First, it is important, as it is attempting to address objective clinical efficacy of a very commonly performed procedure. Unfortunately, I personally have relatively little confidence in the Cochrane conclusions of literature review to direct orthopedic thought or management. The methodology (Table 1) results in virtually every study used to arrive at an opinion are to be one of low quality (Table 4). But, this is not unique to subacromial decompression studies; it is true for all of the orthopedic literature. It really calls into question—what constitutes adequate evidence for effective orthopedic intervention? The intent and goal are spot on; the execution is in question. Finally, it is important to remember absence of evidence is not evidence of absence.

That said, I personally do identify and tend to support the conclusions arrived at with this review.

B. F. Morrey, MD

Injuries Associated with Traumatic Anterior Glenohumeral Dislocations

Robinson CM, Shur N, Sharpe T, et al (Royal Infirmary of Edinburgh, UK)

J Bone Joint Surg Am 94:18-26, 2012

Background.—A number of shoulder girdle injuries are associated with acute anterior glenohumeral dislocations. In the present study we evaluated the prevalence of neurological deficits, greater tuberosity fractures, and rotator cuff injuries in a population of unselected patients who presented with a traumatic anterior glenohumeral dislocation.

Methods.—A prospective trauma database was used to record the demographic details on 3633 consecutive patients (2250 male patients and 1383 female patients with a mean age of 47.6 years) who had sustained a traumatic anterior glenohumeral dislocation between 1995 and 2009. On the basis of these data, we assessed the prevalence of and risk factors for ultrasound-proven rotator cuff tears, tuberosity fractures, and neurological deficits occurring in association with the dislocation.

TABLE 3.—Demographic Features of Patients with Neurological Deficits

Injury Category and Pattern of Neurological Deficit	No. of Patients	Age* (yr)	Male: Female Ratio (No. of Patients)	Mechanism of Injury (No. of Patients) Simple Fall	Fall from Height	Sports Injury	Road Traffic Accident	Other
Dislocation with neurological deficit (Group II)								
Axillary nerve	155	37.2 (33.9 to 40.4)	2.7:1	48 (31%)	19 (12.3%)	77 (49.7%)	8 (5.2%)	3 (1.9%)
Other single nerve	35	54.6 (47.5 to 61.8)	0.7:1	23 (65.7%)	1 (2.9%)	9 (25.7%)	2 (5.7%)	0
Complex nerve/plexus	20	58.0 (49.0 to 66.9)	1.5:1	14 (70%)	3 (15%)	3 (15%)	0	0
All Group II	210	42.5 (39.6 to 45.5)	2.0:1	85 (40.5%)	23 (11%)	89 (42.4%)	10 (4.8%)	3 (1.4%)
Combined injuries (Group IV)								
Axillary nerve	174	54.7 (52.2 to 57.2)	1.3:1	108 (62.1%)	25 (14.4%)	13 (7.5%)	16 (9.2%)	12 (6.9%)
Other single nerve	46	64.6 (60.4 to 68.8)	0.5:1	38 (82.6%)	2 (4.3%)	5 (10.9%)	0	1 (2.2%)
Complex nerve/plexus	62	60.8 (58.5 to 63.0)	0.7:1	47 (75.8%)	7 (11.3%)	2 (3.2%)	2 (3.2%)	4 (6.5%)
All Group IV	282	57.5 (55.5 to 59.5)	1.0:1	193 (68.4%)	34 (12.1%)	20 (7.1%)	18 (6.4%)	17 (6.0%)
All patients with nerve palsy	492	51.5 (49.7 to 53.3)	1.3:1	278 (56.5%)	57 (11.6%)	109 (22.2%)	28 (5.7%)	20 (4.1%)

*The values are given as the mean and the 95% CI.

Results.—Of the 3633 patients who had a dislocation, 492 patients (13.5%) had a neurological deficit following reduction and 1215 patients (33.4%) had either a rotator cuff tear or a greater tuberosity fracture. A dislocation with a neurological deficit alone was found in 210 patients (5.8%), a dislocation with a rotator cuff tear or a greater tuberosity fracture was found in 933 patients (25.7%), and a combined injury pattern was found in 282 patients (7.8%). Female patients with an age of sixty years or older who were injured in low-energy falls were more likely to have a rotator cuff tear or a greater tuberosity fracture. The likelihood of a neurological deficit after an anterior glenohumeral dislocation was significantly increased for patients who had a rotator cuff tear or a greater tuberosity fracture (relative risk, 1.9 [95% confidence interval, 1.7 to 2.1]; $p < 0.001$).

Conclusions.—The prevalence of rotator cuff tear, greater tuberosity fracture, or neurological deficit following primary anterior glenohumeral dislocation is greater than previously appreciated. These associated injuries may occur alone or in combined patterns. Dislocations associated with axillary nerve palsy have similar demographic features to isolated dislocations. Injuries associated with a rotator cuff tear, greater tuberosity fracture, or complex neurological deficit are more common in patients sixty years of age or older. Careful evaluation of rotator cuff function is required for any patient with a dislocation associated with a neurological deficit, and vice versa.

Level of Evidence.—Prognostic Level II. See Instructions for Authors for a complete description of levels of evidence (Table 3).

▶ This is really a useful report, as it should serve to heighten the awareness of the surgeon to the potential presence of associated injury with shoulder dislocation. The constellation of neurologic, osseous, and other co-injuries is well documented. What is important is the recognition that the occurrence is a function of the age on the individual (Table 3). In addition, it is very helpful to know that some of these coexist (Fig 2 in the original article). At the end of the day, note these data and carefully examine your patients for neurologic, cuff, and fracture pathology. It will influence prognosis as well as treatment.

B. F. Morrey, MD

Arthroscopic Bankart Repair Combined With Remplissage Technique for the Treatment of Anterior Shoulder Instability With Engaging Hill-Sachs Lesion: A Report of 49 Cases With a Minimum 2-Year Follow-up

Zhu Y-M, Lu Y, Zhang J, et al (Beijing Ji Shui Tan Hosp, People's Republic of China)

Am J Sports Med 39:1640-1647, 2011

Background.—Engaging Hill-Sachs lesions are known to be a risk factor for recurrence dislocation after arthroscopic repair in patients with anterior shoulder instability. For a large engaging Hill-Sachs lesion, arthroscopic remplissage is a solution.

Hypothesis.—Arthroscopic Bankart repair combined with the Hill-Sachs remplissage technique can achieve good results without significant impairment of shoulder function.

Study Design.—Case Series; Level of evidence, 4.

Methods.—Forty-nine consecutive patients who underwent arthroscopic Bankart repair and Hill-Sachs remplissage for anterior shoulder instability were followed up for a mean duration of 29.0 months (range, 24-35 months). There were 42 males and 7 females with a mean age of 28.4 years (range, 16.7-54.7 years). All patients had diagnosed traumatic unidirectional anterior shoulder instability with a bony lesion of glenoid and an engaging Hill-Sachs lesion. Physical examination, radiographs, and magnetic resonance imaging were performed during postoperative follow-up. The American Shoulder and Elbow Surgeons (ASES) score, Constant score, and Rowe score were used to evaluate shoulder function.

Results.—The active forward elevation increased a mean of 8.0° (range, −10° to 80°) postoperatively. However, the patients lost 1.9° (range, −40° to 30°) of external rotation to the side. Significant improvement was detected with regard to the ASES score (84.7 vs 96.0, $P < .001$), Constant score (93.3 vs 97.8, $P = .005$), and Rowe score (36.8 vs 89.8, $P < .001$). There were 1 redislocation, 2 subluxations, and 1 patient with a positive apprehension test; the overall failure rate was 8.2% (4 of 49). Successful healing of the infraspinatus tendon within the Hill-Sachs lesion was shown by magnetic resonance imaging.

Conclusion.—Arthroscopic Bankart repair combined with Hill-Sachs remplissage can restore shoulder stability without significant impairment of shoulder function in patients with engaging Hill-Sachs lesions.

▶ While arthroscopic repair of the capsule and labrum is now commonplace and the accepted treatment standard, this article was of particular interest to me. It emanates from China, indicating a high level of sophistication and awareness. Although the follow-up period is short, averaging less than 3 years, it adds to the literature by having a relatively large sample of patients with a significant Hill-Sachs lesion treated through the scope by remplissage—affixing the capsule to the defect (Fig 1 in the original article). Hence the finding that the recurrence rate was less than 10% and the loss of motion was negligible is rather impressive.

B. F. Morrey, MD

Glenohumeral Osteoarthritis After Arthroscopic Bankart Repair for Anterior Instability

Franceschi F, Papalia R, Del Buono A, et al (Univ Campus Bio-Medico of Rome, Italy; et al)

Am J Sports Med 39:1653-1659, 2011

Background.—Few data on shoulder arthropathy in patients undergoing arthroscopic repair for glenohumeral instability are available.

TABLE 5.—Logistic Regression Analysis: Arthrogenic Factors

Factor	*P* Value	Odds Ratio	95% Confidence Interval
Time from onset to surgery	.0006	3.3	1.7-6.5
Number of preoperative dislocations	.002	2.3	1.4-3.8
Age at surgery	.0006	1.6	1.2-2.1
Length of follow-up	.006	13.9	2.1-91.2
External rotation of operated side	.09	0.9	0.8-0.97
Number of anchors	.0005	43.5	5.2-363.9
State of labrum	.003	22.9	2.9-183.9

Hypothesis.—Arthroscopic stabilization of Bankart lesions does not prevent the development of postoperative glenohumeral osteoarthritis.

Study Design.—Case series; Level of evidence, 4.

Methods.—Clinical (Rowe and Constant scores) and radiographic preoperative and postoperative data from 60 patients who underwent arthroscopic Bankart repair were compared. Osteoarthritis was graded preoperatively and postoperatively with the Buscayret classification grading system. The average age at surgery was 27.6 years, and follow-up averaged 8.0 years.

Results.—The postoperative incidence of osteoarthritis in patients with no preoperative degenerative changes was 21.8% (12 of 55 patients). The incidence of degenerative joint disease of the glenohumeral joint showed evidence of a statistically significant association with older age at first dislocation and at surgery, increased length of time from the first episode to surgery, increased number of preoperative dislocations, increased length of time from the initial dislocation until surgery, increased number of anchors used at surgery, and more degenerated labrum at surgery. A higher number of preoperative dislocations, a greater length of follow-up, and reduced external rotation in abduction influenced Rowe and Constant scores.

Conclusion.—The number of anchors used and the state of the labrum are the most important factors associated with a higher risk of radiographic degenerative changes. Longer follow-up investigations are needed to draw meaningful conclusions (Table 5).

▶ Long-term implications of chronic shoulder instability are surprisingly poorly documented. It is reasonable to assume, however, that stabilization not only improves function, but also lessens the likelihood of further problems in the future, such as osteoarthritis. Of interest, the logical conclusion has been rarely investigated; hence, this analysis caught my eye. A reasonably large sample was followed up for up to 5 years—still relatively short by most orthopedic standards. Of interest, the authors document the number of dislocations before reconstruction is less important than the age of the patient and duration of the instability (Table 5). The strong correlation with the number of suture anchors may correlate more as a reflection of the degree of instability or of the pathology rather than being directly involved with causing late degenerative changes. However, loose or poorly placed hardware has been well documented to be a source of severe subsequent glenohumeral arthritis.

B. F. Morrey, MD

Factors Affecting Rotator Cuff Healing After Arthroscopic Repair: Osteoporosis as One of the Independent Risk Factors

Chung SW, Oh JH, Gong HS, et al (Seoul Natl Univ Bundang Hosp, Korea)

Am J Sports Med 39:2099-2107, 2011

Background.—The prognostic factors associated with structural outcome after arthroscopic rotator cuff repair have not yet been fully determined.

Hypothesis.—The hypothesis of this study was that bone mineral density (BMD) is an important prognostic factor affecting rotator cuff healing after arthroscopic cuff repair.

Study Design.—Cohort study; Level of evidence, 3.

Methods.—Among 408 patients who underwent arthroscopic repair for full-thickness rotator cuff tear between January 2004 and July 2008, 272 patients were included whose postoperative cuff integrity was verified by computed tomography arthrography (CTA) or ultrasonography (USG) and simultaneously who were evaluated by various functional outcome instruments. The mean age at the time of operation was 59.5 ± 7.9 years. Postoperative CTA or USG was performed at a mean 13.0 ± 5.1 months after surgery, and the mean follow-up period was 37.2 ± 10.0 months (range, 24-65 months). The clinical, structural, and surgery-related factors affecting cuff integrity including BMD were analyzed using both univariate and multivariate analysis. Evaluation of postoperative cuff integrity was performed by musculoskeletal radiologists who were unaware of the present study.

Results.—The failure rate of rotator cuff healing was 22.8% (62 of 272). The failure rate was significantly higher in patients with lower BMD ($P < .001$); older age ($P < .001$); female gender ($P = .03$); larger tear size ($P < .001$); higher grade of fatty infiltration (FI) of the supraspinatus, infraspinatus, and subscapularis (all $P < .001$); diabetes mellitus ($P = .02$); shorter acromiohumeral distance ($P < .001$); and associated biceps procedure ($P < .001$). However, in the multivariate analysis, only BMD ($P = .001$), FI of the infraspinatus ($P = .01$), and the amount of retraction ($P = .03$) showed a significant relationship with cuff healing failure following arthroscopic rotator cuff repair.

Conclusion.—Bone mineral density, as well as FI of the infraspinatus and amount of retraction, was an independent determining factor affecting postoperative rotator cuff healing. Further studies with prospective, randomized, and controlled design are needed to confirm the relationship between BMD and postoperative rotator cuff healing (Table 2).

► I was really impressed with this article. The authors study a massive sample of more than 400 cuff tears and more carefully study more than 200. The hypothesis is sound and the findings novel. The orthopedic community is aware of the relationship of retraction and clinical difficulty, so a correlation to a failure is no surprise. So also, fatty infiltration is an indicator of serious pathology as well as compromised outcome. The additional contribution is that osteoporosis, measured by lower bone mineral density scores, also independently correlates

TABLE 2.—Comparison Between the Healed Cuff Group and the Unhealed Cuff Group[a]

Variables	Healed Cuffs (n = 210)	Unhealed Cuffs (n = 62)	P Value
Gender,[b] n	Men, 101; women, 119	Men, 15; women, 37	.03
Age,[b] y	58.2 ± 7.5 (range, 39-76)	65.0 ± 7.6 (range, 46–80)	<.001
Symptom duration, mo	33.2 ± 54.3	49.0 ± 64.6	.11
Symptom aggravation, mo	5.3 ± 5.7	6.5 ± 12.0	.55
Involvement of dominant side, n (%)	164 (74.5)	44 (84.6)	.15
Smoking, n (%)	34 (15.5)	6 (11.5)	.66
Diabetes,[b] n (%)	25 (11.4)	13 (25.0)	.02
Hypertension or heart disease, n (%)	62 (28.2)	22 (42.3)	.07
Steroid injection history, n (%)	25 (11.4)	4 (7.4)	.19
Traumatic onset, n (%)	34 (15.5)	5 (9.6)	.38
Shoulder stiffness, n (%)	37 (16.8)	9 (17.3)	1
Level of sports activity (high, medium, low), n	49, 95, 74	9, 23, 22	.48
Demand of shoulder activity (high, medium, low), n	59, 105, 55	14, 22, 17	.57
Bone mineral density[b]	−0.92 ± 1.17	−1.94 ± 1.18	<.001
FI of the supraspinatus[b]	2.02 ± 0.99	3.27 ± 0.94	<.001
FI of the infraspinatus[b]	0.96 ± 0.67	2.17 ± 1.10	<.001
FI of the subscapularis[b]	0.74 ± 0.70	1.56 ± 0.85	<.001
Tear size of anteroposterior dimension,[b] cm	1.74 ± 0.72	2.77 ± 1.32	<.001
Amount of retraction,[b] cm	1.82 ± 0.73	2.82 ± 1.18	<.001
Acromiohumeral distance,[b] mm	9.17 ± 1.65	7.73 ± 2.42	<.001
Repair technique, n	SR, 63; DR, 151	SR, 20; DR, 38	.72
Distal clavicle resection, n (%)	24 (11.0)	10 (18.9)	.24
Biceps procedure,[b] n	Tenotomy, 26; tenodesis, 13	Tenotomy, 19; tenodesis, 5	<.001

[a]FI, fatty infiltration; SR, single row; DR, double row.
[b]Statistically significant.

to a poor outcome (Table 2). Unfortunately, the procedures were not uniform, and we do not know the correlation of single or double row fixation of the osteoporotic patient.

B. F. Morrey, MD

Characteristic Retear Patterns Assessed by Magnetic Resonance Imaging After Arthroscopic Double-Row Rotator Cuff Repair

Hayashida K, Tanaka M, Koizumi K, et al (Osaka Police Hosp, Japan)
Arthroscopy 28:458-464, 2012

Purpose.—The purpose of this study was to examine magnetic resonance imaging (MRI) findings and elucidate retear pattern and its characteristics after surgical repair of the rotator cuff using an arthroscopic double-row suture anchor (DRSA) method.

Methods.—Forty-seven patients with complete rotator cuff tears treated by the DRSA method under arthroscopy whose repair condition was assessed by MRI approximately 12 months after the procedure were included in the study. The mean age at treatment was 65 years (range, 42 to 82 years). The mean follow-up period was 26 months (range, 24 to 32 months).

Result.—The repair integrity was classified into 5 groups according to MRI findings. A well-repaired tendon was seen in 34 shoulders. Partial retearing of the deep layer was observed in 2. Partial retearing of the superficial layer around the medial anchors was observed in 3. Complete retearing of the tendon around the medial anchors with a well-preserved footprint was observed in 4. Complete retearing of the tendon from the footprint was observed in 4. The retear patterns involving superficial retearing and complete retearing around the medial anchors were unexpected and unique. These types of retears seem to be characteristic of the DRSA method and were seen in cases with medium-sized tears. The incidence of characteristic retearing was 7 of 47.

Conclusions.—Superficial-side partial tearing and complete tearing around the medial-row anchors with a well-repaired tendon on the footprint could be characteristics of the DRSA method. These retear patterns were observed in 7 of 13 retear cases and 7 of 47 cases overall. The retear rate by the characteristic retear was high. Exploring the causes of this retear and preventing it could lead to better clinical results with the DRSA method.

Level of Evidence.—Level IV, therapeutic case series.

▶ With the ever-increasing interest in arthroscopic intervention coupled with ever-increasing use of the double-row repair, the content of this article offers relevant information. Although the topic is one of failure, and there is no directly useful conclusion, there is merit in understanding the failure pattern of this type of repair for the large tear. If the mechanical basis for the failure could be determined, then the proposition of an improved repair is reasonable. As an aside, as I look back at this year's shoulder selections, I am impressed by the increasing influence and relevance of the scope of study.

B. F. Morrey, MD

Does Platelet-Rich Plasma Accelerate Recovery After Rotator Cuff Repair?: A Prospective Cohort Study

Jo CH, Kim JE, Yoon KS, et al (Seoul Natl Univ College of Medicine, Korea)
Am J Sports Med 39:2082-2090, 2011

Background.—Platelet-rich plasma (PRP) has been recently used to enhance and accelerate the healing of musculoskeletal injuries and diseases, but evidence is still lacking, especially on its effects after rotator cuff repair.

Hypothesis.—Platelet-rich plasma accelerates recovery after arthroscopic rotator cuff repair in pain relief, functional outcome, overall satisfaction, and enhanced structural integrity of repaired tendon.

Study Design.—Cohort study; Level of evidence, 2.

Methods.—Forty-two patients with full-thickness rotator cuff tears were included. Patients were informed about the use of PRP before surgery and decided themselves whether to have PRP placed at the time of surgery. Nineteen patients underwent arthroscopic rotator cuff repair with PRP and 23 without. Platelet-rich plasma was prepared via plateletpheresis and applied in the form of a gel threaded to a suture and placed at the interface between tendon and bone. Outcomes were assessed preoperatively and at 3, 6, 12, and finally at a minimum of 16 months after surgery (at an average of 19.7 ± 1.9 months) with respect to pain, range of motion, strength, and overall satisfaction, and with respect to functional scores as determined using the following scoring systems: the American Shoulder and Elbow Surgeon (ASES) system, the Constant system, the University of California at Los Angeles (UCLA) system, the Disabilities of the Arm, Shoulder and Hand (DASH) system, the Simple Shoulder Test (SST) system, and the Shoulder Pain and Disability Index (SPADI) system. At a minimum of 9 months after surgery, repaired tendon structural integrities were assessed by magnetic resonance imaging.

Results.—Platelet-rich plasma gel application to arthroscopic rotator cuff repairs did not accelerate recovery with respect to pain, range of motion, strength, functional scores, or overall satisfaction as compared with conventional repair at any time point. Whereas magnetic resonance imaging demonstrated a retear rate of 26.7% in the PRP group and 41.2% in the conventional group, there was no statistical significance between the groups ($P = .388$).

Conclusion.—The results suggest that PRP application during arthroscopic rotator cuff repair did not clearly demonstrate accelerated recovery clinically or anatomically except for an improvement in internal rotation. Nevertheless, as the study may have been underpowered to detect clinically important differences in the structural integrity, additional investigations, including the optimization of PRP preparation and a larger randomized study powered for healing rate, are necessary to further determine the effect of PRP (Table 3).

▶ The use of platelet-rich plasma (PRP) is an interesting phenomenon. Its popularity rests primarily in the fact that it is safe; effectiveness is yet to be consistently demonstrated. The question is particularly complex, as there are numerous variations in the active ingredient, the influence of the carrier environment,

TABLE 3.—Comparison of Structural Integrity Evaluated with MRI Between Platelet-Rich Plasma (PRP) and Conventional Groups

		Structural Integrity		
	Tear Size	Healed	Retear	Total
PRP	<30 mm	7 (87.5%)	1 (12.5%)	8
	≥30 mm	4 (57.1%)	3 (42.9%)	7
		11 (73.3%)	4 (26.7%)	15
Conventional	<30 mm	9 (64.3%)	5 (35.7%)	14
	≥30 mm	1 (33.3%)	2 (66.7%)	3
		10 (58.8%)	7 (41.2%)	17

concentration, presence of contaminating cells and molecules, and the like. There appear marked differences referable to these issues as well as pathology and anatomic site. Hence, the perspective of this study that adds an additional variable is the quality, ie, strength, of the repair (Table 3). There is little doubt the value of PRP will emerge with time, largely due to studies such as this.

B. F. Morrey, MD

Arthroscopic Rotator Cuff Repair with and without Acromioplasty in the Treatment of Full-Thickness Rotator Cuff Tears: A Multicenter, Randomized Controlled Trial

MacDonald P, McRae S, Leiter J, et al (Pan Am Clinic and Univ of Manitoba, Winnipeg; Univ of Ottawa, Ontario, Canada)
J Bone Joint Surg Am 93:1953-1960, 2011

Background.—The primary objective of this prospective randomized controlled trial was to compare functional and quality-of-life indices and rates of revision surgery in arthroscopic rotator cuff repair with and without acromioplasty.

Methods.—Eighty-six patients consented and were randomly assigned intraoperatively to one of two study groups, and sixty-eight of them completed the study. The primary outcome was the Western Ontario Rotator Cuff (WORC) index. Secondary outcome measures included the American Shoulder and Elbow Surgeons (ASES) shoulder assessment form and a count of revisions required in each group. Outcome measures were completed preoperatively and at three, six, twelve, eighteen, and twenty-four months after surgery.

Results.—WORC and ASES scores improved significantly in each group over time ($p < 0.001$). There were no differences in WORC or ASES scores between the groups that had arthroscopic cuff repair with or without acromioplasty at any time point. There were no differences in scores on the basis of acromion type, nor were any interaction effects identified between group and acromion type. Four participants (9%) in the group that had arthroscopic cuff repair alone, one with a Type-2 and three with a Type-3 acromion, required additional surgery by the twenty-four-month time point. The number of patients who required additional surgery was greater ($p = 0.05$) in the group that had arthroscopic cuff repair alone than in the group that had arthroscopic cuff repair and acromioplasty.

Conclusions.—Our findings are consistent with previous research reports in which there was no difference in functional and quality-of-life indices for patients who had rotator cuff repair with or without acromioplasty. The higher reoperation rate was found in the group without acromioplasty. Further study that includes follow-up imaging and patient-reported outcomes over a greater follow-up period is needed.

► This is an important study for several reasons. It accepts the hypothesis that arthroscopic rotator cuff repair is accepted, if not the standard of care. That this is a prospective, randomized study is also relatively uncommon in orthopedic circles. For me, the subtle insight of interest that deserves emphasis is the difference between statistical significance and clinical relevance. The conclusion is that acromioplasty shows no statistical value in the setting of rotator cuff tear/repair. Yet, any orthopedic surgeon reviewing the data expressed in Fig 2a and b in the original article would conclude that acromioplasty does offer a marginal value. This is enough for me. Hence I would draw different conclusions than did the authors: acromioplasty is of clinical if not statistical value.

B. F. Morrey, MD

Increasing Incidence of Shoulder Arthroplasty in the United States

Kim SH, Wise BL, Zhang Y, et al (Univ of California at Davis, Sacramento; Musculoskeletal Diseases of Aging Res Group, Sacramento, CA; Boston Univ, MA)

J Bone Joint Surg Am 93:2249-2254, 2011

Background.—The number of total shoulder arthroplasties performed in the United States increased slightly between 1990 and 2000. However, the incidence of shoulder arthroplasty in recent years has not been well described. The purpose of the present study was to examine recent trends in shoulder hemiarthroplasty and total shoulder arthroplasty along with the common reasons for these surgical procedures in the United States.

Methods.—We modeled the incidence of shoulder arthroplasty from 1993 to 2008 with use of the Nationwide Inpatient Sample. On the basis of hemiarthroplasty and total shoulder arthroplasty cases that were identified with use of surgical procedure codes, we conducted a design-based analysis to calculate national estimates.

Results.—While the annual number of hemiarthroplasties grew steadily, the number of total shoulder arthroplasties showed a discontinuous jump ($p < 0.01$) in 2004 and increased with a steeper linear slope ($p < 0.01$) since then. As a result, more total shoulder arthroplasties than hemiarthroplasties have been performed annually since 2006. Approximately 27,000 total shoulder arthroplasties and 20,000 hemiarthroplasties were performed in 2008. More than two-thirds of total shoulder arthroplasties were performed in adults with an age of sixty-five years or more. Osteoarthritis was the primary diagnosis for 43% of hemiarthroplasties and 77% of total shoulder arthroplasties in 2008, with fracture of the humerus as the next most common primary diagnosis leading to hemiarthroplasty.

Conclusions.—The number of shoulder arthroplasties, particularly total shoulder arthroplasties, is growing faster than ever. The use of reverse total arthroplasty, which was approved by the United States Food and Drug Administration in November 2003, may be part of the reason for the greater increase in the number of total shoulder arthroplasties. A long-term follow-up study is warranted to evaluate total shoulder arthroplasty in terms of patient outcomes, safety, and implant longevity.

▶ I have considered including incidence studies such as this one but usually deferred because I wasn't sure of the message. In this instance, I do think there is relevant and thus useful information in this report. The first and most obvious is the exponential increase in the incidence of shoulder replacement in the last 4 years. As the authors accurately point out, this is coincident with the introduction of a new implant philosophy—the reverse shoulder. This truly is an innovation and deserves our admiration. It salvages heretofore unsalvageable conditions. But this would not account for this exponential increase in frequency of replacement (Fig 1 in the original article). The explanation must in part be broadening indications—for primary replacement! This is worrisome for several reasons. First, the reverse shoulder is much more expensive. Possibly more importantly, we see similar trends in hip and knee surgery as well. The concern—can society afford this rate of intervention?

B. F. Morrey, MD

A Complication-based Learning Curve From 200 Reverse Shoulder Arthroplasties

Kempton LB, Ankerson E, Wiater JM (William Beaumont Hosp, MI; William Beaumont Hosp Res Inst, MI)

Clin Orthop Relat Res 469:2496-2504, 2011

Background.—Reported early complication rates in reverse total shoulder arthroplasty have widely varied from 0% to 75% in part due to a lack of standard inclusion criteria. In addition, it is unclear whether revision arthroplasty is associated with a higher rate of complications than primary arthroplasty.

Questions/Purpose.—We therefore (1) determined the types and rates of early complications in reverse total shoulder arthroplasty using defined criteria, (2) characterized an early complication-based learning curve for reverse total shoulder arthroplasty, and (3) determined whether revision arthroplasties result in a higher incidence of complications.

Patients and Methods.—From October 2004 to May 2008, an initial series of 200 reverse total shoulder arthroplasties was performed in 191 patients by a single surgeon. Forty of the 200 arthroplasties were revision arthroplasties. Of these, 192 shoulders were available for minimum 6-month followup (mean, 19.4 months; range, 6–49.2 months). We determined local and systemic complications and distinguished major from minor complications.

Results.—Nineteen shoulders involved local complications (9.9%), including seven major and 12 minor complications. Nine involved perioperative systemic complications (4.7%), including eight major complications and one minor complication. The local complication rate was higher in

TABLE 6.—Complications in Primary Versus Revision Reverse Shoulder Arthroplasties

Type of Complication	Primary Arthroplasty (152 Analyzed)	Revision Arthroplasty (40 Analyzed)	Odds Ratio (95% CI)	p Value*
All local complications	7.9%	17.5%	2.5 (0.9–6.8)	0.080
Major local complications	3.3%	5.0%	1.5 (0.3–8.3)	0.637
Minor local complications	4.6%	12.5%	3.0 (0.9–9.9)	0.133
Transient neuropathies	0.7%	10.0%	16.8 (1.8–154.7)	0.007
Perioperative systemic complications	5.9%	5.0%	0.84 (0.2–4.0)	1.00

*Two-tailed Fisher's exact test; CI = confidence interval.

the first 40 shoulders (23.1%) versus the last 160 shoulders (6.5%). Seven of 40 (17.5%) revision arthroplasties involved local complications, including two major and five minor complications compared to 12 of 152 (7.9%) primary arthroplasties, including five major and seven minor complications. Nerve palsies occurred less frequently in primary arthroplasties (0.6%) compared to revisions (9.8%).

Conclusions.—The early complication-based learning curve for reverse total shoulder arthroplasty is approximately 40 cases. There was a trend toward more complications in revision versus primary reverse total shoulder arthroplasty and more neuropathies in revisions.

Level of Evidence.—Level IV, therapeutic study. See the guidelines online for a complete description of level of evidence (Table 6).

▶ This contribution is both interesting and important because it is rare even to try to document the characteristics of a learning experience. The authors were successful in describing the point at which the complication rate decreased, this being after about 40 cases (Fig 5 in the original article). It is also helpful to see the nature and likelihood of the various complications encountered (Table 6). The authors recognize the shortcomings of this study, specifically the inability to control for confounding variables such as influence of revision cases on the rate and surgeon experience, more than 1 implant design, and a host of pathologic conditions, especially those requiring a revision procedure. Regardless, the work was meticulously performed and clearly presented, making the conclusion of some value to the surgeon undertaking this type of procedure.

B. F. Morrey, MD

6 Total Hip Arthroplasty

Introduction

After decades of successful joint replacement arthroplasty, the topics of today continue to be those of refinement. One of the major controversies known to all is that of the "hard surfaces," specifically metal-on-metal bearings. We may have under-represented the significance of this in the selections this year, but we have made an effort to provide a number of articles that at least characterize the issues. I personally continue to be significantly concerned regarding the implications of the metal ion burden to the solid organs. This is my major reason for never having performed metal-on-metal implants. However, the wear characteristics are so appealing that efforts to mitigate the downside risks will continue. Yet, today the awareness of the usual individual host hyperreaction will continue to dampen the employment of these implants in the near future. The other emphasis of the articles selected this year is that of trends and tendencies of implant usage, much of which is obtained from registry information. It is hoped that you will find value in this section as you determine the best implant and the best approach in your own practice.

Bernard F. Morrey, MD

2010 Mid-America Orthopaedic Association Physician in Training Award: Predictors of Early Adverse Outcomes after Knee and Hip Arthroplasty in Geriatric Patients

Higuera CA, Elsharkawy K, Klika AK, et al (Cleveland Clinic, OH; et al)

Clin Orthop Relat Res 469:1391-1400, 2011

Background.—Geriatric patients experience more adverse events owing to early complications after TKA or THA related to preexisting comorbidities. However, associations between patient and surgery variables, including age, BMI, and comorbidities with complications are unclear. Knowing these relationships is necessary for developing risk stratification, defining contraindications, and predicting complications and adverse outcomes.

Questions/Purposes.—We wished to establish and quantify the associations among age, BMI, comorbidities, and type of surgery and anesthesia with complications and early adverse outcomes including longer length of stay, disposition to an extended care facility, readmission, and reoperation in geriatric patients undergoing TKA and THA.

Patients and Methods.—We prospectively followed a cohort of patients older than 65 years undergoing TKA or THA. Demographics, comorbidities, complications, discharge disposition, readmission, and/or reoperation information within the 90-day postoperative period were collected. Adjusted hierarchical stepwise multivariable regression models were used to analyze associations and relative risks with complications, length of stay, disposition, readmission, and reoperation rates.

Results.—Patients were approximately 40% more likely to have any complication per each subsequent 10 years of age. Patients who underwent bilateral TKAs were 65% more likely to have any type of complication. Patients who had epidural anesthesia were 2.6 times more likely to have a major systemic complication. Patients with coronary artery disease were more likely to have a transfusion, more likely to have major local

TABLE 4.—Regression Models for Complications

Multivariate Predictor	Relative Risk	95% Confidence Interval	p Value
TKA			
All complications			
Age (per 10 years)	1.39	1.17–1.66	0.0003
65–74 years (reference)	1.00	—	—
75–84 years	1.43	1.14–1.80	0.002
85+ years	1.25	0.79–1.98	0.35
Bilateral TKAs (versus TKA)	1.65	1.27–2.15	0.0002
Spinal anesthesia (versus other than spinal)	0.65	0.51–0.81	0.0001
*CCI (per index point)	1.18	1.11–1.26	<0.0001
Coronary artery disease	1.73	1.36–2.21	<0.0001
Minor systemic complications			
Bilateral TKAs (versus TKA)	1.66	1.18–2.35	0.004
Epidural (versus spinal)	1.56	1.12–2.16	0.008
*CCI (per index point)	1.13	1.03–1.24	0.008
Preoperative anemia	1.69	1.25–2.30	0.0007
Major systemic complications			
Epidural (versus other than spinal)	2.65	1.37–5.15	0.004
*CCI (per index point)	1.44	1.24–1.67	<0.0001
Coronary artery disease	2.64	1.38–5.07	0.004
Chronic heart failure	3.15	1.43–6.93	0.005
Major local complications			
Coronary artery disease	5.81	1.27–26.54	0.02
THA			
All complications			
Age (per 10 years)	1.43	1.16–1.77	0.0008
65–74 years (reference)	1.00	—	—
75–84 years	1.45	1.08–1.94	0.01
85 + years	1.79	1.08–2.10	0.02
*CCI (per index point)	1.17	1.07–1.28	0.0006
Coronary artery disease	1.60	1.20–1.40	0.001
Major systemic complications			
*CCI (per index point)	1.73	1.39–2.15	<0.0001
Coronary artery disease	4.31	1.62–11.44	0.003
Chronic heart failure	2.93	1.07–8.05	0.04

*CCI (Charlson Comorbidity Index) evaluated in a separate model without specific comorbidities (ie, coronary artery disease, preoperative anemia, and chronic heart failure).

complications, including joint infection and/or a major systemic complication, and more likely to require a reoperation after TKA.

Conclusions.—Age, type of surgery, anesthesia, and other comorbidities, mainly coronary artery disease and chronic heart failure, were associated with complications and adverse outcomes. We believe these risk factors should be used to counsel patients and make preoperative surgical decisions.

Level of Evidence.—Level II, prognostic study. See Guidelines for Authors for a complete description of levels of evidence (Table 4).

▶ As the reliability of hip and knee replacement continues to improve, or at least stabilize at a very acceptable level, issues such as assessed here are of great importance. Although I do question the relatively small sample size of 550 patients to accurately relate the factors considered, it does have a legitimate statistical analysis that would seem to justify the finding. The categorical risk factors may come as no surprise, but I for one was not expecting coronary artery disease to be the main indicator of potential complications, especially joint infection. It is also of interest that the body mass index has little greater influence on complication than does increased age (Table 4). As the authors indicate, familiarity with these data will assist surgeons in their preoperative counseling of our patients regarding risk/benefit specific to the individual patient.

B. F. Morrey, MD

Assessing patients for joint replacement: can pre-operative Oxford hip and knee scores be used to predict patient satisfaction following joint replacement surgery and to guide patient selection?

Judge A, Arden NK, Price A, et al (Univ of Oxford, UK)

J Bone Joint Surg Br 93-B:1660-1664, 2011

We obtained pre-operative and six-month post-operative Oxford hip (OHS) and knee scores (OKS) for 1523 patients who underwent total hip replacement and 1784 patients who underwent total knee replacement. They all also completed a six-month satisfaction question.

Scatter plots showed no relationship between pre-operative Oxford scores and six-month satisfaction scores. Spearman's rank correlation coefficients were −0.04 (95% confidence interval (CI) −0.09 to 0.01) between OHS and satisfaction and 0.04 (95% CI −0.01 to 0.08) between OKS and satisfaction. A receiver operating characteristic (ROC) curve analysis was used to identify a cut-off point for the pre-operative OHS/OKS that identifies whether or not a patient is satisfied with surgery. We obtained an area under the ROC curve of 0.51 (95% CI 0.45 to 0.56) for hip replacement and 0.56 (95% CI 0.51 to 0.60) for knee replacement, indicating that pre-operative Oxford scores have no predictive accuracy in distinguishing satisfied from dissatisfied patients.

In the NHS widespread attempts are being made to use patient-reported outcome measures (PROMs) data for the purpose of prioritising patients for surgery. Oxford hip and knee scores have no predictive accuracy in relation to post-operative patient satisfaction. This evidence does not support their current use in prioritising access to care.

▶ This interesting article was chosen for review not because of its positive findings but because of the topic. Although it is from the United Kingdom and is oriented to that population, it is not specific to them. If accountable care organizations or some variation do eventually emerge as a required format for practice, outcomes and selection criteria will be required. Hence, the lack of correlation to accepted and validated hip and knee scores serves to caution us, and hopefully administrators, about the difficulty in reliably achieving the expected goal: cost-effective, evidence-based medicine.

B. F. Morrey, MD

Does Ipsilateral Knee Pain Improve after Hip Arthroplasty?

Wang W, Geller JA, Nyce JD, et al (New York-Presbyterian Hosp at Columbia Univ, NY)

Clin Orthop Relat Res 470:578-583, 2012

Background.—Intraarticular hip disease is commonly acknowledged as a cause of ipsilateral knee pain. However, this is based primarily on observational rather than high-quality evidence-based studies, and it is unclear whether ipsilateral knee pain improves when hip disease has been treated.

Questions/Purposes.—We asked whether (1) hip disease was associated with preoperative ipsilateral knee pain and (2) ipsilateral knee pain would improve after hip arthroplasty.

Patients and Methods.—We retrospectively assessed knee pain in 255 patients who underwent hip arthroplasties between 2006 and 2008. The WOMAC pain score of each joint was the primary outcome measure, which was obtained prospectively before surgery and at 3 months and 1 year postoperatively. Of the 255 patients, 245 (96%) had followup data obtained at 3 months or 1 year.

Results.—Preoperatively, ipsilateral knee pain was observed more frequently than contralateral knee pain (55% versus 18%). Preoperative ipsilateral knee pain scores were worse than contralateral knee pain scores (mean, 80 versus 95). Ipsilateral knee pain improved at 3 months and 1 year. When compared with the scores for contralateral knee pain at 3 months (95) and 1 year (96), there were no differences between knees.

Conclusions.—Our observations suggest hip disease is associated with ipsilateral knee pain and that it improves after hip arthroplasty. This should be considered during preoperative evaluation for patients with hip and knee pain.

Level of Evidence.—Level III, diagnostic study. See Guidelines for Authors for a complete description of levels of evidence.

▶ I really like these kinds of studies. A simple, clinically relevant question is addressed, and answered. The investigators have adequate power and follow-up data to conclude that yes, ipsilateral knee pain is statistically significantly improved by hip replacement. This improvement persists for at least a year (Fig 2 in the original article). In my practice, the more common question has been, in the setting of bilateral involvement, are the contralateral joint symptoms made better or worse with replacement of the more severe joint? My experience is this can go either way, but because patients experience such pain relief, they more often than not request the contralateral joint be addressed sooner rather than later.

B. F. Morrey, MD

Does cementing the femoral component increase the risk of peri-operative mortality for patients having replacement surgery for a fracture of the neck of femur? Data from the National Hip Fracture Database

Costa ML, Griffin XL, Pendleton N, et al (Natl Hip Fracture Database, UK)
J Bone Joint Surg Br 93-B:1405-1410, 2011

Concerns have been reported to the United Kingdom National Patient Safety Agency, warning that cementing the femoral component during hip replacement surgery for fracture of the proximal femur may increase peri-operative mortality.

The National Hip Fracture Database collects demographic and outcome data about patients with a fracture of the proximal femur from over 100 participating hospitals in the United Kingdom. We conducted a mixed effects logistic regression analysis of this dataset to determine whether peri-operative mortality was increased in patients who had undergone either hemiarthroplasty or total hip replacement using a cemented femoral component. A total of 16 496 patients from 129 hospitals were included in the analysis, which showed a small but significant adjusted survival benefit associated with cementing (odds ratio 0.83, 95% confidence interval 0.72 to 0.96). Other statistically significant variables in predicting death at discharge, listed in order of magnitude of effect, were gender, American Society of Anesthesiologists grade, age, walking accompanied outdoors and arthroplasty. Interaction terms between cementing and these other variables were sequentially added to, but did not improve, the model.

This study has not shown an increase in peri-operative mortality as a result of cementing the femoral component in patients requiring hip replacement following fracture of the proximal femur.

► We remember the well-worn phrase "nothing interferes with good outcomes like accurate data." With the ever-increasing tendency, at least in the United States, to manage all femoral pathology with uncemented devices, this study is refreshing. It also continues to demonstrate the strength of national registries. This assessment of 16 500 procedures not only fails to reveal a higher failure rate or an increase in mortality of the cemented femoral stem for acute fracture in the older patient, it actually reveals a slightly but meaningfully lower complication rate in the cemented group of patients.

Although this study will not reverse the trend, it should make us stop and think. Sadly, an increasing number of surgeons do not even know how to cement a femoral stem!

B. F. Morrey, MD

Comparative Survival of Uncemented Acetabular Components Following Primary Total Hip Arthroplasty

Howard JL, Kremers HM, Loechler YA, et al (London Health Sciences Centre, Ontario, Canada; Mayo Clinic, Rochester, MN)

J Bone Joint Surg Am 93:1597-1604, 2011

Background.—Since their initial introduction in the early 1980s, uncemented acetabular components have become the preferred implant type for the majority of hip arthroplasties performed in the United States. The purpose of the present study was to compare differences in the survival of uncemented acetabular components following primary total hip arthroplasty.

Methods.—The study population included 7989 patients who had undergone 9584 primary total hip arthroplasties with twenty different types of uncemented acetabular components at the Mayo Clinic from January 1984 to December 2004. The overall rate of survival as well as the rate of survival free of revision for specific reasons (aseptic loosening, wear, osteolysis) were compared among the different components using age and sex-adjusted Cox proportional hazards regression models.

Results.—The risk of acetabular cup revision was significantly higher for beaded and hydroxyapatite-coated designs as compared with titanium wire mesh designs. Cross-linked polyethylene performed better than conventional polyethylene, but this finding did not reach significance. Elevated liners were associated with a significantly higher risk of cup revision due to aseptic loosening.

Conclusions.—There are significant differences in the long-term survival of different types of uncemented acetabular components following total hip arthroplasty. The increased risk of revisions in the second decade after the initial total hip arthroplasty is a concern and is largely due to a steady increase in revisions because of polyethylene wear, osteolysis, and component loosening more than ten years after the time of the index arthroplasty.

▶ This is a really good article. This is not because it came from my department and was written by my partners. It assesses an important question with almost 10 000 procedures followed over a 20-year period! The findings are truly relevant. First, longevity is design specific (Fig 1A in the original article). Second, the more recent designs are better than the first generation (Fig 1B in the original article). Third, differences in design of current implants will not be seen before 10 years (Fig 1B in the original article). The authors provide extensive detail. The article must be read in its entirety, but, note the increased incidence of problems with the elevated liner. We had hypothesized this in the past, but only long-term surveillance of large numbers was able to confirm the theoretical concern. The message, among many, is that elevated liners are not free. Use when, but only when, needed.

B. F. Morrey, MD

A comparison of a less invasive piriformis-sparing approach *versus* the standard posterior approach to the hip: A randomised controlled trial

Khan RJK, Maor D, Hofmann M, et al (Sir Charles Gairdner Hosp, Nedlands, Australia)

J Bone Joint Surg Br 94-B:43-50, 2012

We undertook a randomised controlled trial to compare the piriformis-sparing approach with the standard posterior approach used for total hip replacement (THR). We recruited 100 patients awaiting THR and randomly allocated them to either the piriformis-sparing approach or the standard posterior approach. Pre- and post-operative care programmes and rehabilitation regimes were identical for both groups. Observers were blinded to the allocation throughout; patients were blinded until the two-week assessment. Follow-up was at six weeks, three months, one year and two years. In all 11 patients died or were lost to follow-up.

There was no significant difference between groups for any of the functional outcomes. However, for patients in the piriformis-sparing group there was a trend towards a better six-minute walk test at two weeks and greater patient satisfaction at six weeks. The acetabular components were less anteverted ($p = 0.005$) and had a lower mean inclination angle ($p = 0.02$) in the piriformis-sparing group. However, in both groups the mean component positions were within Lewinnek's safe zone. Surgeons perceived the piriformis-sparing approach to be significantly more difficult than the standard approach ($p = 0.03$), particularly in obese patients.

In conclusion, performing THR through a shorter incision involving sparing piriformis is more difficult and only provides short-term benefits compared with the standard posterior approach.

► As the orthopedic community continues to consider and even struggle with the issue of optimum exposure for hip replacement, studies such as this are rather few and far between. I was attracted to this contribution, as it represented a true prospective, randomized study, with objective and discrete endpoints. Hence, the findings are of no real difference, other than that in the short term. With considerably more difficulty is the piriformis-sparing approach accomplished, which would lead one to conclude there is limited value in the more difficult exposure. Enough said.

B. F. Morrey, MD

Patient Experiences as Knowledge for the Evidence Base: A Qualitative Approach to Understanding Patient Experiences Regarding the Use of Regional Anesthesia for Hip and Knee Arthroplasty

Webster F, Bremner S, McCartney CJL (Univ of Toronto, Ontario, Canada)
Reg Anesth Pain Med 36:461-465, 2011

Background and Objectives.—It is reported that patients continue to have misgivings about regional anesthesia (RA) despite strong evidence to support its use for hip and knee replacement surgery. To date, no one has had an opportunity to study the experiences of patients who have undergone both types of anesthesia for these procedures.

Methods.—Using descriptive qualitative methods, 12 patients who had hip or knee replacements under both RA and GA at two different time points (excluding revisions) were interviewed using purposeful sampling until saturation had been reached. Following transcription of each tape, a small study team met over the course of several months to read and discuss each transcript. A coding template was developed, and emerging themes noted.

Results.—For the majority of patients, RA was either well tolerated or preferred. Having a previous negative experience with general anesthesia was common and was strongly associated with a patient's satisfaction with RA. Patients also described being highly influenced by the preference of their surgeon.

Conclusions.—These findings have important implications. First, many patients were surprisingly neutral about the procedure and seemed more fearful of anesthesia in general rather than of either technique specifically. This finding, combined with patient's influence by clinician preference, underscores the importance of physician support for RA. Some participants identified one of their misgivings about RA as being fear of being awake, which is consistent with the medical literature. Our findings also support the idea that from a patient's perspective, appropriate sedation while undergoing RA may be important.

▶ I didn't see that coming! How often have we heard that. I found myself thinking this when I read this article. Trends in health care will continue to place emphasis on outcomes and on subjective satisfaction. I do think there is value in surgeons realizing that fear of anesthesia exceeds fear of the surgery itself. The take-home issues are 2-fold.

First, there are considerations we do not appreciate that are beyond our control and that influence our intervention. Second, be aware and sensitive to number 1.

B. F. Morrey, MD

A Short Tapered Stem Reduces Intraoperative Complications in Primary Total Hip Arthroplasty

Molli RG, Lombardi AV Jr, Berend KR, et al (Joint Implant Surgeons Inc, New Albany, OH; et al)

Clin Orthop Relat Res 470:450-461, 2012

Background.—While short-stem design is not a new concept, interest has surged with increasing utilization of less invasive techniques. Short stems are easier to insert through small incisions. Reliable long-term results including functional improvement, pain relief, and implant survival have been reported with standard tapered stems, but will a short taper perform as well?

Questions/Purposes.—We compared short, flat-wedge, tapered, broach-only femoral stems to standard-length, double-tapered, ream and broach femoral stems in terms of intraoperative complications, short-term survivorship, and pain and function scores.

Patients and Methods.—We retrospectively reviewed the records of 606 patients who had 658 THAs using a less invasive direct lateral approach from January 2006 to March 2008. Three hundred sixty patients (389 hips) had standard-length stems and 246 (269 hips) had short stems. Age averaged 63 years, and body mass index averaged 30.7 kg/m^2. We recorded complications and pain and function scores and computed short-term survival. Minimum followup was 0.8 months (mean, 29.2 months; range, 0.8–62.2 months).

Results.—We observed a higher rate of intraoperative complications with the standard-length stems (3.1%; three trochanteric avulsions, nine femoral fractures) compared with the shorter stems (0.4%; one femoral fracture) and managed all complications with application of one or more cerclage cables. There were no differences in implant survival, Harris hip score, and Lower Extremity Activity Scale score between groups.

Conclusions.—Fewer intraoperative complications occurred with the short stems, attesting to the easier insertion of these devices. While longer followup is required, our early results suggest shortened stems can be used with low complication rates and do not compromise the survival and functional outcome of cementless THA.

Level of Evidence.—Level III, therapeutic study. See the Guidelines for Authors for a complete description of levels of evidence (Table 2).

▶ Right up front I must admit to my potential conflict as we designed a non-stemmed metaphyseal implant in 1983 (the Mayo Conservative Hip TM). Since the patent has died, there has been a plethora of metaphyseal implants appearing on the market. Although there is a growing body of evidence to document their effectiveness, the perspective of this article is a bit different. It focuses on complications. The sample size is reasonable and the comparison is with a similar design, just stemmed. That the stemless implant, at least in this experience, had rather markedly fewer complications (Table 2) should at least prompt the reader to consider this option, the main reason being that outcome results are

TABLE 2.—Results for Standard-Length Taper and Short Taper Stem Groups

Parameter	Standard-Length Stem Group	Short-Stem Group	p Value
Intraoperative complications (number)	12 (3.1%)	1 (0.4%)	0.013
Avulsion of trochanter	3	0	
Femoral fracture Type I	7	1	
Femoral fracture Type II	0	0	
Femoral fracture Type III	2	0	
Average operative time (minutes)	69.5	67.4	0.162
Average estimated blood loss (mL)	146.8	140.9	0.332
Average hemoglobin at discharge (g/dL)	11.1	11.0	0.328
Average length of acute stay (days)	2.1	2.0	0.184
Discharge disposition (number)			0.181
Not available	21 (5.4%)	15 (5.6%)	
Home	263 (67.6%)	189 (70.3%)	
Home with home health or therapy	14 (3.6%)	15 (5.6%)	
Home with outpatient therapy	2 (0.5%)	4 (1.5%)	
Skilled nursing facility	87 (22.4%)	44 (16.4%)	
Transferred to acute care	2 (0.5%)	2 (0.7%)	
Average clinical preoperative (points)			
HHS pain (0–44)	13.8	13.0	0.077
HHS total (0–100)	50.0	49.9	0.980
LEAS score (1–18)	9.1	9.3	0.772
Average clinical at 6 weeks postoperatively (points)			
HHS pain (0–44)	37.6	38.5	0.181
HHS total (0–100)	75.8	75.4	0.674
LEAS score (1–18)	7.7	7.8	0.784
Average clinical at most recent followup (points)			
HHS pain (0–44)	38.5	38.0	0.496
HHS total (0–100)	83.8	83.1	0.570
LEAS score (1–18)	10.1	9.8	0.384
Reoperations (number)	5 (1.3%)	6 (2.2%)	0.156
Incision and débridement, wound issue	0	3 (1.1%)	0.068
Cup revision, loosening	3 (0.8%)	2 (0.7%)	0.347
Cup revision, metal sensitivity	1	0	0.591
Stem revision, fracture	1	0	0.591
Full revision, sepsis	0	1	0.409

HHS = Harris hip score; LEAS = Lower Extremity Activity Scale.

also similar, at least. Time will tell, but as noted here, and as performed in my practice, if the shaft does not need to be accessed, a less-invasive approach may be used. This has been my practice for more than 20 years.

B. F. Morrey, MD

Birmingham hip resurfacing at a mean of ten years: Results from an independent centre

Coulter G, Young DA, Dalziel RE, et al (Melbourne Orthopaedic Group, Australia)

J Bone Joint Surg Br 94-B:315-321, 2012

We report the findings of an independent review of 230 consecutive Birmingham hip resurfacings (BHRs) in 213 patients (230 hips) at a mean follow-up of 10.4 years (9.6 to 11.7). A total of 11 hips underwent revision; six patients (six hips) died from unrelated causes; and 13 patients (16 hips) were lost to follow-up. The survival rate for the whole cohort was 94.5% (95% confidence interval (CI) 90.1 to 96.9). The survival rate in women was 89.1% (95% CI 79.2 to 94.4) and in men was 97.5% (95% CI 92.4 to 99.2). Women were 1.4 times more likely to suffer failure than men. For each millimetre increase in component size there was a 19% lower chance of a failure. The mean Oxford hip score was 45.0 (median 47.0, 28 to 48); mean University of California, Los Angeles activity score was 7.4 (median 8.0, 3 to 9); mean patient satisfaction score was 1.4 (median 1.0, 0 to 9). A total of eight hips had lysis in the femoral neck and two hips had acetabular lysis. One hip had progressive radiological changes around the peg of the femoral component. There was no evidence of progressive neck narrowing between five and ten years.

Our results confirm that BHR provides good functional outcome and durability for men, at a mean follow-up of ten years. We are now reluctant to undertake hip resurfacing in women with this implant.

▶ Debate regarding the metal-on-metal bearing continues unabated. We do know that not all such articulations are created equal. To find truth, large samples followed up for long periods reported by nonconflicted surgeons are essential elements of the report. This may satisfy those criteria. Hence, the findings are useful. It is truly rare to find men outperforming women in joint replacement survival, but this does appear to be the case with this design (Fig 4 in the original article). The authors report a modest 10 of 155 having radiographic osteolysis at 10 years, 8 of which are on the femoral side of the joint. The finding of better outcomes with larger implants is also worthwhile information. Overall this is a well-done study and can serve as a benchmark for others.

B. F. Morrey, MD

Cobalt and Chromium Levels in Blood and Urine Following Hip Resurfacing Arthroplasty with the Conserve Plus Implant

Kim PR, Beaulé PE, Dunbar M, et al (The Ottawa Hosp—General Campus, Ontario, Canada; QEII Health Sciences Centre, Halifax, Nova Scotia, Canada; et al)

J Bone Joint Surg Am 93:107-117, 2011

Background.—The purpose of the present study was to determine cobalt and chromium ion levels in the blood and urine of patients in whom a modern-generation metal-on-metal hip resurfacing device had been implanted.

Methods.—A total of ninety-seven patients with a Conserve Plus metal-on-metal hip resurfacing implant were followed prospectively for two years. Cobalt and chromium levels in erythrocytes, serum, and urine were measured preoperatively as well as three, six, twelve, and twenty-four months postoperatively.

Results.—The median serum cobalt and chromium ion levels were 1.04 μg/L (range, 0.31 to 7.42 μg/L) and 2.00 μg/L (range, 0.28 to 10.49 μg/L), respectively, at one year after surgery and 1.08 μg/L (range, 0.44 to 7.13 μg/L) and 1.64 μg/L (range, 0.47 to 10.95 μg/L), respectively, at two years after surgery. The corresponding mean levels (and standard deviations) of serum cobalt and chromium were 1.68 ± 1.66 μg/L and 2.70 ± 2.22 μg/L, respectively, at one year after surgery and 1.79 ± 1.66 μg/L and 2.70 ± 2.37 μg/L, respectively, at two years after surgery.

Conclusions.—These levels compare favorably with other published ion results for metal-on-metal hip resurfacing and replacement implants. No pseudotumors or other adverse soft-tissue reactions were encountered in our study population. Further research is needed to determine the clinical importance of increased cobalt and chromium ion levels in serum and urine following metal-on-metal hip resurfacing (Table 2).

▶ The issue of metal-on-metal bearing is well recognized by all. I'm not sure this article changes anything but is included to make the point that these bearings

TABLE 2.—Median and Mean Cobalt and Chromium Ion Levels in Erythrocytes, Serum, and Urine Prior to Surgery and at Three, Six, Twelve, and Twenty-four Months After Surgery

	Chromium					
	N*	Erythrocyte Level *(μg/L)*	N*	Serum Level *(μg/L)*	N*	Urine Level *(μg/L)*
Median (range)						
Preop	97	1.00 (0.50 to 4.10)	71	0.19 (0.10 to 0.93)	61	0.19 (0.01 to 1.26)
3 months	83	1.30† (0.40 to 3.50)	63	1.62† (0.10 to 20.16)	50	2.39† (0.04 to 20.00)
6 months	79	1.10 (0.40 to 3.40)	66	1.98† (0.46 to 17.31)	55	3.05† (1.09 to 12.71)
12 months	73	1.30 (0.40 to 2.90)	64	2.00†‡ (0.28 to 10.49)	51	3.42†‡ (0.61 to 21.10)
24 months	47	1.10 (0.40 to 2.60)	41	1.64†‡ (0.47 to 10.95)	35	4.21†§ (1.02 to 12.82)
Mean (standard deviation)						
Preop.	97	1.19 (0.68)	71	0.23 (0.16)	61	0.25 (0.22)
3 months	83	1.40 (0.65)	63	2.14 (2.61)	50	3.75 (3.78)
6 months	79	1.34 (0.68)	66	2.79 (2.87)	55	4.10 (3.03)
12 months	73	1.30 (0.56)	64	2.70 (2.22)	51	4.58 (3.96)
24 months	47	1.20 (0.57)	41	2.70 (2.37)	35	4.91 (3.14)

Cobalt					
Erythrocyte N*	Level (mg/L)	Serum N*	Level (mg/L)	Urine N*	Level (mg/L)
97	0.10 (0.04 to 0.41)	71	0.08 (0.03 to 0.86)	60	0.27 (0.03 to 3.48)
83	0.64† (0.26 to 16.50)	63	0.92† (0.09 to 49.05)	50	7.86† (0.01 to 74.49)
79	0.63† (0.25 to 37.80)	67	1.04† (0.36 to 12.78)	55	7.38† (0.54 to 41.48)
73	0.78†‡§ (0.25 to 5.32)	64	1.04†‡ (0.31 to 7.42)	51	8.52† (0.62 to 61.44)
48	0.75†‡ (0.21 to 2.98)	41	1.08†‡ (0.44 to 7.13)	35	9.88† (0.98 to 78.84)
97	0.11 (0.05)	71	0.11 (0.10)	60	0.46 (0.59)
83	0.92 (1.79)	63	1.94 (6.11)	50	11.63 (13.89)
79	1.29 (4.21)	67	1.63 (1.86)	55	11.47 (10.53)
73	1.07 (1.02)	64	1.68 (1.66)	51	11.94 (11.52)
48	1.02 (0.75)	41	1.79 (1.66)	35	12.72 (13.62)

*N = number of subjects available for calculating the mean or median levels of chromium and cobalt.
†Significantly different from preoperative level ($p < 0.05$; Wilcoxon signed-rank test).
‡Significantly different from postoperative level at three months ($p < 0.05$; Wilcoxon signed-rank test).
§Significantly different from postoperative level at six months ($p < 0.05$; Wilcoxon signed-rank test).

do cause increased ion concentrations in the serum, erythrocytes, and urine (Table 2). Others have shown similar findings with elevated concentrations in the solid organs. Although the sample is small, less than 100, and moderate dropout occurred at the 24-month period, the fact that no clinical adverse effects were documented is worthy of note. This suggests the problems may be design specific, to some extent. The extreme reactions and documented toxicity would seem to further implicate marked individual host variation in sensitivity to ion exposure.

B. F. Morrey, MD

Accelerating failure rate of the ASR total hip replacement

Langton DJ, Jameson SS, Joyce TJ, et al (Univ Hosp of North Tees, Stockton, UK)

J Bone Joint Surg [Br] 93-B:1011-1016, 2011

There is widespread concern regarding the incidence of adverse soft-tissue reactions after metal-on-metal (MoM) hip replacement. Recent National Joint Registry data have shown clear differences in the rates of failure of different designs of hip resurfacing. Our aim was to update the failure rates related to metal debris for the Articular Surface Replacement (ASR). A total of 505 of these were implanted.

Kaplan-Meier analysis showed a failure rate of 25% at six years for the ASR resurfacing and of 48.8% for the ASR total hip replacement (THR). Of 257 patients with a minimum follow-up of two years, 67 (26.1%) had a serum cobalt concentration which was greater than 7 µg/l. Co-ordinate measuring machine analysis of revised components showed that all patients suffering adverse tissue reactions in the resurfacing group had abnormal wear of the bearing surfaces. Six THR patients had relatively low rates of articular wear, but were found to have considerable damage at the trunion-taper interface. Our results suggest that wear at the modular junction is an important factor in the development of adverse tissue reactions after implantation of a large-diameter MoM THR.

▶ While it may seem inclusion of this study is an expression of jumping on the metal bearing bashing bandwagon, I have long expressed my reservation regarding the metal-on-metal bearing, whether resurfacing or modular in design. It is encouraging to see the National-Registry performing in the manner desired—identity of uncommon problems by aggregating data and sources. The findings are rather striking, confirmatory but with an added twist. The failure rates seen with both resurfacing and modular metal articular designs are striking (Fig 2 in the original article). The study also seems to define a critical head size for the modular design to be no more than 53 mm in diameter (Fig 3 in the original article). Finally, the authors note that some of the adverse reaction and debris originate from the trunion, not just from the articular interface. Regardless, there are continued worrisome findings for the metal articular implant.

B. F. Morrey, MD

A MRI classification of periprosthetic soft tissue masses (pseudotumours) associated with metal-on-metal resurfacing hip arthroplasty

Hauptfleisch J, Pandit H, Grammatopoulos G, et al (Oxford Univ Hosps NHS Trust, UK; Univ of Oxford, UK)

Skeletal Radiol 41:149-155, 2012

Objective.—Metal-on-metal hip resurfacing arthroplasty (MoMHRA) has become a popular option for young patients requiring hip replacement. A recognised complication is the formation of a symptomatic reactive periprosthetic soft tissue mass (pseudotumour). We present a radiological classification system for these reactive masses, dividing them into three groups: Type I are thin-walled cystic masses (cyst wall <3 mm), Type II are thick-walled cystic masses (cyst wall >3 mm, but less than the diameter of the cystic component) and Type III are predominantly solid masses.

Materials and Methods.—We reviewed all MRI performed over a 4-year period in patients with primary MoMHRA referred to our institution. In all cases the masses were assessed on MRI according to size, anatomical position, signal intensity and involvement of bone, muscle or neighbouring neurovascular bundles.

Results.—Periprosthetic masses were seen in 33 hips in 17 female (7 bilateral) and 8 male patients (1 bilateral). The Type I lesions were the most common and more likely to be posterior to the hip joint. The Type III masses were significantly larger than the cystic lesions and were more likely to be located anterior to the hip joint. To date 22 patients have undergone revision surgery with conversions to total hip replacement. Severity of symptoms and revision rates were lowest in the Type I group and highest in the Type III group.

Conclusion.—Solid anterior pseudotumours were most likely to have the more severe symptoms and require revision surgery.

▶ There are several important insights from this study. It documents a fairly large number (33) of symptomatic hips with metal bearings, 22 of which resulted in a revision. While the incidence of the indication for magnetic resonance imaging, symptomatic painful total hip arthroplasty, is not stated, the literature places this at 1% to 4%. The classification into type 1 (Fig 1 in the original article), type 2 (Fig 2 in the original article), and type 3 (Fig 3 in the original article) is helpful, first to realize that type 1 is usually asymptomatic, and second that type 3 will typically require revision. Unfortunately, we do not have good insight as to the nature or rate of progression from one type to another. Regardless, this does offer further insight as to the nature and management of this ever more worrisome complication of the metal articulated hip.

B. F. Morrey, MD

Allergic complications from orthopaedic joint implants: the role of delayed hypersensitivity to benzoyl peroxide in bone cement

Bircher A, Friederich NF, Seelig W, et al (Univ Basel, Switzerland; Kantonsspital Bruderholz, Bottmingen, Switzerland; Hirslanden Klinik Birshof, Münchenstein, Switzerland)

Contact Dermatitis 66:20-26, 2012

Background.—Orthopaedic implants and osteosynthesis materials are increasingly being used. Complications include mainly physical–mechanical problems and infections. Uncommonly, an allergic reaction towards an alloy metal or a bone cement component has been implicated. Potential bone cement allergens include acrylates, benzoyl peroxide, *N,N*-dimethyl-*p*-toluidine, and gentamicin. Typical symptoms are pain, swelling, inflammatory skin reactions, implant loosening, and fistula formation.

Objectives.—To report on 5 patients with complications from a knee or a shoulder joint implant in whom a relevant sensitization to benzoyl peroxide was shown.

Methods.—Patch tests were performed with the European baseline series, an extended metal series, and a bone cement series. Patch tests with benzoyl peroxide were performed twice in all patients. A bone cement-free replacement was chosen in sensitized patients.

Results.—In 4 patients sensitized to benzoyl peroxide, a bone cement-free replacement resulted in a considerable decrease or disappearance of pain and swelling, and complete clearing of cutaneous symptoms.

Conclusions.—Components of bone cement, such as benzoyl peroxide, may rarely cause allergic complications. However, because of the irritant potential of these substances, careful performance, reading and interpretation of the patch tests is required.

► This is a case study, which I rarely review for the YEAR BOOK. However, this is an important contribution because it reports, confirms, and discusses a hot topic in hip replacement: allergic reaction. Years ago, I was concerned that a few of my patients may have been allergic to the cement, but I could not prove it. This simple report confirms that this is possible and does rarely occur, with benzoyl peroxide being primarily implicated.

Sadly, even cementing an implant in place does not guarantee against host reaction.

B. F. Morrey, MD

Measurement of leg length discrepancy after total hip arthroplasty. The reliability of a plain radiographic method compared to CT-scanogram

Kjellberg M, Al-Amiry B, Englund E, et al (Sundsvall Hosp, Sweden; Karolinska Univ Hosp, Huddinge, Stockholm, Sweden; Västernorrland County, Sundsvall, Sweden)

Skeletal Radiol 41:187-191, 2012

Objective.—To measure the interobserver reliability and intraobserver reproducibility of post total hip arthroplasty (THA) leg length discrepancy (LLD) measurement on radiographs as well as to evaluate its accuracy by comparing it with LLD measurement on computed tomographic scanogram (CT-scanogram).

Materials and Methods.—In this prospective study, postoperative LLD measurements in ten THA patients were made by four observers on anteroposterior radiographs of the pelvis (inter-teardrop line to the tip of lesser trochanter) and compared to LLD measurements made on CT-scanogram scout views of the lower limb. Two observers repeated the LLD measurements on radiographs 8 weeks after the first measurements. The interobserver reliability of the LLD measurement on plain radiographs was evaluated by comparing the measurements of the four observers and the intraobserver reproducibility by comparing the two repeated measurements made by the two observers.

Results.—We found excellent interobserver reliability (mean ICC 0.83) and intraobserver reproducibility (ICC 0.90 and 0.88) of the LLD measurements on plain radiographs. There was a moderate to excellent agreement, but with wide variation of measurements among the four observers, when plain radiographic measurement was compared with CT-scanogram (ICC 0.58, 0.60, 0.71, and 0.82).

Conclusion.—Despite the excellent interobserver reliability and intraobserver reproducibility of LLD measurement on radiographs, clinicians

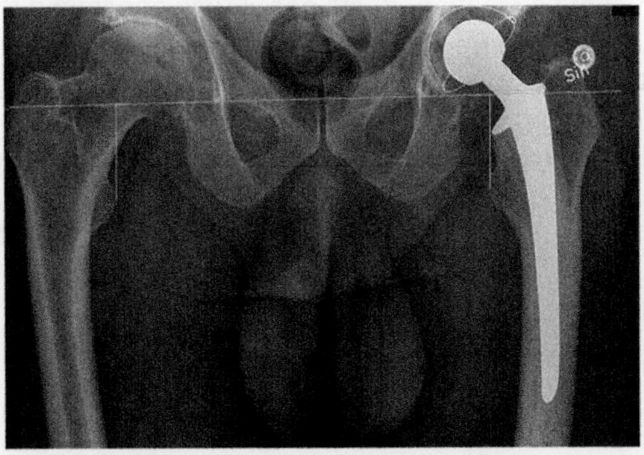

FIGURE 1.—Radiographic measurement method. The LLD was defined as the difference in perpendicular distance in millimeters between a line passing through the lower edge of the teardrop points to the corresponding tip of the lesser trochanter. (Reprinted from Kjellberg M, Al-Amiry B, Englund E, et al. Measurement of leg length discrepancy after total hip arthroplasty. The reliability of a plain radiographic method compared to CT-scanogram. *Skeletal Radiol.* 2012;41:187-191, with permission from ISS.)

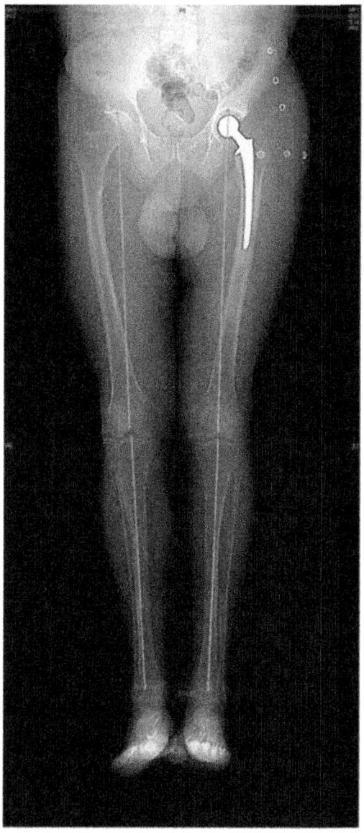

FIGURE 2.—CT-scanogram measurement method. The LLD was defined as the difference in millimeters between the sum of the femoral and tibial lengths on the operated leg versus the contralateral side. The femoral length at the operated side was measured from the upper edge of the acetabular cup to the lower edge of the intercondylar notch and on the contralateral side from the top of the femoral head to the lower edge of the intercondylar notch. On both sides, the tibial length was measured from the center of the intercondylar eminence to the center of the tibial plafond. (Reprinted from Kjellberg M, Al-Amiry B, Englund E, et al. Measurement of leg length discrepancy after total hip arthroplasty. The reliability of a plain radiographic method compared to CT-scanogram. *Skeletal Radiol.* 2012;41:187-191, with permission from ISS.)

should be aware of its limited accuracy when compared to CT-scanogram (Fig 1 and 2).

▶ Leg length inequality (LLD) seems to be much less discussed lately. This is good, since in the past LLD has been a major cause of lawsuits after hip replacement. There are numerous ways to ensure accurate technique preoperatively or intraoperatively, but once the procedure is finished, the clinician faces the issue of the patient's perception of LLD based on what is seen on the images. The issue is of course complex and involves preoperative LLD, fixed pelvic obliquity, and similar issues. This study is useful in that it allows the clinician some confidence when using the plane anteroposterior pelvis radiograph to estimate leg lengths (Fig 1), with the same statistical confidence as that rendered by the gold standard, the scanogram (Fig 2). This has been my practice, and now it has scientific validity.

B. F. Morrey, MD

COX-2 Inhibitors for the Prevention of Heterotopic Ossification After THA

Vasileiadis GI, Sioutis IC, Mavrogenis AF, et al (Athens Univ Med School, Greece; Asklipieion General Hosp, Voula, Athens, Greece)

Orthopedics 34:467, 2011

Nonsteroidal anti-inflammatory drugs (NSAIDs) may prevent heterotopic ossification after total hip arthroplasty (THA). Cyclooxygenase 2 (COX-2) inhibitors may minimize side effects. The goal of this review was to compare the effectiveness and side effects of the perioperative use of selective COX-2 inhibitors with those of conventional NSAIDs in patients undergoing THA. We followed the systematic reviews' updated methods of the Cochrane Collaboration Back Review Group and searched MEDLINE, EMBASE, and Cochrane Central Register of Controlled Trials. We identified all randomized controlled trials until April 2009 enrolling THA patients and comparing COX-2 inhibitors to NSAIDs. We assessed their methodological quality and extracted data. Five randomized controlled trials were included. Prevention of heterotopic ossification and side effects with COX-2 inhibitors were significant in 2 studies. Discontinuation for side effects was not significant. COX-2 inhibitors do not prevent heterotopic ossification after THA significantly better than conventional NSAIDs, while they are advantageous regarding side effects.

▶ The presence of heterotopic ossification (HO) after total hip arthroplasty is variable, reported as 10% to 50%. The key is the extent and significance. Regardless, it is, or can be, a problem in approximately 5% of patients. Prevention is a source of debate. The use of nonsteroidal anti-inflammatory drugs (NSAIDs) has been regularly discussed. The question is refined in this study, specifically using a COX-2 inhibitor. The Cochrane reports and methodology are of questionable value to orthopedics, in my opinion. Regardless, the COX-2 appears ineffective, but safe. Who knows? I personally do not use NSAIDs for HO prevention and favor radiation.

B. F. Morrey, MD

An Articulating Antibiotic Spacer Controls Infection and Improves Pain and Function in a Degenerative Septic Hip

Fleck EE, Spangehl MJ, Rapuri VR, et al (Mayo Clinic Arizona, Phoenix)

Clin Orthop Relat Res 469:3055-3064, 2011

Background.—Treating septic arthritis of the hip with coexisting advanced degenerative disease is challenging. The use of primary total hip arthroplasty (THA) has led to postoperative infection rates as high as 22%. Insertion of antibiotic spacers with subsequent reimplantation of a THA controls infection and improves pain and function in patients with periprosthetic infections.

Questions/Purposes.—We asked whether two-stage exchange for patients with degenerative joint disease (DJD) and coexisting septic arthritis would control infection and improve pain relief and function both during the period after insertion of the spacer and after conversion to THA.

Methods.—We retrospectively reviewed 14 patients with severe DJD and either active or recent septic arthritis treated with débridement and insertion of a primary antibiotic-loaded cement spacer between 1996 and 2008. Ten patients underwent subsequent exchange to a permanent hip arthroplasty. Four patients did not undergo exchange to a permanent THA: two died from unrelated causes and two elected not to proceed with exchange because their spacer provided adequate function. We obtained a modified Harris hip score. The minimum clinical followup was 7 months (average, 28 months; range, 7–65 months) after insertion of the spacer.

Results.—Mean pain scores improved from 6 to 34, and overall Harris hip scores improved from 11 to 67 at last followup with the spacer. Those who underwent definitive THA had further improvement in their mean Harris hip scores to 93.

Conclusions.—Articulating antibiotic spacers offer acceptable pain relief and function while the infection is treated in this unique group of patients.

Level of Evidence.—Level IV, therapeutic study. See Guidelines for Authors for a complete description of levels of evidence.

► Although the numbers are relatively small and this type contribution would be classified as a technique, it has great merit. I personally have used the treatment philosophy of low-friction antibiotic spacers for years and have a clinical impression that they work extremely well to maintain motion and lessen postoperative pain. Because the success of treating joint infection is regarded to be quite reliable today with staged reimplantation, the greatest gain is to maintain function and reduce pain after the infection is controlled. This technique, pioneered by the senior author (CB), is shown here to do just that. Although this report is for the hip (Figs 3 and 4 in the original article), we have found it quite helpful for the knee as well.

B. F. Morrey, MD

Meta-analysis of cause of death following total joint replacement using different thromboprophylaxis regimens

Poultsides LA, Gonzalez Della Valle A, Memtsoudis SG, et al (Hosp for Special Surgery, NY)

J Bone Joint Surg Br 94-B:113-121, 2012

We performed a meta-analysis of modern total joint replacement (TJR) to determine the post-operative mortality and the cause of death using different thromboprophylactic regimens as follows: 1) no routine chemothromboprophylaxis (NRC); 2) Potent anticoagulation (PA) (unfractionated or low-molecular-weight heparin, ximelagatran, fondaparinux or rivaroxaban);

3) Potent anticoagulation combined (PAC) with regional anaesthesia and/or pneumatic compression devices (PCDs); 4) Warfarin (W); 5) Warfarin combined (WAC) with regional anaesthesia and/or PCD; and 6) Multimodal (MM) prophylaxis, including regional anaesthesia, PCDs and aspirin in low-risk patients. Cause of death was classified as autopsy proven, clinically certain or unknown. Deaths were grouped into cardiopulmonary excluding pulmonary embolism (PE), PE, bleeding-related, gastrointestinal, central nervous system, and others (miscellaneous). Meta-analysis based on fixed effects or random effects models was used for pooling incidence data.

In all, 70 studies were included (99 441 patients; 373 deaths). The mortality was lowest in the MM (0.2%) and WC (0.2%) groups. The most frequent cause of death was cardiopulmonary (47.9%), followed by PE (25.4%) and bleeding (8.9%). The proportion of deaths due to PE was not significantly affected by the thromboprophylaxis regimen (PA, 35.5%; PAC, 28%; MM, 23.2%; and NRC, 16.3%). Fatal bleeding was higher in groups relying on the use of anticoagulation (W, 33.8%; PA, 9.4%; PAC, 10.8%) but the differences were not statistically significant.

Our study demonstrated that the routine use of PA does not reduce the overall mortality or the proportion of deaths due to PE.

▶ The conclusions of this article are unbelievable. Is there no evidence the most popular regimens used in the United States are of any value? A review of this article should be placed within the context that the UK practice style has never fully embraced chemical prophylaxis as universally as has the US practice. Regardless, this is a pretty objective assessment of the issue. I must say I fully agree. Why? For the past 20 years I have used the least expensive regimen with the lowest complication rate, and, according to this assessment, most successful regime: warfarin with compressive stockings! Regardless, the message from my perspective is simple: keep it simple, inexpensive, and effective. This study directs the surgeon to the options that fulfill these criteria.

B. F. Morrey, MD

7 Total Knee Arthroplasty

Introduction

I have long felt that the knee arthritis was "solved" with the introduction of the generic condylar implants. I am referring to the total condylar that was introduced in the late 1970s. Since then it is difficult to identify a major breakthrough other than that of Hungerford emphasizing the need for accurate instrumentation based on osseous fixation. This being the case we have tried to characterize the current state-of-the-art, the expectations of the outcome, as well as the areas of lingering controversy. Certainly the management of the patellofemoral component remains one of these areas of debate, and this is discussed in this year's selections. Bilateral replacements continue to be a source of discussion, and this topic is also represented in this year's selections. Overall, the knee joint and hip joint replacements are so successful. The key in my mind is to define the articles that truly provide value to the surgeon today, as opposed to offering possibilities of only marginal improvement. The reason for this is well known to the orthopedic surgeon, specifically all changes in our progress, and in many instances change has resulted in degradation in these results rather than in enhancement. It is hoped that the selection of articles in the knee section this year will be of value to the reader.

Bernard F. Morrey, MD

Factors Influencing Health-related Quality of Life after TKA in Patients who are Obese

Nuñez M, Lozano L, Nuñez E, et al (Univ of Barcelona, Spain; Institut Catalá de la Salut, Barcelona, Spain)
Clin Orthop Relat Res 469:1148-1153, 2011

Background.—Although the health-related quality of life (HRQL) for patients who are obese seems to improve after TKA, the magnitude of improvement and the associated factors remain controversial. We previously found body mass index was not associated with changes in HRQL after TKA.

TABLE 2.—Variables Independently Associated with WOMAC Dimension Scores at 12 Months

	Dependent Variables* WOMAC Scores at 12 Months								
	Pain R^2 Adjusted 0.369			Stiffness R^2 Adjusted 0.185			Function R^2 Adjusted 0.307		
Independent Variables	Coefficients	95% CI	p Value	Coefficients	95% CI	p Value	Coefficients	95% CI	p Value
Number of preexisting comorbidities							5.4	1.2–9.6	0.012
Infrapatellar index less than 75%	22.4	8.2–36.5	0.021				14.9	2.2–27.6	0.023
IOD (grade 2)	15.5	2.5–28.4	0.021						
Number of complications after discharge	28.5	13.1–43.9	0.001	25.79	9.94–41.64	0.002	23.0	9.1–36.8	0.002

SD = Standard deviation; CI = confidence interval; IOD = degree of intraoperative difficulty.

*The coefficients of regression models indicate if an increase in the independent variables is related with worse (positive coefficient) or better (negative coefficient) WOMAC dimension score. R^2 adjusted is the proportion of variance in the dependent variable explained by the relevant independent variables shown. N = number; WOMAC = Western Ontario and McMaster Universities Osteoarthritis Index. The three WOMAC scales were normalized to a 0–100 scale for each separate WOMAC dimension, where 0 represents the best health status and 100 the worse health status.

Questions/Purposes.—The purposes of this secondary analysis were to determine which patient characteristics and surgical factors were associated with worse health status after TKA in patients who are severe or morbidly obese.

Methods.—We assessed 60 patients (53 females; mean age, 70 years) 12 months after surgery. The mean number of comorbidities was 2.5. Mean lower limb anthropometric index scores were: suprapatellar, 1.6; infrapatellar, 2; and suprapatellar/infrapatellar, 1.2. Intraoperative difficulty (IOD) was Grade 0, 40%; Grade 1, 48%; and Grade 2, 12%. Ten patients (17%) had complications. We measured HRQL using the disease-specific WOMAC questionnaire. Patient characteristics (sociodemographic variables, BMI, comorbidity, lower limb anthropometry) and surgical factors (IOD, complications, postoperative medical data) were collected. Associations between WOMAC dimension scores at 12 months and patient characteristics and surgical factors were analyzed using linear regression models.

Results.—Factors associated with worse WOMAC dimension scores in patients who were obese included the number of comorbidities, an infrapatellar index percentile less than 75, IOD Grade 2, and the number of complications after discharge.

Conclusions.—For patients with knee osteoarthritis who were severe or morbidly obese, various lower limb anthropometric features, degree of IOD, and postoperative complications negatively influenced postoperative WOMAC scores.

Level of Evidence.—Level II Prognostic Study. See Guidelines for a complete description of levels of evidence (Table 2).

► The subject of body mass index (BMI) and its influence on the execution and success of joint replacement has been extensively studied. After earlier series failed to show the anticipated adverse association, more recent, more stratified investigations had clearly defined the adverse effect of marked (BMI > 35) and morbid (BMI > 40) obesity with intraoperative and postoperative outcome. However, what is also true is that these patients do markedly improve from the replacement, albeit at a cost. The correlations shown here with a lower Western Ontario and McMaster Universities Osteoarthritis Index based on the association of comorbidities is not surprising or new. The infrapatellar measurement as an indicator, however, is new and possibly worth noting. Because obesity is endemic, the message is we can't change the country's demographics or eating habits, but we can be aware of the implications.

B. F. Morrey, MD

Acute primary total knee arthroplasty for peri-articular knee fractures in patients over 65 years of age

Malviya A, Reed MR, Partington PF (Northumbria Healthcare NHS Foundation Trust, UK)

Injury 42:1368-1371, 2011

Peri-articular knee fractures in osteoporotic or osteoarthritic bone present a challenge to fixation, mobilisation or non-operative management. We present a series of 15 proximal tibial and 11 distal femoral fractures treated with total knee arthroplasty at over mean follow-up period of 38.8 months. The mean age of the patients was 80 years. The choice of the implant and level of constraint was determined as per the nature of injury and preference of the surgeon dealing with the fracture. Patients were allowed rapid mobilisation with immediate full weight-bearing. Good clinical results were achieved with fracture healing, sound fixation and well-aligned flexible knees. Mean Knee Society knee score was 90.2; Knee Society function score was 35.5; Oxford Knee score was 39.5; and Short Form (SF)-36 physical function score was 37.3 and mental score 50.6. Good correlation was noted between Knee society knee score and SF-36 physical function score (Pearson's 0.76, $p = 0.001$), suggesting that generic health would dictate the final function achieved, whilst high knee scores suggest the satisfactory results of the operation. Analogous to arthroplasty for hip fractures, this technique should be considered as a treatment option in elderly peri-articular knee fractures with osteoporosis and/or osteoarthritis (Fig 2).

▶ Prosthetic replacement for acute fractures about the knee is not commonly used. The patients in this report were older, averaging 80 years, and all had

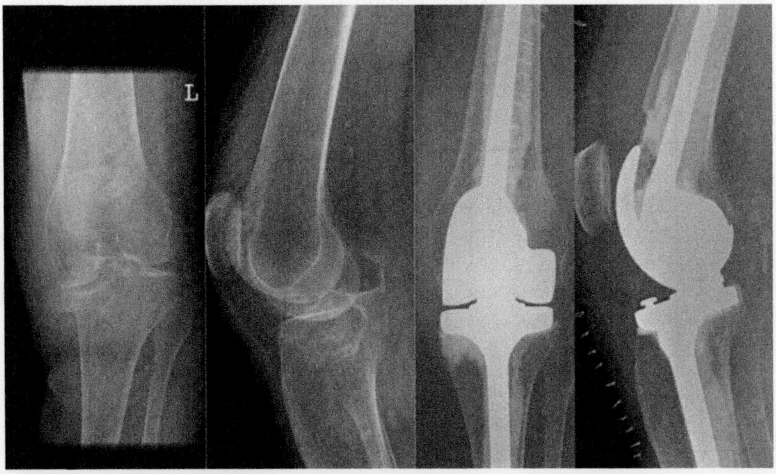

FIGURE 2.—Proximal tibial fracture with poor bone quality and postoperative radiograph showing reconstruction with the rotating hinge knee replacement. (Reprinted from Malviya A, Reed MR, Partington PF. Acute primary total knee arthroplasty for peri-articular knee fractures in patients over 65 years of age. *Injury.* 2011;42:1368-1371, Copyright 2011, with permission from Elsevier.)

prefracture symptoms of arthritis of the knee (Fig 2). That 80% returned to their preinjury state and 90% were satisfied with their status is a reasonable outcome for this type of injury in this type of patient. Of note is the low complication rate and that all had retained their implant, although the follow-up is short, averaging only about 3 years. The one issue I would raise is the necessity to use a linked, hinged device in 17 of the 26 procedures. Certainly, stemmed devices with greater articular stability are a must, but the routine need for a linked implant has not been my experience.

B. F. Morrey, MD

Failure of total knee arthroplasty with or without patella resurfacing: A study from the Norwegian Arthroplasty Register with 0–15 years of follow-up

Lygre SHL, Espehaug B, Havelin LI, et al (Haukeland Univ Hosp, Bergen, Norway; et al)

Acta Orthop 82:282-292, 2011

Background and Purpose.—Patella resurfacing during primary total knee arthroplasty (TKA) is disputed and new prosthesis designs have been introduced without documentation of their survival. We assessed the impact on prosthesis survival of patella resurfacing and of prosthesis brand, based on data from the Norwegian Arthroplasty Register.

Patients and Methods.—5 prosthesis brands in common use with and without patella resurfacing from 1994 through 2009 were included $n = 11{,}887$. The median follow-up times were 9 years for patella-resurfaced implants and 7 years for implants without patella resurfacing. For comparison of prosthesis brands, also brands in common use with only one of the two treatment options were included in the study population ($n = 25{,}590$). Cox regression analyses were performed with different reasons for revision as endpoints with adjustment for potential confounders.

Results.—We observed a reduced overall risk of revision for patella resurfaced (PR) TKAs, but the statistical significance was borderline ($RR = 0.84$, $p = 0.05$). At 15 years, 92% of PR and 91% of patella non resurfaced (NR) prostheses were still unrevised. However, PR implants had a lower risk of revision due to pain alone ($RR = 0.1$, $p < 0.001$), but a higher risk of revision due to loosening of the tibial component ($RR = 1.4$, $p = 0.03$) and due to a defective polyethylene insert ($RR = 3.2$, $p < 0.001$).

At 10 years, the survival for the reference NR brand AGC Universal was 93%. The NR brands Genesis I, Duracon, and Tricon ($RR = 1.4–1.7$) performed statistically significantly worse than NR AGC Universal, while the NR prostheses e.motion, Profix, and AGC Anatomic ($RR = 0.1–0.7$), and the PR prostheses NexGen and AGC Universal ($RR = 0.4–0.5$) performed statistically significantly better. LCS, NexGen, LCS Complete (all NR), and Tricon, Genesis I, LCS, and Kinemax (all PR) showed no differences in this respect from the reference brand. A lower risk of revision (crude) was found for TKAs performed after 2000 as compared to those performed earlier (RR = 0.8, p = 0.001).

Interpretation.—Although revision risk was similar for PR and NR TKAs, we found important differences in reasons for revision. Our results also indicate that survivorship of TKAs has improved.

▶ Again, we turn to a national registry to answer a lingering question regarding knee replacement: include the patella or not? The findings are, frankly, more difficult to interpret than one might think. The reason is that long-term data are needed to answer such a question, but the implants used today are different from those being studied. Regardless, the findings have been known but not necessarily quantified. Marginally better results are seen when the patella is resurfaced (Fig 3 in the original article) and the failure is mechanical as opposed to pain for the unresurfaced patella. What is not emphasized here is the revision of a failed resurfacing patella is much more difficult and less rewarding than salvage of a painful unresurfaced patella. The trend to leave the patella alone is very interesting (Fig 2 in the original article).

B. F. Morrey, MD

Does Preoperative Patellofemoral Joint State Affect Medial Unicompartmental Arthroplasty Survival?

Berend KR, Lombardi AV Jr, Morris MJ, et al (The Ohio State Univ, New Albany)

Orthopedics 34:e494-e496, 2011

One contested contraindication to medial unicompartmental knee arthroplasty (UKA) has been status of the patellofemoral joint. Surgeons have avoided UKA when the patellofemoral joint has radiographic evidence of arthritic changes. However, recent studies advocate ignoring patellofemoral joint status when considering UKA. The purpose of this study was to compare the failure rate of mobile-bearing, medial UKA in patients with and without preoperative radiographic evidence of patellofemoral joint degeneration. Preoperative radiographs from a random selection of 503 patients (638 knees) treated with UKA for anteromedial osteoarthritis were assessed by an observer blinded to clinical outcome. The patellofemoral joint was graded using the modified Altman classification from 0 to 3 with 0 being no evidence of changes and 3 being severe, and identified 396 grade 0, 168 grade 1, 65 grade 2, and 9 grade 3 knees. At 1- to 7-year follow-up, there have been 17 revisions for overall survivorship of 97.3%. Kaplan-Meier analysis predicted 97.9% survival in knees with patellofemoral joint disease and 93.8% survival in knees without patellofemoral joint disease at 70 months ($P = .1$). Failure requiring revision occurred in 3.5% (14/396) of grade 0 knees, 1.2% (2/168) of grade 1, 1.5% (1/65) of grade 2, and 0% (0/9) of grade 3. No survival difference was noted between knees with medial or lateral patellofemoral joint disease ($P = .1$). No knees were revised for progression of disease in the patellofemoral joint or anterior knee pain. In light of this investigation and the work of others, preoperative radiographic changes in the patellofemoral joint can be safely ignored when considering patients for medial UKA without compromising survivorship.

► Use of the unicompartmental knee replacement remains somewhat controversial. Of the various considerations for its use are patient age, extent of disease, angular alignment, implant design, anticipated activity, and precise surgical technique. One additional consideration is that the universally recognized patellofemoral involvement is considered a contraindication, at least a relative contraindication. This study reports a large clinical practice of more than 600 procedures and demonstrates no correlation with any degree of patellofemoral disease (Fig 1 in the original article). While it is unclear if selection factors regarding the patella existed in the early years of this procedure being adopted, it does appear to support other reports arriving at a similar conclusion. Regardless, it would seem there is good reason to avoid a symptomatic patellofemoral component when selecting the unicompartment replacement.

B. F. Morrey, MD

Cemented All-Polyethylene and Metal-Backed Polyethylene Tibial Components Used for Primary Total Knee Arthroplasty: A Systematic Review of the Literature and Meta-Analysis of Randomized Controlled Trials Involving 1798 Primary Total Knee Implants

Voigt J, Mosier M (Med Device Consultants of Ridgewood, NJ; Washburn Univ, Topeka, KS)

J Bone Joint Surg Am 93:1790-1798, 2011

Background.—The cost of the implant as part of a total knee arthroplasty accounts for a substantial portion of the costs for the overall procedure: all-polyethylene tibial components cost considerably less than cemented metal-backed tibial components. We performed a systematic review of the literature to determine whether the clinical results of lower-cost all-polyethylene tibial components were comparable with the results of a more expensive metal-backed tibial component.

Methods.—We searched The Cochrane Library, MEDLINE, EMBASE, EBSCO CINAHL, the bibliographies of identified articles, orthopaedic meeting abstracts, health technology assessment web sites, and important orthopaedic journals. This search was performed for the years 1990 to the present. No language restriction was applied. We restricted our search to Level-I studies involving participants who received either an all-polyethylene or a metal-backed tibial implant. The primary outcome measures were durability, function, and adverse events. Two reviewers independently screened the papers for inclusion, assessed trial quality, and extracted data. Effects estimates were pooled with use of fixed and random-effects models of risk ratios, calculated with 95% confidence intervals. Heterogeneity was assessed with the I^2 statistic. Forest plots were also generated.

Results.—Data on 1798 primary total knee implants from twelve studies were analyzed. In all studies, the median or mean age of the participants was greater than sixty-seven years, with a majority of the patients being female. There was no difference between patients managed with an all-polyethylene tibial component and those managed with a metal-backed tibial component in terms of adverse events. There was no significant difference between the two groups in terms of the durability of the implants at two, ten, and fifteen years postoperatively, regardless of the year or how durability was defined (revision or radiographic failure). Finally, with use of a variety of validated measures, there was no difference between the two groups in terms of functional status at two, eight, and ten years, regardless of the measure used.

Conclusion.—A less expensive all-polyethylene component as part of a total knee arthroplasty has results equivalent to those obtained with a cemented metal-backed tibial component. Using a total knee implant with a cemented all-polyethylene tibial component could save the health-care system substantial money while obtaining equivalent results to more expensive cemented designs and materials.

▶ Again, I gravitate toward those topics in which I have a special interest. I returned to the all-polyethylene (all-poly) tibial tray more than 15 years ago. My experience and interpretation of the literature tended to support this choice. This rigorous analysis of the literature, including 9 studies and more than 1700 patients, confirms that choice. Regardless of the hype, at the end of the day, the all-poly tibial tray is as good as, if not better than, the metal-backed, modular design (Fig 8 in the original article). These findings are not design specific. If and when we finally accept that controlling the cost of care is on us, we will, or should, drift again to the cemented all-poly component for primary total knee arthroplasty.

B. F. Morrey, MD

Metal-backed versus all-polyethylene tibial components in primary total knee arthroplasty: A meta-analysis and systematic review of randomized controlled trials

Cheng T, Zhang G, Zhang X (Shanghai Jiao Tong Univ School of Medicine, People's Republic of China; Wenzhou Med College, People's Republic of China)

Acta Orthop 82:589-595, 2011

Background and Purpose.—The choice of either all-polyethylene (AP) tibial components or metal-backed (MB) tibial components in total knee arthroplasty (TKA) remains controversial. We therefore performed a meta-analysis and systematic review of randomized controlled trials that have evaluated MB and AP tibial components in primary TKA.

Methods.—The search strategy included a computerized literature search (Medline, EMBASE, Scopus, and the Cochrane Central Register of Controlled Trials) and a manual search of major orthopedic journals. A meta-analysis and systematic review of randomized or quasi-randomized trials that compared the performance of tibial components in primary TKA was performed using a fixed or random effects model. We assessed the methodological quality of studies using Detsky quality scale.

Results.—9 randomized controlled trials (RCTs) published between 2000 and 2009 met the inclusion quality standards for the systematic review. The mean standardized Detsky score was 14 (SD 3). We found that the frequency of radiolucent lines in the MB group was significantly higher than that in the AP group. There were no statistically significant differences between the MB and AP tibial components regarding component positioning, knee score, knee range of motion, quality of life, and postoperative complications.

Interpretation.—Based on evidence obtained from this study, the AP tibial component was comparable with or better than the MB tibial component in TKA. However, high-quality RCTs are required to validate the results.

▶ I seem to be in a rut selecting topics in which I have a special interest. But, I do try to be sure they are of interest to our readership. Whether to use an all poly- or metal-backed component is re-emerging as a legitimate question for the joint replacement surgeon. The key to the questions, as reflected in this article, is follow the data. The data say no difference (Fig 1 in the original article). What is not reflected here is the impact of ease or value of revision—and our own studies at Mayo and others answer this question. The potential value of the metal-backed implant has not been realized in reality. There is great value in modular trials to determine the proper thickness of the implant. Once this is decided, cost and outcomes favor the all-poly device, according to my interpretation of this and other studies.

B. F. Morrey, MD

Comparison of Patient-Reported and Clinician-Assessed Outcomes Following Total Knee Arthroplasty

Khanna G, Singh JA, Pomeroy DL, et al (Univ of Minnesota Med School, Minneapolis; The Kirklin Clinic, Birmingham, AL; Univ of Louisville Med College, KY; et al)

J Bone Joint Surg Am 93:e117.1-e117.7, 2011

Background.—Although the necessity of long-term follow-up after total knee arthroplasty is unquestioned, this task may become burdensome as greater numbers of total knee arthroplasties are performed. We sought to use comparisons with clinician-assessed values to determine whether patients could reliably assess their own outcome with use of a combination of American Knee Society Score and Oxford Knee Score questionnaires and self-reported knee motion. We hypothesized that patients would self-report worse pain and function and a similar range of knee motion than clinicians would.

Methods.—One hundred and forty patients (181 knees) scheduled for routine follow-up at two centers after primary total knee arthroplasty were mailed American Knee Society Score and Oxford Knee Score questionnaires, a set of photographs illustrating knee motion in 5° increments for comparison with the patient's range of knee motion, and a goniometer with instructions. The patient's American Knee Society Score, Oxford Knee Score, and knee motion were then independently assessed within two weeks of the self-evaluation by one of three clinicians who had not been involved with the surgery. Patient-reported and clinician-assessed measures were compared with use of a paired-sample t test and the Spearman correlation coefficient.

Results.—The mean patient-reported American Knee Society pain subscore was 4 points worse than the clinician-assessed score, and the function subscore was 10 points worse ($p < 0.001$ for both). The mean Oxford Knee Score did not differ significantly between the patient self-assessment and the clinician assessment ($p = 0.05$). The mean maximum flexion reported by the patient with use of the photographs differed by <1° from the mean value reported by the patient with use of the goniometer or the mean value measured by the clinician; these differences were not clinically important.

Conclusions.—Patients' self-reported American Knee Society pain and function subscores were worse than the corresponding clinician assessments, but the two Oxford Knee Scores were similar. Range of knee motion may reasonably be self-assessed by comparison with photographs. Long-term follow-up of patients after total knee arthroplasty may be possible with use of patient-reported measures, alleviating the burden of clinic visits yet maintaining contact, but further studies involving other validated instruments is warranted.

▶ The topic of whether patients and physicians view outcomes similarity has been long considered. The issue is increasingly relevant, as outcomes are now considered to be primarily based on patient, not physician, perception. The fact that patients increasingly cannot return for assessment also is an important component of the equation. Hence, the finding that the correlation of outcome perception is a function of the tool used for the measurement is important (Fig 1 in the original article). That the Oxford instrument does accurately resolve the 2 frames of reference is encouraging. Going forward, much more outcome documentation will be based on these measurement tools, and the patient will emerge as the primary source of outcome truth.

B. F. Morrey, MD

Increased Long-Term Survival of Posterior Cruciate-Retaining Versus Posterior Cruciate-Stabilizing Total Knee Replacements

Abdel MP, Morrey ME, Jensen MR, et al (Mayo Clinic, Rochester, MN)

J Bone Joint Surg Am 93:2072-2078, 2011

Background.—Considerable debate remains regarding the use of posterior cruciate-retaining or posterior cruciate-stabilizing designs for total knee arthroplasty. Multiple studies have investigated kinematic, radiographic, and clinical outcomes of both. Nevertheless, long-term survivorship analyses directly comparing the two designs have not been performed, to our knowledge. Our goal was to analyze the fifteen-year survival of posterior cruciate-retaining and posterior cruciate-stabilizing total knee replacements at our institution.

Methods.—A retrospective review identified 8117 total knee arthroplasties (5389 posterior cruciate-retaining and 2728 posterior cruciate-stabilizing) that had been performed from 1988 to 1998. This range was chosen because both designs were used in high volumes at our institution during this period. Patients were followed via our total joint registry at one, two, and five years after the arthroplasty and every five years thereafter. Aseptic revision surgery was the primary end point of our analysis. Implant survival was estimated with Kaplan-Meier curves.

Results.—Survival at fifteen years was 90% for posterior cruciate-retaining total knee replacements, compared with 77% for posterior cruciate-stabilizing total knee replacements ($p < 0.001$). In knees with preoperative deformity, the fifteen-year survival was 90% for posterior cruciate-retaining total knee replacements, compared with 75% for posterior cruciate-stabilizing total knee replacements ($p < 0.04$). Likewise, in knees without preoperative deformity, the fifteen-year survival was 88% for posterior cruciate-retaining total knee replacements, compared with 78% for posterior cruciate-stabilizing total knee replacements ($p < 0.001$). After adjustment for age, sex, preoperative diagnosis, and preoperative deformity, the risk of revision was significantly lower in knees with a posterior cruciate-retaining total knee replacement ($p < 0.001$; hazard ratio = 0.5; 95% confidence interval, 0.4 to 0.6).

Conclusions.—In evaluating the implants used at our institution for total knee arthroplasty during the study period, posterior cruciate-retaining prostheses had significantly improved survival in comparison with posterior cruciate-stabilizing prostheses at fifteen years. Furthermore, this significant difference remained when accounting for age, sex, diagnosis, and deformity.

▶ This important article was included, not because I was involved, but because of the message. The orthopedic community, like the Mayo Clinic, has accepted the design philosophy of posterior cruciate substituting implant designs (Fig 1 in the original article). The original indications to use this in the presence of deformity have given way to becoming the accepted first-line implant design. We simply studied our institutional experience with the 2 designs. Note in the review that the cruciate retaining device, at Mayo and in the years studied, outperformed the cruciate substituting implants. Note that this is true when stratifying the patients by deformity as well! The Kaplan-Meier curves are dramatic but were edited out of the article by the journal (you can find them in the appendix). You draw your own conclusions. This is not a perfect study, and it is possible the designs of today are better than those in the past. If so, this should be proven by data, not promise.

B. F. Morrey, MD

Perioperative Morbidity and Mortality of 2-team Simultaneous Bilateral Total Knee Arthroplasty

Dimitris CN, Taylor BC, Mowbray JG, et al (Mount Carmel West Hosp, Columbus, OH; et al)
Orthopedics 34:e841-e846, 2011

Total knee arthroplasty (TKA) has a well-established track record for relieving pain associated with arthritis of the knee joint. The total rate of bilateral TKA has doubled over the past 2 decades, and the rate in women has tripled over that same time period. In patients with bilateral knee arthritis, a decision must be made whether to operate at 2 different settings (staged), a single setting with 1 surgeon (sequential simultaneous), or a single setting with 2 surgeons (2-team simultaneous). The purpose of this study was to examine the perioperative morbidity and mortality of 2-team simultaneous bilateral TKA. Two hundred twenty-seven consecutive 2-team simultaneous bilateral TKA and 216 consecutive unilateral TKA

TABLE 1.—Demographic and Perioperative Data

	Bilateral TKA Group (n=227)[a]	Unilateral TKA Group (n=216)[b]	*P*
Mean±SD age, y	65.7±4.1	66.0±4.1	.238
Sex, M:F (M%)	83:144 (36.6)	71:145 (32.9)	
Mean±SD BMI, kg/m^2 (range)	34.0±7.1 (19.2-61.4)	33.7±7.5 (19.8-67.8)	.646
ASA class			
ASA 4, n (%)	14 (6.2)	18 (8.3)	
ASA 3, n (%)	126 (55.5)	131 (60.6)	
ASA 2, n (%)	68 (30.0)	59 (27.3)	
ASA 1, n (%)	3 (1.3)	3 (1.4)	
Mean±SD tourniquet time, min	114.4±18.0	109.4±17.6	.004
Mean±SD estimated blood loss, mL	161.7±214.2	105.0±154.1	.002
Patients transfused, n (%)	148 (65.0)	31 (14.4)	
Mean±SD units transfused	1.4±1.3	0.3±0.8	<.001
Mean±SD length of hospital stay, d	3.71±1.3	3.38±0.98	.002
Discharged to extended care facility, n (%)	168 (76)	60 (27)	<.001

Abbreviations: ASA, American Society of Anesthesiologists; BMI, body mass index; SD, standard deviations; TKA, total knee arthroplasty.

[a]The ASA operative documentation could not be found for 16 patients.

[b]The ASA operative documentation could not be found for 5 patients.

patients were reviewed. Major (deep infection, death, cerebrovascular accident, myocardial infarction, pulmonary embolism, revision within the 1-year follow-up) and minor (all other) complications were compared. No deaths occurred, and the major and minor complication rates were not statistically significantly different between the 2 groups, but a trend toward higher rates of both major and minor complications existed in the bilateral TKA group. Two-team simultaneous bilateral TKA offers the potential benefits of decreased overall recovery time, decreased overall cost, decreased number of anesthetic administrations, and simultaneous correction of significant deformity. It remains an appropriate option in select patients (Table 1).

► In a way, this study does not prove anything—definitively. This topic is one of the most frequently studied in knee replacement today. It is easy to find conclusions on both sides of the question: for or against this practice. But, because there is a high patient preference for the simultaneous procedure, and because of the obvious cost advantages, any conclusions that favor this approach are of value (Table 1).

B. F. Morrey, MD

Bilateral Total Knee Arthroplasty: Risk Factors for Major Morbidity and Mortality

Memtsoudis SG, Ma Y, Chiu Y-L, et al (Weill Cornell Med College, NY)
Anesth Analg 113:784-790, 2011

Background.—Bilateral total knee arthroplasty (BTKA) performed during the same hospitalization carries increased risk for morbidity and mortality compared with the unilateral approach. However, no evidence-based stratifications to identify patients at risk for major morbidity and mortality are available. Our objective was to determine the incidence and patient-related risk factors for major morbidity and mortality among patients undergoing BTKA.

Methods.—Nationwide Inpatient Survey data collected for the years 1998 to 2007 were analyzed and cases of elective BTKA procedures were included. Patient demographics, including comorbidities, were analyzed and frequencies of mortality and major complications were computed. Subsequently, a multivariate analysis was conducted to determine independent risk factors for major morbidity and mortality.

Results.—Included were 42,003 database entries, representing an estimated 206,573 elective BTKAs. The incidence of major in-hospital complications and mortality was 9.5%. Risk factors for adverse outcome included advanced age (odds ratios [ORs] for age groups 65–74 and >75 years were 1.88 [confidence interval, CI: 1.72, 2.05] and 2.66 [CI: 2.42, 2.92], respectively, compared with the 45–65 years group), male gender (OR: 1.54 [CI: 1.44, 1.66]), and a number of comorbidities. The presence of congestive

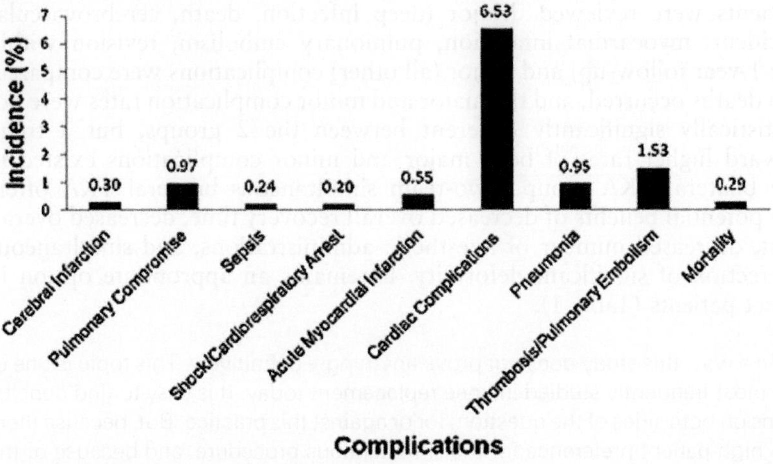

FIGURE 1.—Depicted is the incidence of major complications and mortality among cases of bilateral total knee arthroplasty. (Reprinted from Memtsoudis SG, Ma Y, Chiu Y-L, et al. Bilateral total knee arthroplasty: risk factors for major morbidity and mortality. *Anesth Analg*. 2011;113:784-790, with permission from International Anesthesia Research Society.)

TABLE 2.—The Prevalence of Comorbidities in Cases with and without Major Complications/Mortality

Comorbidity	Complications, Weighted *n* (%)	No Complications, Weighted *n* (%)	*P* Value*	Total
Alcohol abuse	143 (0.73%)	985 (0.53%)	0.11	1128 (0.55%)
Chronic lung disease	2832 (14.41%)	19,711 (10.55%)	<0.001	22,543 (10.91%)
Congestive heart failure	2317 (11.78%)	2943 (1.57%)	<0.001	5259 (2.55%)
Uncomplicated diabetes mellitus	2882 (14.66%)	25,817 (13.81%)	0.15	28,699 (0.17%)
Complicated diabetes mellitus	229 (1.16%)	1689 (0.90%)	0.11	1918 (0.93%)
Liver dysfunction	127 (0.65%)	814 (0.44%)	0.07	940 (0.46%)
Coagulopathy	881 (4.48%)	2772 (1.48%)	<0.001	3653 (1.77%)
Neurologic disorders	517 (2.63%)	3039 (1.63%)	<0.001	3556 (1.72%)
Obesity	2397 (12.19%)	25,135 (13.45%)	0.03	27,532 (13.33%)
Peripheral vascular disease	449 (2.28%)	2176 (1.16%)	<0.001	2625 (1.27%)
Renal disease	505 (2.57%)	1305 (0.70%)	<0.001	1810 (0.88%)
Pulmonary hypertension	335 (1.70%)	462 (0.25%)	<0.001	797 (0.39%)
Cardiac valvular disorders	1777 (9.04%)	6464 (3.46%)	<0.001	8241 (0.10%)
Electrolyte/fluid abnormalities	3709 (18.87%)	14,276 (7.64%)	<0.001	17,986 (8.71%)
Metastatic cancer	17 (0.09%)	79 (0.04%)	0.25	96 (0.05%)
Cancer	100 (0.51%)	858 (0.46%)	0.65	959 (0.46%)

Prevalence of comorbidities in cases with and without major complications/mortality. Shown are the weighted *n* and percentage of cases with and without major complications and mortality.
*P value was calculated from χ^2 tests from PROC SURVEYFREQ.

heart failure (OR: 5.55 [CI: 4.81, 6.39]) and pulmonary hypertension (OR: 4.10 [CI: 2.72, 6.10]) were the most significant risk factors associated with increased odds for adverse outcome.

Conclusions.—We identified patient-related risk factors for major morbidity and mortality in patients undergoing BTKA. Our data can be used to aid in the selection of patients for this procedure (Fig 1, Table 2).

► This article addresses an issue that is a source of continued debate, and it probably should be. The fact that this originates from the anesthesia literature probably explains the lack of awareness that the orthopedic surgeon has of the findings reported here . The major additional risks of age and especially of coronary artery disease have been repeatedly and well demonstrated. However, it is of value for the surgeon to review the findings here, as they have merit if discussing this option with your patient (Fig 1, Table 2). The large database used in this study does not allow one to distinguish the influence of doing the procedure concurrently or in tandem, nor does it allow understanding of the manner in which the tourniquet was employed and whether intra- or extramedullary alignment techniques were used. These are all technical considerations for those who still perform bilateral procedures because there is a high patient preference for such surgery.

B. F. Morrey, MD

A Population-Based Comparison of the Incidence of Adverse Outcomes After Simultaneous-Bilateral and Staged-Bilateral Total Knee Arthroplasty

Meehan JP, Danielsen B, Tancredi DJ, et al (Univ of California, Davis, Sacramento)

J Bone Joint Surg Am 93:2203-2213, 2011

Background.—It is unclear whether simultaneous-bilateral total knee arthroplasty is as safe as staged-bilateral arthroplasty is. We are aware of no randomized trials comparing the safety of these surgical strategies. The purpose of this study was to retrospectively compare these two strategies, with use of an intention-to-treat approach for the staged-bilateral arthroplasty cohort.

Methods.—We used linked hospital discharge data to compare the safety of simultaneous-bilateral and staged-bilateral knee arthroplasty procedures performed in California between 1997 and 2007. Estimates were generated to take into account patients who had planned to undergo staged-bilateral arthroplasty but never underwent the second procedure because of death, a major complication, or elective withdrawal. Hierarchical logistic regression modeling was used to adjust the comparisons for patient and hospital characteristics. The principal outcomes of interest were death, a major complication involving the cardiovascular system, and a periprosthetic knee infection or mechanical malfunction requiring revision surgery.

Results.—Records were available for 11,445 simultaneous-bilateral arthroplasty procedures and 23,715 staged-bilateral procedures. On the basis of an intermediate estimate of the number of complications that occurred after the first procedure in a staged-bilateral arthroplasty, patients who underwent simultaneous-bilateral arthroplasty had a significantly higher adjusted odds ratio (OR) of myocardial infarction (OR = 1.6, 95% confidence interval [CI] = 1.2 to 2.2) and of pulmonary embolism (OR = 1.4, 95% CI = 1.1 to 1.8), similar odds of death (OR = 1.3, 95% CI = 0.9 to 1.9) and of ischemic stroke (OR = 1.0, 95% CI = 0.6 to 1.6), and significantly lower odds of major joint infection (OR = 0.6, 95% CI = 0.5 to 0.7) and of major mechanical malfunction (OR = 0.7, 95% CI = 0.6 to 0.9) compared with patients who planned to undergo staged-bilateral arthroplasty. The unadjusted thirty-day incidence of death or a coronary event was 3.2 events per thousand patients higher after simultaneous-bilateral arthroplasty than after staged-bilateral arthroplasty, but the one-year incidence of major joint infection or major mechanical malfunction was 10.5 events per thousand lower after simultaneous-bilateral arthroplasty.

Conclusions.—Simultaneous-bilateral total knee arthroplasty was associated with a clinically important reduction in the incidence of periprosthetic joint infection and malfunction within one year after arthroplasty, but it was associated with a moderately higher risk of an adverse cardiovascular outcome within thirty days. If patients who are at higher risk for cardiovascular complications can be identified, simultaneous-bilateral knee arthroplasty may be the preferred surgical strategy for the remaining lower-risk patients.

▶ Here it is again—possibly my favorite knee subject. I almost didn't include this article because so much has been written on the subject. However, it is a well-done study, and I liked the authors' conclusion. They confirm that those with serious cardiovascular disease are at risk for simultaneous bilateral replacements (Fig 2 in the original article). However, they then demonstrate even greater differences and advantages, with the bilateral cohort being associated with fewer infections and less mechanical failure (Fig 3 in the original article). They conclude that the bilateral option is viable if those at risk are screened and not offered the bilateral procedure. I completely agree, and this has been my practice.

B. F. Morrey, MD

Flexion Contracture Following Primary Total Knee Arthroplasty: Risk Factors and Outcomes

Goudie ST, Deakin AH, Ahmad A, et al (Golden Jubilee Natl Hosp, Scotland, UK)

Orthopedics 34:e855-e859, 2011

Function and satisfaction after total knee arthroplasty (TKA) are partially linked to postoperative range of motion (ROM). Fixed flexion contracture is a recognized complication of TKA that reduces ROM and is a source of morbidity for patients. This study aimed to identify preoperative risk factors for developing fixed flexion contracture following TKA and to quantify the effect of fixed flexion contracture on outcomes (Oxford knee score 12-60 and patient satisfaction) at 2 years. Pre-, intra-, and postoperative data for 811 TKAs were retrospectively reviewed. At 2 years postoperatively, the incidence of fixed flexion contracture was 3.6%. Men were 2.6 times more likely than women to have fixed flexion contracture ($P = .012$), and patients with preimplant fixed flexion contracture were 2.3 times more likely than those without to have fixed flexion contracture ($P = .028$). Increasing age was associated with an increased rate of fixed flexion contracture ($P = .02$). Body mass index was not a risk factor ($P = .968$). Incidence of fixed flexion contracture for those undergoing computer navigated TKA was 3.9% compared with 3.4% for those having conventional surgery ($P = .711$). Patients with fixed flexion contracture had poorer outcomes with a median [interquartile range] Oxford Knee Score of 25 [15] compared with 20 [11] for those without ($P = .003$) and lower patient satisfaction ($P = .036$). These results support existing literature for incidence of fixed flexion contracture after TKA, risk factors, and outcomes, indicating that these figures can be extrapolated to a wide population. They also clarify a previously contentious point by excluding body mass index as a risk factor.

▶ In fact there really is nothing new in this article. But the topic is important and the finding worth noting and re-emphasizing. As the authors readily acknowledge, the finding simply supports the observations of Ritter, which have been previously published. It is known that the presence of a postoperative contracture is correlated to preoperative contracture. This is known to be correlated with advanced age, and known, but possibly less appreciated, to be associated with increasing body mass index. The authors confirm the correlation of residual contracture of greater than 5° to be correlated to poorer outcomes and functional results. All observations are valid and worth remembering when performing the procedure.

B. F. Morrey, MD

A prospective study comparing the functional outcome of computer-assisted and conventional total knee replacement

Hoffart H-E, Langenstein E, Vasak N (Kreiskrankenhaus, Jugenheim, Germany)
J Bone Joint Surg Br 94-B:194-199, 2012

The aim of this prospective single-centre study was to assess the difference in clinical outcome between total knee replacement (TKR) using computerised navigation and that of conventional TKR. We hypothesised that navigation would give a better result at every stage within the first five years. A total of 195 patients (195 knees) with a mean age of 70.0 years (39 to 89) were allocated alternately into two treatment groups, which used either conventional instrumentation (group A, 97 knees) or a navigation system (group B, 98 knees). After five years, complete clinical scores were available for 121 patients (62%). A total of 18 patients were lost to follow-up. Compared with conventional surgery, navigated TKR resulted in a better mean Knee Society score ($p = 0.008$). The difference in mean Knee Society scores over time between the two groups was not constant ($p = 0.006$), which suggests that these groups differed in their response to surgery with time. No significant difference in the frequency of malalignment was seen between the two groups.

In summary, computerised navigation resulted in a better functional outcome at five years than conventional techniques. Given the similarity in mechanical alignment between the two groups, rotational alignment may prove to be a better method of identifying differences in clinical outcome after navigated surgery.

▶ As the use of navigation continues to be an active topic of discussion, if not debate, I have tried to carefully survey the literature to help elucidate the current reality. This prospective, randomized study deserves to be read and considered. It is one of the very few that focuses on functional outcome rather than on alignment. The sample size is adequate, although not robust. The measurement parameters are standard and accepted. The surveillance period is very limited. Yet the authors show a difference in pain and functional outcome (Fig 2a, c in the original article) favoring the computerized procedure. It might be noted there was no difference in complications (Table 2 in the original article). I cannot offer this as proof of the superiority of navigated total knee arthroplasty. It is extremely difficult for me to understand how pain is less in the navigated knee. Because of this, I have difficulty understanding the outcome reported. The message? Stay tuned; the answer remains elusive in my mind. The cost effectiveness will be the ultimate trump card.

B. F. Morrey, MD

Effect of Polyethylene Component Thickness on Range of Motion and Stability in Primary Total Knee Arthroplasty

Lanting BA, Snider MG, Chess DG (St Joseph's Health Care, London, Ontario, Canada; Grand River Hosp, Kitchener, Ontario, Canada)
Orthopedics 35:e170-e174, 2012

Total knee arthroplasty (TKA) is a common procedure with good survivorship and functional results. Optimal results are dependent on proper osseous cuts and soft tissue balancing. Soft tissue tensioning via the polyethylene spacer thickness is an important component of soft tissue balancing. Increased thickness increases soft tissue tension and, therefore, has the potential to increase stability but decrease range of motion (ROM). Decreased polyethylene thickness may decrease soft tissue tension and has the potential to increase ROM but decrease stability.

Using computer-based navigation, the intraoperative effect of increasing and decreasing polyethylene thickness in 1-mm increments on ROM and coronal stability throughout the ROM of 35 patients was examined. It was found that increasing the polyethylene thickness by 1-mm increments had a statistically significant impact on the ability to achieve full extension but had no impact on flexion. Increased polyethylene thickness decreased coronal plane motion. Coronal plane laxity increased with increased flexion irrespective of polyethylene thickness. In this patient cohort, lateral laxity became >1° when the knee was flexed. However, medial structures prevented valgus angulation of >1° in all scenarios except when the polyethylene was diminished by 2 mm.

Changes in polyethylene thickness had an impact on the ability to gain full extension and coronal plane motion.

▶ One of the most common decisions made by the surgeon during knee replacement is the thickness of the tibial tray. The most important consideration heretofore is to avoid a critical thinness because surface stress increases with decreased poly thickness.

While we know thicker poly influences range of motion, especially in extension, this has uncommonly been studied. The disclaimer in this study is that the results will vary as a function of the initial preparation extension gap. That said, I was surprised that in this study, 4-mm variation in poly thickness only changed extension by about 6°, or about 1.5° per millimeter (Fig 1 in the original article). This isn't much, and is less than my surgical experience would suggest.

B. F. Morrey, MD

Can Computer Assistance Improve the Clinical and Functional Scores in Total Knee Arthroplasty?

Hernández-Vaquero D, Suarez-Vazquez A, Iglesias-Fernandez S (Univ of Oviedo, Spain; Hosp St Agustin, Aviles, Spain; Apartado de Correos, Aviles, Oviedo, Spain)

Clin Orthop Relat Res 469:3436-3442, 2011

Background.—Surgical navigation in TKA facilitates better alignment; however, it is unclear whether improved alignment alters clinical evolution and midterm and long-term complication rates.

Questions/Purposes.—We determined the alignment differences between patients with standard, manual, jig-based TKAs and patients with navigation-based TKAs, and whether any differences would modify function, implant survival, and/or complications.

Patients and Materials.—We retrospectively reviewed 97 patients (100 TKAs) undergoing TKAs for minimal preoperative deformities. Fifty TKAs were performed with an image-free surgical navigation system and the other 50 with a standard technique. We compared femoral angle (FA), tibial angle (TA), and femorotibial angle (FTA) and determined whether any differences altered clinical or functional scores, as measured by the Knee Society Score (KSS), or complications. Seventy-three patients (75 TKAs) had a minimum followup of 8 years (mean, 8.3 years; range, 8–9.1 years).

Results.—All patients included in the surgical navigation group had a FTA between 177° and 182°. We found no differences in the KSS or implant survival between the two groups and no differences in complication rates, although more complications occurred in the standard technique group (seven compared with two in the surgical navigation group).

Conclusions.—In the midterm, we found no difference in functional and clinical scores or implant survival between TKAs performed with and without the assistance of a navigation system.

Level of Evidence.—Level II, therapeutic study. See the Guidelines online for a complete description of levels of evidence.

▶ This study was included to convey the general message: nothing has changed. By that I mean, navigation lessens the variation, at least in the AP plane of the femoral tibial alignment (Fig 1A and B in the original article). This finding has been shown by every investigator that has ever assessed this question. The problem, once again, is the investigators cannot find that this variation influences long-term outcome. Maybe with larger numbers, and longer surveillance, a difference will be demonstrated, but not to date. Then we will have to factor in the costs. So, for me, the answer is clear: it's just not worth it. And the data, to date, support that position.

B. F. Morrey, MD

Femoral component loosening in high-flexion total knee replacement: An *in vitro* comparison of high-flexion *versus* conventional designs

Bollars P, Luyckx J-P, Innocenti B, et al (European Centre for Knee Res, Leuven, Belgium)

J Bone Joint Surg Br 93-B:1355-1361, 2011

High-flexion total knee replacement (TKR) designs have been introduced to improve flexion after TKR. Although the early results of such designs were promising, recent literature has raised concerns about the incidence of early loosening of the femoral component. We compared the minimum force required to cause femoral component loosening for six high-flexion and six conventional TKR designs in a laboratory experiment.

Each TKR design was implanted in a femoral bone model and placed in a loading frame in 135° of flexion. Loosening of the femoral component was induced by moving the tibial component at a constant rate of displacement while maintaining the same angle of flexion. A stereophotogrammetric system registered the relative movement between the femoral component and the underlying bone until loosening occurred.

Compared with high-flexion designs, conventional TKR designs required a significantly higher force before loosening occurred ($p < 0.001$). High-flexion designs with closed box geometry required significantly higher loosening forces than high-flexion designs with open box geometry ($p = 0.0478$). The presence of pegs further contributed to the fixation strength of components.

TABLE 1.—List of the Total Knee Replacement Designs Used in This Study, with Their Characteristics

Design	Prosthesis	Company*	Type	Internal Femoral Component Geometry	Pegs	Site of Design Modification	Mean (SD) Loosening Force (N)
A	Journey	Smith & Nephew	High-flexion	Closed	No	Femoral component	185 (87.3)
B	NexGen LPS-flex	Zimmer	High-flexion	Open	Yes	Femoral component	32 (17.3)
C	PFC Sigma HF	DePuy	High-flexion	Open	No	Femoral component	127 (54.5)
D	Scorpio HF	Stryker Howmedica	High-flexion	Parallel	Yes	Tibial insert	228 (65.0)
E	Genesis II HF	Smith & Nephew	High-flexion	Parallel	No	Tibial insert	148 (37.2)
F	Genesis II HF	Smith & Nephew	High-flexion	Parallel	Yes	Tibial insert	222 (18.9)
G	Genesis II	Smith & Nephew	Conventional	Parallel	No		218 (9.6)
H	Genesis II	Smith & Nephew	Conventional	Parallel	Yes		259 (11.2)
I	NexGen LPS	Zimmer	Conventional	Open	Yes		190 (28.2)
J	PFC Sigma	DePuy	Conventional	Open	No		383 (59.8)
K	Scorpio	Stryker Howmedica	Conventional	Parallel	Yes		370 (48.8)
L	Plus knee	Smith & Nephew	Conventional	Open	No		443 (95.7)

*Smith & Nephew (Memphis, Tennessee), Zimmer (Warsaw, Indiana), DePuy (Warsaw, Indiana), Stryker & Howmedica (Mahwah, New Jersey).

We conclude that high-flexion designs have a greater risk for femoral component loosening than conventional TKR designs. We believe this is attributable to the absence of femoral load sharing between the prosthetic component and the condylar bone during flexion (Table 1).

▶ In spite of my interest and background in biomechanics, I find myself selecting few biomechanical studies for the YEAR BOOK. This exception addresses a clinically relevant question, uses a straightforward methodology, and offers practical observations based on the data. The article emphasizes not all designs are the same, and a subtle design feature can have a marked effect on the tendency for the implant to loosen (Fig 1 in the original article). In fact, most large companies now offer the high flexed knee design (Table 1). However, the authors demonstrate the design variables of contour, stabilizing pegs, and box geometry all contribute to more stable femoral components (Fig 4 in the original article).

B. F. Morrey, MD

Can Implant Retention be Recommended for Treatment of Infected TKA?

Choi H-R, von Knoch F, Zurakowski D, et al (Massachusetts General Hosp, Boston; et al)

Clin Orthop Relat Res 469:961-969, 2011

Background.—Retention treatment is reportedly associated with lower infection control rates than two-stage revision. However, the studies on which this presumption are based depend on comparisons of historical rather than concurrent controls.

Questions/purposes.—We (1) asked whether the infection control rates, number of additional procedures, length of hospital stay, and treatment duration differed between implant retention and two-stage revision treatment; and (2) identified risk factors that can contribute to failure of infection control.

Methods.—We reviewed the records of 60 patients treated for 64 infected TKA from 2002 to 2007. Twenty-eight patients (32 knees) underwent débridement with retention of component, and 32 patients (32 knees) were treated with component removal and two-stage revision surgery. We determined patients' demographics, type of infection, causative organisms, and outcome of treatment. Mean followup was 36 months (range, 12–84 months).

Results.—Infection control rate was 31% in retention and 59% in the removal group after initial surgical treatment, and 81% and 91% at latest followup, respectively. Treatment duration was shorter in the retention group and there was no difference in number of additional surgeries and length of hospital stay. Type of treatment (retention versus removal) was the only factor associated with infection control; subgroup analysis in the retention group showed Staphylococcus aureus infection and polyethylene nonexchange as contributing factors for failure of infection control.

Conclusions.—Although initial infection control rate was substantially lower in the retention group than the removal group, final results were comparable at latest followup. We believe retention treatment can be selectively considered for non-S. aureus infection, and when applied in selected patients, polyethylene exchange should be performed.

Level of Evidence.—Level III, therapeutic study. See the Guidelines for Authors for a complete description of levels of evidence (Table 4).

▶ Infection remains a major problem following total knee arthroplasty. The frequency is low, but implications are profound. I was interested in this article because we wrote one of the first papers advocating debridement and retention in selected patients. This article confirms the validity of the approach for some patients. As in our original study, infection with *Staphylococcus aureus* remains

TABLE 4.—Factors Associated with Infection Control After Postoperative Infection Index Procedure: Entire Cohort (N = 64 knees)

Variable	Infection Controlled (N = 29)	Infection not Controlled (N = 35)	Multivariable p Value (Logistic Regression)
Age at PIIP (years)			0.64
≤ 65	16 (55)	17 (49)	
> 65	13 (45)	18 (51)	
Gender			0.74
Female	16 (55)	17 (49)	
Male	13 (45)	18 (51)	
Host factor			0.16
Uncompromised	15 (52)	12 (34)	
Compromised	14 (48)	23 (66)	
Diabetes mellitus			0.62
Yes	9 (31)	9 (26)	
No	20 (69)	26 (74)	
Pre-PIIP number of operations			0.16
One	16 (55)	15 (43)	
Two or more	13 (45)	20 (57)	
Pre-PIIP treatment for infection			0.55
Yes	11 (38)	10 (29)	
No	18 (62)	25 (71)	
Pre-PIIP implant			0.07
Primary	25 (86)	24 (69)	
Revision	4 (14)	11 (31)	
Type of infection			0.88
Early postoperative	2 (7)	4 (12)	
Acute hematogenous	10 (34)	19 (54)	
Chronic	17 (59)	12 (34)	
Microorganism			0.18
Staphylococcus aureus	9 (31)	17 (49)	
Other	20 (69)	18 (51)	
Number of microorganisms			0.52
Polybacterial	2 (7)	4 (11)	
Monobacterial	27 (93)	31 (89)	
PIIP			0.02*
Retention	10 (35)	22 (63)	
Removal	19 (65)	13 (37)	

Percentages are shown in parentheses. PIIP = postoperative infection index procedure.
*Statistically significant predictor.

a major confounding variable. When one factors the morbidity and costs associated with staged reimplantation, retention is clearly a viable option. The key is to understand the variables that correlate to outcome, which, as noted, is primarily that of organism type (Table 4).

B. F. Morrey, MD

Comparison of articulating and static spacers regarding infection with resistant organisms in total knee arthroplasty

Chiang E-R, Su Y-P, Chen T-H, et al (Veterans General Hosp, Taipei, Taiwan)
Acta Orthop 82:460-464, 2011

Introduction.—The result of treatment of infections involving antibiotic-resistant organisms in total knee arthroplasty (TKA) is often poor. We evaluated the efficacy of 2-stage revision in TKAs infected with resistant organisms and compared the clinical outcomes with articulating and conventional static spacers, in terms of both infection control and function.

Methods.—In a prospective manner, from June 2003 to January 2007 selected patients with a TKA infected with resistant organisms were enrolled and treated with 2-stage re-implantation. The 45 patients were divided into 2 groups: group A (23 patients) implanted with the articulating spacers and group S (22 patients) implanted with static spacers. All patients followed the same antibiotic protocols and had the same re-implantation criteria. The efficacy of infection control was evaluated using re-implantation rate, recurrence rate, and overall success rate. The functional and radiographic results were interpreted with the Hospital of Special Surgery (HSS) knee score and the Insall-Salvati ratio.

Results.—With mean 40 (24–61) months of follow-up, 22 of 23 knees were re-implanted in group A and 21 of 22 were re-implanted in group S. Of these re-implanted prostheses, 1 re-infection occurred in group A and 2 occurred in group S. Range of motion after re-implantation, the final functional scores, and the satisfaction rate were better in group A. One third of the patients in group S, and none in group A, had a patella baja.

Interpretation.—After 2-stage re-implantation of TKAs originally infected with resistant organisms, the clinical outcome was satisfactory—and similar to that reported after treatment of TKAs infected with low-virulence strains. Treatment with an articulating spacer resulted in better functional outcome and lower incidence of patella baja (Table 2).

▶ This important study provides credence to an ever-emerging practice of articulating spacers as a staged treatment for infected total knees (Fig 2 in the original article). The problem of motion altering the effectiveness of the treatment would be especially of concern in the highly virulent infections—hence, the focus of this study. It is reassuring that these investigators found the articulated spacer group to have equal effective control of infection with better motion (Table 2). What is important from my perspective is the lower frequency of

TABLE 2.—Clinical Results

	Articulating Spacer (n = 23)	Static Spacer (n = 2)
Re-infection rate	1/22	2/21
Success rate	21/23	19/22
ROM at spacer stage (°)	84 (50–105)	0
Post-revision ROM (°)	113 (95–125)	85 (70–100)[b]
Post-revision HSS score	90 (86–94)	82 (81–88)[b]
Patella baja		
Preoperative (%)	0	0
Mean ISR[a]	0.98	0.95
Postoperative (%)	0	33[b]
Mean ISR[a]	0.93	0.81[b]
Satisfaction rate	21/23	7/22[b]

[a]Insall-Salvati ratio.
[b]$p < 0.05$

patella infra in the articulated spacer group. This is particularly true when one considers the difficulty of subsequent revisions in the patient with a low-riding patella.

B. F. Morrey, MD

8 Sports Medicine

Introduction

It seems as though every year I mention that a review of the sports literature is synonymous with a review of the literature dealing with the anterior cruciate ligament. The same is true this year. I have made a major effort to select articles that relate to topics other than anterior cruciate ligament. Hence, in this section interventions regarding the ankle, shoulder, and knee are included. I have made some effort to select anterior cruciate topics that I think are most relevant and pick the articles I consider to be of the highest quality, thus providing the best data by which to make a decision in your own practice management of these patients. The sports medicine area has become extremely sophisticated and quite successful. It is exciting to see the advances being made in this area.

Bernard F. Morrey, MD

Epidemiology of Injuries Requiring Surgery Among High School Athletes in the United States, 2005 to 2010

Rechel JA, Collins CL, Comstock RD (The Res Inst at Nationwide Children's Hosp, Columbus, OH)

J Trauma 71:982-989, 2011

Background.—The proportion of high school sports-related injuries requiring surgery, which pose monetary and time loss burdens, has significantly increased during the last decade. The objective was to investigate the epidemiology of high school athletic injuries requiring surgery.

Methods.—High school sports-related injury data were collected for nine sports from 2005 to 2010 from 100 nationally representative US high schools.

Results.—Athletes sustained 1,380 injuries requiring surgery for a rate of 1.45 injuries per 10,000 athlete exposures. Boys' football had the highest injury rate (2.52) followed by boys' wrestling (1.64). Among gender comparable sports, girls' sports has a higher injury rate (1.20) than boys' (0.94) (rate ratio, 1.28; 95% confidence interval, 1.08–1.51; $p = 0.004$). The rate of injuries was higher in competition (3.23) than practice (0.79) (rate ratio, 4.08; 95% confidence interval, 3.67–4.55; $p < 0.001$) overall and in each sport. Commonly injured body sites were the knee (49.4%), head/face/mouth (9.7%), and shoulder (8.7%). Common diagnoses were complete ligament strain (32.1%) and fracture (26.4%). Nearly half (48.0%) resulted in medical disqualification for the season.

Conclusions.—Rates and patterns of injuries requiring surgery differ by sport, type of exposure, and gender. Future studies should identify sport-specific risk factors to drive effective interventions to decrease the incidence and severity of such injuries (Tables 1-3).

▶ As survey data, the main value is the numbers; the interpretation is more difficult and less relevant. Hence, we include all 3 tables. The first (Table 1) gives

TABLE 1.—Rates of Injuries Requiring Surgery per 10,000 Athlete Exposures by Sport and Type of Exposure, National High School Sports-Related Injury Surveillance Study, United States, 2005 to 2010 School Years

Sport	Type of Exposure	No. Injuries Requiring Surgery	National Estimate	AE*	Rates per 10,000 AE	RR (95% CI)†
Boys' football	Overall	648	179,958	2,569,733	2.52	
	Competition	376	109,728	434,561	8.65	6.79 (5.81–7.94)
	Practice	272	70,230	2,135,172	1.27	
Boys' soccer	Overall	92	45,607	917,409	1.00	
	Competition	73	36,130	274,833	2.66	8.98 (5.42–14.88)
	Practice	19	9,477	642,576	0.30	
Girls' soccer	Overall	120	63,467	811,324	1.48	
	Competition	98	51,142	242,324	4.04	10.46 (6.59–16.61)
	Practice	22	12,325	569,000	0.39	
Girls' volleyball	Overall	32	12,106	797,059	0.40	
	Competition	21	8,789	269,642	0.78	3.73 (1.80–7.74)
	Practice	11	3,317	527,417	0.21	
Boys' basketball	Overall	107	29,046	1,111,213	0.96	
	Competition	48	13,705	324,870	1.48	1.97 (1.35–2.88)
	Practice	59	15,341	786,343	0.75	
Girls' basketball	Overall	130	34,960	916,177	1.42	
	Competition	87	22,491	272,234	3.20	4.79 (3.32–6.90)
	Practice	43	12,469	643,943	0.67	
Boys' wrestling	Overall	138	32,775	840,881	1.64	
	Competition	67	16,748	219,136	3.06	2.68 (1.92–3.74)
	Practice	71	16,027	621,745	1.14	
Boys' baseball	Overall	75	24,272	876,299	0.86	
	Competition	38	13,166	312,425	1.22	1.85 (1.18–2.91)
	Practice	37	11,106	563,874	0.66	
Girls' softball	Overall	38	16,145	663,546	0.57	
	Competition	25	9,827	231,656	1.08	3.59 (1.83–7.01)
	Practice	13	6,318	431,890	0.30	
Boys' sports	Overall	1,060	311,658	6,315,535	1.68	
	Competition	602	189,477	1,565,825	3.84	3.99 (3.53–4.50)
	Practice	458	122,181	4,749,710	0.96	
Girls' sports	Overall	320	126,678	3,188,106	1.00	
	Competition	231	92,249	1,015,856	2.27	5.55 (4.35–7.09)
	Practice	89	34,429	2,172,250	0.41	
All sports	Overall	1,380	438,336	9,503,641	1.45	
	Competition	833	281,726	2,581,681	3.23	4.08 (3.67–4.55)
	Practice	547	156,610	6,921,960	0.79	

*AE is athletic exposure. One athlete participating in one practice or competition represents one AE.
†Rate ratios compare the competition rate of injuries requiring surgery with the practice rate of injuries requiring surgery.

TABLE 2.—Body Sites of Injuries Requiring Surgery by Sport, National High School Sports-Related Injury Surveillance Study, United States, 2005 to 2010 School Years*

Sport	Head/Face/ Mouth (%)	Shoulder (%)	Hand/Finger (%)	Knee (%)	Lower Leg (%)	Ankle (%)	Other† (%)
Boys' football‡	3.1	12.9	12.2	44.9	5.8	4.3	16.7
Boys' soccer‡	23.3	2.0	8.1	38.4	7.3	1.6	19.4
Girls' soccer	5.3	0.0	1.5	74.4	4.0	5.1	9.7
Girls' volleyball	9.0	2.1	2.3	79.2	0.0	3.2	4.2
Boys' basketball‡	19.8	5.7	9.8	47.3	1.3	5.4	10.6
Girls' basketball‡	12.2	1.9	2.9	68.8	3.5	3.6	7.0
Boys' wrestling‡	7.2	16.6	11.5	34.4	1.1	5.0	24.3
Boys' baseball‡	22.7	13.9	10.3	24.6	10.3	3.8	14.5
Girls' softball	25.3	6.9	7.7	38.5	7.0	13.0	1.6
Boys' sports‡	9.6	11.1	11.2	41.5	5.5	4.0	17.2
Girls' sports	10.1	1.6	2.8	68.7	3.9	5.5	7.4
All sports‡	9.7	8.3	8.7	49.4	5.0	4.5	14.3

*These proportions reflect national estimates of injuries requiring surgery.
†Other includes elbow, forearm, wrist, etc.
‡Does not sum to 100.0% due to rounding.

TABLE 3.—Diagnoses of Injuries Requiring Surgery by Sport, National High School Sports-Related Injury Surveillance Study, United States, 2005 to 2010 School Years*

Sport	Dislocation (%)	Fracture (%)	Ligament Sprain, Complete (%)	Ligament Sprain, Incomplete (%)	Torn Cartilage (%)	Other† (%)
Boys' football‡	10.0	28.5	28.3	5.4	11.5	16.2
Boys' soccer	1.8	37.2	19.0	10.0	8.1	23.9
Girls' soccer	0.0	18.1	60.5	2.5	8.7	10.2
Girls' volleyball	0.0	14.9	74.9	0.0	3.9	6.3
Boys' basketball‡	7.9	30.6	17.4	6.3	15.7	22.2
Girls' basketball	1.8	13.9	47.3	4.9	16.1	16.0
Boys' wrestling	14.7	22.4	14.7	5.4	21.5	21.3
Boys' baseball	10.0	37.1	11.8	2.6	15.4	23.1
Girls' softball	4.9	24.9	28.1	8.9	9.7	23.5
Boys' sports	9.1	30.0	23.2	5.9	12.8	19.0
Girls' sports‡	1.1	17.5	54.1	3.7	10.4	13.1
All sports	6.8	26.4	32.1	5.3	12.1	17.3

*These proportions reflect national estimates of injuries requiring surgery.
†Other includes hernia, muscle strain, separation, etc.
‡Does not sum to 100.0% due to rounding.

the incidence data, the second (Table 2) the anatomic distribution, and the third (Table 3) the pathologic distribution. I found the logic difficult to follow. In addition, this would be much more helpful if the trends, that is change over time, could have been identified. Regardless, this is a massive study, and the data are absolutely of interest.

B. F. Morrey, MD

Arthroscopic Stabilization of the Shoulder in Adolescent Athletes Participating in Overhead or Contact Sports

Castagna A, Rose GD, Borroni M, et al (IRCCS Istituto Clinico Humanitas, Milan, Italy; et al)
Arthroscopy 28:309-315, 2012

Purpose.—To investigate the outcome of arthroscopic capsular repair for shoulder instability in an active adolescent population participating in overhead or contact sports.

Methods.—We identified 67 patients (aged 13 to 18 years) with post-traumatic recurrent shoulder instability for inclusion in the study from our computer database. Of these patients, 65 (96%) were available for clinical review. There were 44 male and 21 female patients, with a mean age of 16 years at the time of surgery. All patients participated in overhead or contact sports at a competitive level. Arthroscopic capsulolabral repair was performed after at least 6 months of failed nonoperative treatment. The mean follow-up was 63 months. Shoulder range of motion and functional outcomes were measured preoperatively and postoperatively with Single Assessment Numeric Evaluation (SANE), Rowe, and American Shoulder and Elbow Surgeons (ASES) scores. Furthermore, type of sport, time until surgery, and number of dislocations were analyzed from our database to find any correlation with the recurrence rate.

Results.—At final follow-up, the mean SANE score was 87.23% (range, 30% to 100%) (preoperative mean, 46.15% [range, 20% to 50%]); the mean Rowe score was 85 (range, 30 to 100) (preoperative mean, 35.9 [range, 30 to 50]); and the mean ASES score was 84.12 (range, 30 to 100) (preoperative mean, 36.92 [range, 30 to 48]). The mean forward flexion and external rotation with the arm at 90° abduction did not change from preoperative values; 81% of the patients returned to their preinjury level of sport, and the rate of failure was 21%. The recurrence rate was not related to the postoperative scores ($P = .556$ for SANE score, $P = .753$ for Rowe score, and $P = .478$ for ASES score), the number of preoperative episodes of instability ($P = .59$), or the time from the first instability episode to the time of surgery ($P = .43$). There was a statistically significant relation ($P = .0021$) between recurrence and the type of sport practiced. Recurrence rate was related to the type of sport practiced.

Conclusions.—Arthroscopic stabilization is a reasonable surgical option even in an adolescent population performing sports activities. However, it must be emphasized to the patients and their relatives that the recurrence rate that could be expected after an arthroscopic procedure is higher than in the adult population.

Level of Evidence.—Level IV, therapeutic case series.

▶ The value of arthroscopic versus open reconstruction for the unstable shoulder continues to be widely discussed. This study is not a comparative one, but, in addition to several accepted scoring systems, focuses on age, maturity, and activity type as key parameters of success. What I found of interest is the correlation of overall recurrence with the type of sport, specifically, contact versus noncontact. This association has been previously reported from the United States, and this report from Italy finds the same correlation. The important message from my perspective, is, as previously reported, an open procedure may be better in those planning to return to a contact sport.

B. F. Morrey, MD

Articular Cartilage Treatment in High-Level Male Soccer Players: A Prospective Comparative Study of Arthroscopic Second-Generation Autologous Chondrocyte Implantation Versus Microfracture

Kon E, Filardo G, Berruto M, et al (Rizzoli Orthopaedic Inst, Bologna, Italy; Gaetano Pini Orthopaedic Inst, Milano, Italy; et al)

Am J Sports Med 39:2549-2557, 2011

Background.—Soccer is a highly demanding sport for the knee joint, and chondral injuries can cause disabling symptoms that may jeopardize an athlete's career. Articular cartilage lesions are difficult to treat, and the increased mechanical stress produced by this sport makes their management even more complex.

Hypothesis.—To evaluate whether the regenerative cell-based approach allows these highly demanding athletes a better functional recovery compared with the bone marrow stimulation approach.

Study Design.—Cohort study; Level of evidence, 2.

Methods.—Forty-one professional or semiprofessional male soccer players were treated from 2000 to 2006 and evaluated prospectively at 2 years and at a final 7.5-year mean follow-up (minimum, 4 years). Twenty-one patients were treated with arthroscopic second-generation autologous chondrocyte implantation (Hyalograft C) and 20 with the microfracture technique. The clinical outcome of all patients was analyzed using the cartilage standard International Cartilage Repair Society (ICRS) evaluation package. The sport activity level was evaluated with the Tegner score, and the recovery time was also recorded.

Results.—A significant improvement in all clinical scores from preoperative to final follow-up was found in both groups. The percentage of patients who returned to competition was similar: 80% in the microfracture group and 86% in the Hyalograft C group. Patients treated with microfracture needed a median of 8 months before playing their first official soccer game, whereas the Hyalograft C group required a median time of 12.5 months ($P = .009$). The International Knee Documentation Committee (IKDC) subjective score showed similar results at 2 years' follow-up but significantly better results in the Hyalograft C group at the final evaluation ($P = .005$). In fact, in the microfracture group, results decreased over time (from 86.8 ± 9.7 to 79.0 ± 11.6, $P < .0005$), whereas the Hyalograft C group presented a more durable outcome with stable results (90.5 ± 12.8 at 2 years and 91.0 ± 13.9 at the final follow-up).

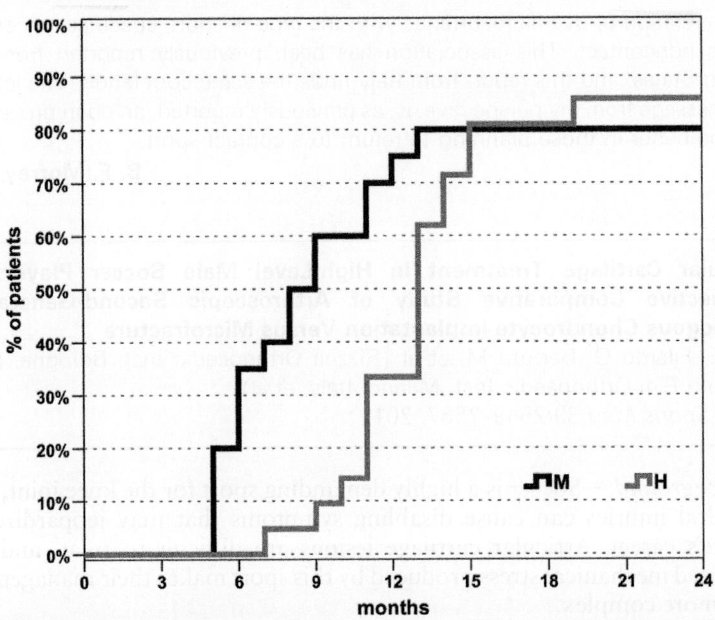

FIGURE 6.—The curves show the time needed to return to competitive sport activity level (first official soccer game) in the microfracture and Hyalograft C group, respectively. (Reprinted from Kon E, Filardo G, Berruto M, et al. Articular cartilage treatment in high-level male soccer players: a prospective comparative study of arthroscopic second-generation autologous chondrocyte implantation versus microfracture. *Am J Sports Med*. 2011;39:2549-2557, with permission from The Author(s).)

Conclusion.—Despite similar success in returning to competitive sport, microfracture allows a faster recovery but present a clinical deterioration over time, whereas arthroscopic second-generation autologous chondrocyte implantation delays the return of high-level male soccer players to competition but can offer more durable clinical results (Fig 6).

▶ The debate continues. This nicely done study is important because it compares 2 accepted treatment modalities for high-demand patients, that is, those playing competitive soccer (football). The sample is large enough to make valid comparisons. It may come as only a slight surprise that microfractures allowed an earlier return to full-out sport (Fig 6). However, it seems equally true, if not more relevant, that with longer follow-up, those with allograft transplants did significantly better than those with microfractures. It should be noted that both interventions were successful in more than 70% of the patients treated.

B. F. Morrey, MD

A Prospective Multicenter Study on the Outcome of Type I Collagen Hydrogel–Based Autologous Chondrocyte Implantation (CaReS) for the Repair of Articular Cartilage Defects in the Knee

Schneider U, Rackwitz L, Andereya S, et al (Arthro Nova Clinic, Ringsee, Germany; Univ of Würzburg, Germany; Univ of Aachen, Germany; et al)

Am J Sports Med 39:2558-2565, 2011

Background.—The Cartilage Regeneration System (CaReS) is a novel matrix-associated autologous chondrocyte implantation (ACI) technique for the treatment of chondral and osteochondral lesions (Outerbridge grades III and IV). For this technology, no expansion of the chondrocytes in a monolayer culture is needed, and a homogeneous cell distribution within the gel is guaranteed.

Purpose.—To report a prospective multicenter study of matrix-associated ACI of the knee using a new type I collagen hydrogel (CaReS).

Study Design.—Case series; Level of evidence, 4.

Methods.—From 2003 to 2008, 116 patients (49 women and 67 men; mean age, 32.5 ± 8.9 years) had CaReS implantation of the knee in 9 different centers. On the basis of the International Cartilage Repair Society (ICRS) Cartilage Injury Evaluation Package 2000, the International Knee Documentation Committee (IKDC) score, pain score (visual analog scale [VAS]), SF-36 score, overall treatment satisfaction and the IKDC functional status were evaluated. Patient follow-up was performed at 3, 6, and 12 months after surgery and annually thereafter. Mean follow-up was 30.2 ± 17.4 months (range, 12-60 months). There were 67 defects of the medial condyle, 14 of the lateral, 22 of the patella/trochlea, and 3 of the tibial plateau, and 10 patients had 2 lesions. The mean defect size was 5.4 ± 2.4 cm^2. Thirty percent of the defects were <4 cm^2 and 70% were >4 cm^2.

Results.—The IKDC score improved significantly from 42.4 ± 13.8 preoperatively to 70.5 ± 18.7 ($P < .001$) at latest follow-up. Global pain level significantly decreased ($P < .001$) from 6.7 ± 2.2 preoperatively to 3.2 ± 3.1 at latest follow-up. There also was a significant increase of both components of the SF-36 score. The overall treatment satisfaction was judged as very good or good in 88% by the surgeon and 80% by the patient. The IKDC functional knee status was grade I in 23.4%, II in 56.3%, III in 17.2%, and IV in 3.1% of the patients.

Conclusion.—Matrix-associated ACI employing the CaReS technology for the treatment of chondral or osteochondral defects of the knee is a safe and clinically effective treatment that yields significant functional improvement and improvement in pain level. However, further investigation is necessary to determine the long-term viability and clinical outcome of this procedure (Fig 2).

▶ The sports medicine community appropriately continues to search for a solution to the treatment of knees that have significant cartilage defects of grade III and IV. This study presents a relatively large sample of 119 patients treated by

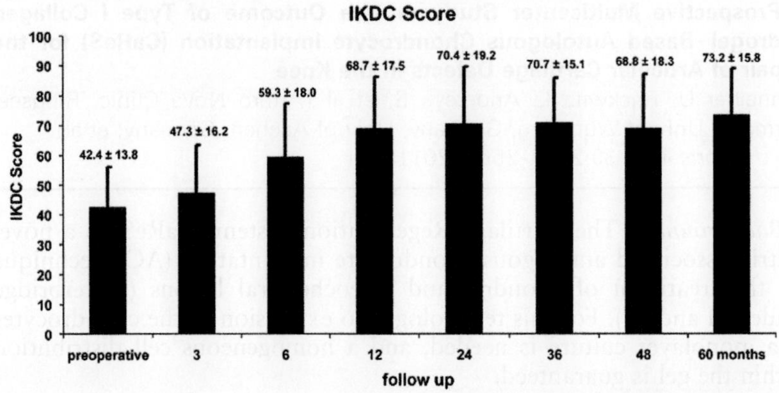

FIGURE 2.—Time course of the International Knee Documentation Committee (IKDC) score in 116 patients up to 60 months. (Reprinted from Schneider U, Rackwitz L, Andereya S, et al. A prospective multicenter study on the outcome of type I collagen hydrogel–based autologous chondrocyte implantation (CaReS) for the repair of articular cartilage defects in the knee. *Am J Sports Med.* 2011;39:2558-2565, with permission from The Author(s).)

the Cartilage Regeneration System. The advantage of the methodology is the maintenance of the chondrocytes within the defective knee via a hydrogel technology. An additional advantage of the method is that of precisely tailoring the size of the gel patch to the defect. The ability to treat large lesions is indeed attractive. As with all such studies, the key is long-term durability. While the average surveillance is only 30 months, some patients were followed up for as long as 2 years. The data concerning these patients suggest little deterioration in outcome after the third year (Fig 2). This seems to be a viable approach to addressing cartilage defects, even in those with large deficiencies.

B. F. Morrey, MD

Clinical Outcome of Autologous Chondrocyte Implantation for Failed Microfracture Treatment of Full-Thickness Cartilage Defects of the Knee Joint

Pestka JM, Bode G, Salzmann G, et al (Freiburg Univ Hosp, Germany)
Am J Sports Med 40:325-331, 2012

Background.—Although various factors have been identified that influence outcome after autologous chondrocyte implantation (ACI), the relevance of prior treatment of the cartilage defect and its effect concerning the outcome of second-line ACI have not been evaluated to a full extent.

Hypothesis.—Autologous chondrocyte implantation used as a second-line treatment after failed arthroscopic microfracturing is associated with a higher failure rate and inferior clinical results compared with ACI as a first-line treatment.

Study Design.—Cohort study; Level of evidence, 3.

Methods.—A total of 28 patients with isolated cartilage defects at the knee joint were treated with ACI after microfracture as a first-line treatment had failed (failure defined as the necessity of reintervention). These patients were assigned to group A and compared with a matched-pair cohort of patients of identical age, defect size, and defect location (group B) in which ACI was used as a first-line treatment. Failure rates in both groups were assessed. Postoperative knee status was evaluated with the International Knee Documentation Committee (IKDC) score and Knee injury and Osteoarthritis Outcome Score (KOOS), and sporting activity was assessed by use of the Activity Rating Scale. Mean follow-up times were 48.0 months (range, 15.1-75.1 months) in group A and 41.4 months (range, 15.4-83.6 months) in group B. Differences between groups A and B were analyzed by Student *t* test.

Results.—Group A had significantly greater failure rates (7 of 28 patients) in comparison with group B (1 of 28 patients; $P = .0241$). Mean (SD) postoperative IKDC scores revealed 58.4 (22.4) points in group A with a trend toward higher score results (69.0 [19.1] points) for patients in group B ($P = .0583$). Significantly different results were obtained for KOOS pain and activity of daily living subscales, whereas the remaining KOOS subscales did not show significant differences. Despite the significantly higher failure rate observed in group A, those patients did not participate in fewer activities or perform physical activity less frequently or at a lower intensity.

Conclusion.—Autologous chondrocyte implantation after failed microfracturing appears to be associated with a significantly higher failure rate and inferior clinical outcome when compared with ACI as a first-line treatment (Table 2).

▶ This is a very interesting study of considerable value. It addresses the issue of prioritization of decision making when several viable options are available. I am

TABLE 2.—Postoperative Knee Status Surveyed by the International Knee Documentation Committee (IKDC) Score and Knee Injury and Osteoarthritis Outcome Score (KOOS)[a]

Parameter	Group A	Group B	*P* Value
Number of patients	27	28	NA
IKDC score, mean ± SD	58.4 ± 22.4	69.0 ± 19.1	.058
KOOS score, mean ± SD			
Symptoms	72.7 ± 22.3	80.0 ± 16.7	.088
Pain	69.2 ± 25.6	80.1 ± 16.4	.034[b]
Sports/recreation	43.7 ± 31.3	56.4 ± 28.4	.061
ADL	78.5 ± 19.3	86.3 ± 14.3	.024[b]
QOL	41.5 ± 24.5	48.9 ± 23.7	.133
$KOOS_4$	56.8 ± 23.6	66.3 ± 19.0	.053
VAS subjective pain before ACI (0-10), mean ± SD	3.4 ± 1.9	4.4 ± 2.5	.014[b]
VAS subjective knee function after ACI (0-10), mean ± SD	6.2 ± 2.3	6.9 ± 2.2	.032[b]

[a]ACI, autologous chondrocyte implantation; ADL, activities of daily living; NA, not applicable; QOL, quality of life. $KOOS_4$ was calculated as (KOOS-P + KOOS-S + KOOS-SR + KOOS-Q)/4; VAS (visual analog scale) was assessed for knee pain before ACI and knee function after ACI on a scale ranging from 0 (no knee pain, poor knee function after ACI) to 10 (maximum pain, excellent knee function after ACI).

[b]Indicates statistically significant differences ($P \leq .05$).

particularly interested in this study, as it reinforces a point I have long tried to make—incorrect initial decisions and improper or inadequate treatment is not free.

That is, the best chance for a good outcome is at the initial treatment. Not profound, but no less true. Hence, this nice, clean study clearly demonstrates (Table 2) failed microfracture adversely affects the subsequent ability to salvage with autologous chondrocyte transplantation in the ACL-deficient knee. This gives clear direction in the decision making of the cartilage/anterior cruciate ligament–deficient knee.

B. F. Morrey, MD

Former Male Elite Athletes Have a Higher Prevalence of Osteoarthritis and Arthroplasty in the Hip and Knee Than Expected

Tveit M, Rosengren BE, Nilsson J-Å, et al (Lund Univ, Malmö, Sweden)
Am J Sports Med 40:527-533, 2012

Background.—Intense exercise has been reported as one risk factor for hip and knee osteoarthritis (OA).

Purpose.—This study aimed to evaluate (1) whether this is true for both former impact and nonimpact athletes, (2) if the risk of a hip or knee arthroplasty due to OA is higher than expected, and (3) if joint deterioration is associated with knee injuries.

Study Design.—Cohort study; Level of evidence, 3.

Methods.—The prevalence of OA and arthroplasty in the hip and knee were registered in 709 former male elite athletes with a median age of 70 years (range, 50-93 years), retired from sports for a median 35 years (range, 1-63 years), and compared with 1368 matched controls. Odds ratios (ORs) are presented as means with 95% confidence intervals (95% CIs).

Results.—The risk of hip or knee OA was higher in former athletes (OR, 1.9; 95% CI, 1.5-2.3), as was arthroplasty based on OA in either of these joints (OR, 2.2; 95% CI, 1.6-3.1). The risk of hip OA was doubled (OR, 2.0; 95% CI, 1.5-2.8) and hip arthroplasty was 2.5 times higher (OR, 2.5; 95% CI, 1.6-3.7) in former athletes than in controls, predominantly driven by a higher risk in former impact athletes. Also, the risk of knee OA was higher (OR, 1.6; 95% CI, 1.3-2.1), as was knee arthroplasty (OR, 1.6; 95% CI, 0.9-2.7), driven by a higher risk in both former impact and nonimpact athletes. Knee OA in impact athletes was associated with knee injury.

Conclusion.—Hip and knee OA and hip and knee arthroplasty are more commonly found in former male elite athletes than expected. A previous knee injury is associated with knee OA in former impact athletes but not in nonimpact athletes (Tables 3 and 4).

► The orthopedic surgeon has known for years that there is some relation between prior injury and development of joint arthritis. The European data document these quantitative findings—sport participation doubles the likelihood of subsequent arthritis for both the hip (Table 3) and the knee (Table 4). What I

TABLE 3.—Prevalence of Hip Osteoarthritis and Hip Arthroplasty[a]

	N[b]	Participants With Osteoarthritis/Arthroplasty, Unadjusted n (%)	P Value	Adjusted for Age OR (95% CI)	Adjusted for Age, BMI, and Occupational Load OR (95% CI)	Adjusted for Age, BMI, Occupational Load, and Soft Tissue Knee Injury OR (95% CI)
Hip osteoarthritis						
All athletes	662	**94 (14.2)**	<.0001	**2.03 (1.51-2.76)**	**2.18 (1.53-3.10)**	**2.18 (1.52-3.13)**
Controls	1247	98 (7.9)	—	1.00	1.00	1.00
Nonimpact sport	90	8 (8.9)	.73	1.35 (0.63-2.92)	0.90 (0.34-2.39)	0.94 (0.35-2.52)
Impact sport	572	**86 (15.0)**	<.0001	**2.14 (1.57-2.92)**	**2.37 (1.65-3.38)**	**2.35 (1.62-3.40)**
Soccer	366	**52 (14.2)**	<.001	**2.01 (1.40-2.89)**	**2.19 (1.40-3.29)**	**2.14 (1.40-3.25)**
Handball	141	**21 (14.9)**	.005	**2.09 (1.25-3.47)**	**2.41 (1.38-4.22)**	**2.65 (1.50-4.67)**
Ice hockey	65	**13 (20.0)**	<.001	**3.13 (1.64-5.98)**	**3.41 (1.72-6.76)**	**3.24 (1.58-6.65)**
Hip arthroplasty						
All athletes	663	**55 (8.3)**	<.0001	**2.47 (1.64-3.70)**	**2.71 (1.67-4.38)**	**2.94 (1.78-4.85)**
Controls	1247	47 (3.8)	—	1.00	1.00	1.00
Nonimpact sport	90	5 (5.6)	.40	1.87 (0.71-4.90)	1.75 (0.57-5.35)	1.90 (0.61-5.91)
Impact sport	573	**50 (8.7)**	<.0001	**2.56 (1.69-3.87)**	**2.83 (1.74-4.61)**	**3.05 (1.84-5.07)**
Soccer	368	**32 (8.7)**	<.001	**2.54 (1.59-4.06)**	**2.83 (1.65-4.85)**	**3.02 (1.72-5.28)**
Handball	141	**12 (8.5)**	.008	**2.48 (1.27-4.82)**	**2.91 (1.37-6.16)**	**3.29 (1.53-7.07)**
Ice hockey	64	**6 (9.4)**	.03	**2.95 (1.20-7.27)**	**3.25 (1.26-8.40)**	**3.50 (1.32-9.27)**

[a]Data are presented as number of individuals with proportions (%) in parentheses or as odds ratios (ORs) with 95% confidence intervals (95% CIs) in parentheses in different models adjusted for combinations of age, body mass index (BMI), occupational load, and soft tissue knee injury. Statistically significant differences are highlighted in bold.

[b]Excluded in the analyses were 29 individuals with a history of hip fracture, and, depending on the specific estimation, those who had not answered whether they had been diagnosed with hip osteoarthritis and/or whether they had undergone a hip replacement surgery.

TABLE 4.—History of Soft Tissue Knee Injury and Prevalence of Knee Osteoarthritis and Knee Arthroplasty[a]

	N[b]	Participants With Soft Tissue Knee Injury/ Osteoarthritis/ Arthroplasty, Unadjusted n (%)	*P* Value	Adjusted for Age OR (95% CI)	Adjusted for Age, BMI, and Occupational Load OR (95% CI)	Adjusted for Age, BMI, Occupational Load, and Soft Tissue Knee Injury OR (95% CI)
Soft tissue knee injury						
All athletes	678	**245 (36.1)**	<.0001	**1.66 (1.35-2.02)**	**1.53 (1.23-1.92)**	—
Controls	1316	332 (25.2)	—	1.00	1.00	—
Nonimpact sport	92	22 (23.9)	.79	0.89 (0.54-1.46)	0.80 (0.47-1.37)	—
Impact sport	586	**223 (38.1)**	<.0001	**1.81 (1.47-2.23)**	**1.67 (1.33-2.10)**	—
Soccer	378	**139 (36.8)**	<.0001	**1.71 (1.34-2.18)**	**1.59 (1.22-2.07)**	—
Handball	140	**50 (35.7)**	.007	**1.65 (1.14-2.38)**	**1.47 (1.00-2.17)**	—
Ice hockey	68	**34 (50.0)**	<.0001	**2.93 (1.79-4.79)**	**2.68 (1.60-4.49)**	—
Knee osteoarthritis						
All athletes	664	**129 (19.4)**	<.001	**1.64 (1.27-2.11)**	**1.56 (1.17-2.07)**	1.31 (0.93-1.85)
Controls	1258	163 (13.0)	—	1.00	1.00	1.00
Nonimpact sport	90	18 (20.0)	.06	**1.81 (1.04-3.14)**	1.65 (0.90-3.02)	**3.19 (1.47-6.91)**
Impact sport	574	**111 (19.3)**	<.001	**1.62 (1.25-2.12)**	**1.55 (1.16-2.08)**	1.19 (0.83-1.71)
Soccer	368	**67 (18.2)**	.01	**1.52 (1.11-2.07)**	**1.46 (1.04-2.05)**	1.13 (0.75-1.72)
Handball	141	**30 (15.8)**	.007	**1.82 (1.18-2.81)**	**1.86 (1.16-3.00)**	1.62 (0.89-2.94)
Ice hockey	65	**14 (21.5)**	.05	**1.88 (1.01-3.47)**	1.51 (0.77-2.95)	0.92 (0.42-1.98)
Knee arthroplasty						
All athletes	658	24 (3.6)	.12	1.58 (0.91-2.73)	1.32 (0.73-2.40)	1.51 (0.58-3.93)
Controls	1245	30 (2.4)	—	1.00	1.00	1.00
Nonimpact sport	91	1 (1.1)	.42	0.49 (0.07-3.71)	0.46 (0.06-3.54)	0.59 (0.11-3.26)
Impact sport	567	**23 (4.1)**	.05	**1.74 (1.00-3.02)**	1.45 (0.79-2.64)	1.67 (0.64-4.35)
Soccer	363	12 (3.3)	.35	1.40 (0.71-2.77)	1.15 (0.56-2.39)	1.21 (0.38-3.84)
Handball	141	7 (5.0)	.07	2.12 (0.91-4.92)	1.93 (0.75-4.94)	1.71 (0.33-8.88)
Ice hockey	63	4 (6.3)	.05	2.81 (0.96-8.27)	2.29 (0.75-6.93)	**4.50 (1.02-19.79)**

[a]Data are presented as numbers of individuals with proportions (%) in parentheses or as odds ratios (ORs) with 95% confidence intervals (95% CIs) in parentheses in different models adjusted for combinations of age, body mass index (BMI), occupational load, and soft tissue knee injury. Statistically significant differences are highlighted in bold.

[b]Excluded in the analyses were 11 individuals with a history of knee fracture, and, depending on the specific estimation, those who had not answered whether they had been diagnosed with a soft tissue knee injury or knee osteoarthritis and/or whether they had undergone a knee replacement surgery.

found interesting is the even higher frequency for impact sports, not to be confused with contact sports. Impact means running or gliding (eg, soccer and ice hockey). Who knows how much greater this would be for contact sports, such as football or rugby. Study the tables; they are revealing.

B. F. Morrey, MD

Does Anterior Cruciate Ligament Reconstruction Lead to Degenerative Disease?: Thirteen-Year Results After Bone–Patellar Tendon–Bone Autograft

Murray JRD, Lindh AM, Hogan NA, et al (AOC Southmead Hosp, Westbury on Trym, Bristol, UK; Southmead Hosp, Bristol, Avon, UK; Australian Inst of Musculoskeletal Res, Sydney, Australia)

Am J Sports Med 40:404-413, 2012

Background.—Reporting of long-term outcome of anterior cruciate ligament (ACL) reconstruction with the patellar tendon (bone–patellar tendon–bone [BTB]) autograft is limited. There are concerns that degenerative joint disease is common in the long term, which may be associated with the procedure itself.

Hypotheses.—(1) ACL reconstruction with BTB provides good long-term outcome. (2) There are additional factors to surgical reconstruction that can be associated with the development of degenerative disease.

Study Design.—Case series; Level of evidence, 4.

Methods.—Of 161 patients, 114 were eligible. Patient-centered outcome was by Lysholm and subjective International Knee Documentation Committee (IKDC) score; objective outcome measures were clinical examination and IKDC radiological grade.

Results.—Mean average follow-up was 13 years. The IKDC radiological grades in the worst compartment were A = 15%, B = 51%, C = 19%, and D = 14% (n = 83). There was a significant difference between the injured versus contralateral uninjured knee (n = 42, P = .003). In a subgroup with no meniscal or chondral injury the IKDC grades were A = 38%, B = 55%, C = 7%, and D = 0% (n = 29). The mean subjective scores were 89 ± 11 (Lysholm) and 83 ± 15 (IKDC) (n = 114). Poor IKDC subjective outcome was associated with chondral injury (P = .001), previous surgery (P = .022), return to sport (P = .013), and poor radiological grade in the ipsilateral medial compartment (P = .004). A poor IKDC radiological grade was associated with chondral injury (P = .002), meniscal injury (P = .010) and meniscectomy (P = .012), an IKDC subjective score of <85 (P = .01), and poor radiological grade in the contralateral medial compartment (P = .041).

Conclusion.—At 13 years, BTB ACL reconstruction provides a good outcome. Chondral and meniscal damage at surgery were associated with a poor radiological outcome, indicating that injuries sustained during

TABLE 5.—International Knee Documentation Committee (IKDC) Radiological Grading of the Worst-Graded Compartment in the Injured and Uninjured Knee in Patients With No Chondral or Meniscal Injury[a]

IKDC Grade of Worst Compartment	Ipsilateral ACLR Knee	Contralateral Knee
A	12 (41)	7 (58)
B	14 (48)	4 (34)
C	3 (7)	1 (8)
D	0 (0)	0 (0)

[a]The values are given as n (%). ACLR, anterior cruciate ligament-reconstructed.

ACL rupture may be the main predictors of degenerative bone disease (Table 5).

▶ The article is of great interest by topic and intent. Unfortunately, without a true control group we continue our quest to truly understand the indications for anterior cruciate ligament (ACL) reconstruction. The study does validate what is known, that is, the profound impact of associated injury, especially when involving the articular surface. The increased frequency of radiographic changes in the ACL reconstructed knee (Table 5) is attributed to the associated injuries. The study covers 13 years and has a large number of patients (more than 100) and hence does offer considerable insight. It does seem reasonable to conclude the ACL reconstruction, as such, does not cause the progressive disease. What is not clear is the role of the reconstruction in preventing the progression.

B. F. Morrey, MD

Clinical Results and Risk Factors for Reinjury 15 Years After Anterior Cruciate Ligament Reconstruction: A Prospective Study of Hamstring and Patellar Tendon Grafts

Leys T, Salmon L, Waller A, et al (North Sydney Orthopaedic and Sports Medicine Centre, Sydney, New South Wales, Australia; et al)
Am J Sports Med 40:595-605, 2012

Background.—There is a lack of prospective studies comparing the long-term outcome of endoscopic anterior cruciate ligament (ACL) reconstruction with either a patellar tendon or hamstring tendon autograft.

Purpose.—This prospective longitudinal study compared the results of isolated endoscopic ACL reconstruction utilizing a 4-strand hamstring tendon (HT) or patellar tendon (PT) autograft over a 15-year period with respect to reinjury, clinical outcomes, and the development of osteoarthritis.

Study Design.—Cohort study; Level of evidence, 2.

Methods.—Ninety consecutive patients with isolated ACL rupture were reconstructed with a PT autograft, and 90 patients received an HT autograft, with an identical surgical technique. Patients were assessed at 2,

5, 7, 10, and 15 years. Assessment included the International Knee Documentation Committee (IKDC) knee ligament evaluation including radiographic evaluation, KT-1000 arthrometer testing, and Lysholm knee score.

Results.—Patients who received the PT graft had significantly worse outcomes compared with those who received the HT graft at 15 years for the variables of radiologically detectable osteoarthritis (grade A: 46% in PT and 69% in HT; $P = .04$), motion loss (extension deficit <3°: 79% in PT and 94% in HT; $P = .03$), single-legged hop test (grade A: 65% in PT and 92% in HT; $P = .001$), participation in strenuous activity (very strenuous or strenuous: 62% of PT and 77% of HT; $P = .04$), and kneeling pain (moderate or greater pain: 42% of PT and 26% of HT; $P = .04$). There was no significant difference between the HT and PT groups in overall IKDC grade (grade A: 47% of PT and 57% of HT; $P = .35$). An ACL graft rupture occurred in 17% of the HT group and 8% of the PT group ($P = .07$). An ACL graft rupture was associated with nonideal tunnel position (odds ratio [OR], 5.0) and male sex (OR, 3.2). Contralateral ACL rupture occurred in significantly more PT patients (26%) than HT patients (12%) ($P = .02$) and was associated with age ≤18 years (OR, 4.1) and the PT graft (OR, 2.6).

Conclusion.—Anterior cruciate ligament reconstruction using ipsilateral autograft continues to show excellent results in terms of patient satisfaction, symptoms, function, activity level, and stability. The use of HT autograft does, however, show better outcomes than the PT autograft in all of these outcome measures. Additionally, at 15 years, the HT graft–reconstructed ACLs have shown a lower rate of radiological osteoarthritis (Figs 4, 12, and 13).

▶ I found this to be a truly worthwhile study. It is a true prospective assessment of the bone tendon bone versus the hamstring autograft reconstruction for anterior cruciate ligament (ACL) deficiency.

The assessment tools were rigorous, including objective clinical and radiographic data as well as subjective information. The conclusions are difficult to

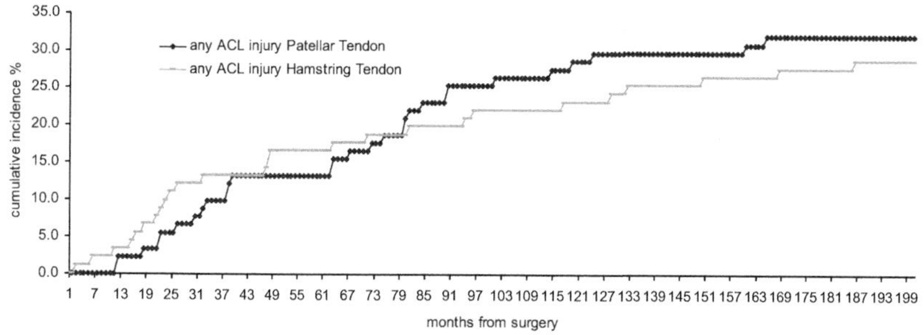

FIGURE 4.—Incidence of any anterior cruciate ligament (ACL) rupture after surgery. Percentage of patients with either ACL graft rupture or contralateral ACL rupture in the patellar tendon and hamstring tendon groups over a 15-year period. (Reprinted from Leys T, Salmon L, Waller A, et al. Clinical results and risk factors for reinjury 15 years after anterior cruciate ligament reconstruction: a prospective study of hamstring and patellar tendon grafts. *Am J Sports Med.* 2012;40:595-605, with permission from The Author(s).)

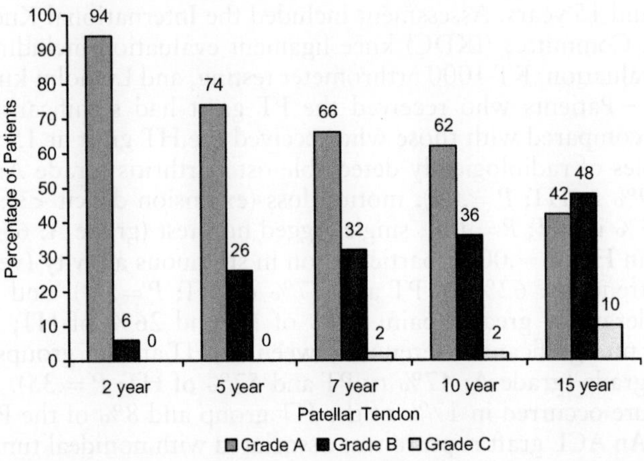

FIGURE 12.—Patellar tendon radiographic grade over time. Percentage of patients from the patellar tendon group with radiographic grades A, B, or C over time. (Reprinted from Leys T, Salmon L, Waller A, et al. Clinical results and risk factors for reinjury 15 years after anterior cruciate ligament reconstruction: a prospective study of hamstring and patellar tendon grafts. *Am J Sports Med.* 2012;40:595-605, with permission from The Author(s).)

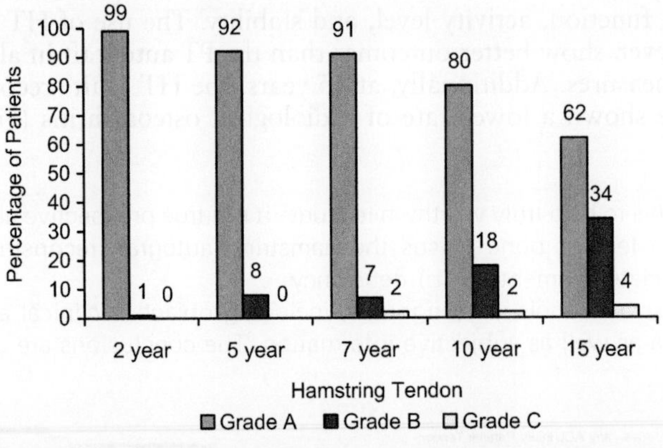

FIGURE 13.—Hamstring tendon radiographic grade over time. Percentage of patients from the hamstring tendon group with radiographic grades A, B, or C over time. (Reprinted from Leys T, Salmon L, Waller A, et al. Clinical results and risk factors for reinjury 15 years after anterior cruciate ligament reconstruction: a prospective study of hamstring and patellar tendon grafts. *Am J Sports Med.* 2012;40:595-605, with permission from The Author(s).)

criticize: hamstring reconstruction, at least in these surgeons' hands and with their technique is superior to bone patella bone as a graft tissue. With the exception of rerupture (Fig 4), all other assessments favor using the hamstring. The interesting finding for me was the increased incidence of contralateral ACL injury, which I don't really understand, in the bone tendon cohort. The radiographic finding of greater arthrosis with the bone tendon graft (Fig 12) compared with the hamstring reconstruction (Fig 13), however, is almost enough to compel one to use the hamstring tissue. My confession, I have always been an advocate and user of the bone tendon bone!

B. F. Morrey, MD

Amount of Meniscal Resection After Failed Meniscal Repair

Pujol N, Barbier O, Boisrenoult P, et al (Versailles-Saint Quentin Univ, Le Chesnay, France)

Am J Sports Med 39:1648-1652, 2011

Background.—The failure rate after arthroscopic meniscal repair ranges from 5% to 43.5% (mean, 15%) in the literature. But little is known about the amount of meniscal tissue removed after failed meniscal repair.

Hypothesis.—The volume of subsequent meniscectomy after failed meniscal repair is not increased when compared with the volume of meniscectomy that would have been performed if not initially repaired.

Study Design.—Case series; Level of evidence, 4.

Methods.—From January 2000 to December 2009, 295 knees underwent arthroscopic meniscal repair for unstable peripheral vertical tears. When present (219 cases), all anterior cruciate ligament (ACL) tears underwent reconstruction. Patients with multiple ligament injuries and posterior cruciate ligament injuries were excluded from the analysis. Thirty-two medial and 5 lateral menisci underwent subsequent meniscectomy after failed repair at a mean of 26 months postoperatively (range, 3-114 months). Five parameters were specifically evaluated: the amount of meniscectomy related to the initial tear, the ACL status, the appearance of chondral lesions, the time from the initial injury to meniscal repair, and the time from repair to meniscectomy.

Results.—The posterior segment of the meniscus was involved in all tears and retears. Among failures, resection of the meniscal segments primarily repaired occurred for 17 medial and 2 lateral meniscal tears (52%); the tear extended in 5 cases (all medial menisci), and healing of some repaired segments led to a partial resection of the initial lesion in 35% of cases (10 medial menisci, 3 lateral menisci). The time from injury to meniscal repair was correlated with an increasing volume of meniscus removed ($P < .05$) and with the presence of stage 2 or 3 chondral lesions at revision ($P < .03$). All knees with extended tears (5 cases) and/or with significant chondral degeneration (8 cases) occurred in ACL-reconstructed knees. Among them, 50% (6 of 12) of ACL-reconstructed knees were ACL deficient.

Conclusion.—There are few detrimental effects when repairing a repairable meniscal lesion, even if it fails. The amount of meniscectomy is rarely increased when compared with the initial lesion. This study supports the hypothesis that the meniscus can be partially saved and that a risk of a partial failure should be taken when possible.

▶ This is my kind of study. It has asked a simple, but clinically relevant question that has not been studied, at least to any significant extent. If one repairs a torn meniscus, is it free? By that I mean, other than another operation, has the initial decision compromised future treatment of prognosis? For the meniscus, the question is most relevant, as the status of the meniscus is so closely related to subsequent degenerative arthritis. The simple answer—no. Unsuccessful repair of a torn meniscus does not result in greater resection to address the failure. Helpful and encouraging.

B. F. Morrey, MD

Are Meniscus and Cartilage Injuries Related to Time to Anterior Cruciate Ligament Reconstruction?

Chhadia AM, Inacio MCS, Maletis GB, et al (Kaiser Permanente, Irvine, CA; Kaiser Permanente, San Diego, CA; Kaiser Permanente, Baldwin Park, CA)

Am J Sports Med 39:1894-1899, 2011

Background.—Functional instability after anterior cruciate ligament injury can be successfully treated with ligament reconstruction. However, the associated meniscus and cartilage lesions often cannot be repaired and may have long-term detrimental effects on knee function.

Purpose.—The authors used the large database within the Kaiser Permanente Anterior Cruciate Ligament Reconstruction Registry to evaluate time to surgery, age, and gender as risk factors for meniscus and cartilage injury and associations with meniscus repair rates in patients.

Study Design.—Cross-sectional study; Level of evidence, 3.

Methods.—A retrospective review of the Kaiser Permanente Anterior Cruciate Ligament Reconstruction Registry was performed. The associations between time to surgery, age, and gender with meniscus and cartilage lesions and meniscus repair were analyzed using binary logistic regression modeling to calculate odds ratios (ORs) while adjusting for potential confounding variables.

Results.—A total of 1252 patients met the inclusion criteria. The risk of medial meniscus injury increased only with time to surgery (6—12 months: OR = 1.81, 95% confidence internal [CI] 1.29-2.54, $P = .001$; and >12 months: OR = 2.19, 95% CI 1.58-3.02, $P < .001$). The risk of lateral meniscus injury decreased only with female gender (OR = 0.65, 95% CI 0.51-0.83, $P = .001$). The risk of cartilage injury increased with age (OR = 1.05 per year, 95% CI 1.04-1.07, $P < .001$) and time to surgery >12 months (OR = 1.57, 95% CI 1.12-2.20, $P = .009$), but decreased with female gender (OR = 0.71, 95% CI 0.54-0.92, $P = .009$). Medial meniscus repairs relative to medial meniscus injury decreased with increasing time to surgery (3-6 months: OR = 0.61, 95% CI 0.37-1.00, $P = .050$; and >12 months: OR = 0.41, 95% CI 0.25-0.67, $P < .001$) and increasing age (OR = 0.96 per year, 95% CI 0.94-0.98, $P < .001$).

Conclusion.—Increased risk of medial meniscus injury and decreased repair rate were strongly associated with increasing time to surgery.

TABLE 2.—Study Population Average Age by Time to Surgery and Gender[a]

Gender	Time to Surgery	Mean	SD	*P* Value
Male	0-3 months	26.5	9.9	.001
	3-6 months	27.8	10.8	
	6-12 months	27.6	10.3	
	>12 months	29.6	8.7	
	Total	28.0	10.0	
Female	0-3 months	21.9	10.0	<.001
	3-6 months	24.4	11.8	
	6-12 months	25.5	12.0	
	>12 months	30.4	11.1	
	Total	24.7	11.4	

[a]SD, standard deviation.

Increased risk of cartilage injury was associated with increasing age, increasing time to surgery, and male gender (Table 2).

▶ From our perspective, protection of the knee from subsequent injury is a major indication for anterior cruciate ligament (ACL) reconstruction. The meniscus is known to be both vulnerable to tear in the unstable knee and strongly correlated to subsequent arthritis if removed. Hence the central question addressed here is critical. Is the patient at risk the longer the delay from injury to surgery from the perspective of subsequent meniscus and cartilage damage? Using the massive Kaiser Permanente database, the question is cleanly answered: delay to reconstruction and male gender are both major risk factors (Table 2). This study should be considered when advising our patients on the matter and importance of timing. What is not known is the subtleties of the specific findings, such as pivot shift status. Regardless, this is a useful contribution.

B. F. Morrey, MD

Bone Contusion and Associated Meniscal and Medial Collateral Ligament Injury in Patients with Anterior Cruciate Ligament Rupture

Yoon KH, Yoo JH, Kim K-I (Kyung Hee Univ, Dongdaemun-gu, Seoul, South Korea)

J Bone Joint Surg Am 93:1510-1518, 2011

Background.—The present study examined the prevalence of bone contusions in patients with anterior cruciate ligament (ACL) injury as well as its association with tears of the lateral meniscus, medial meniscus, and medial collateral ligament (MCL).

Methods.—Eighty-one patients with an arthroscopy-proven ACL rupture for whom magnetic resonance images (MRI) were acquired within six weeks after the initial trauma were examined. The bone contusions on the lateral femoral condyle, lateral aspect of the tibial plateau, medial femoral condyle, and medial aspect of the tibial plateau were documented. The injury to MCL was also observed with MRI. The tears of the lateral meniscus and medial meniscus were detected during arthroscopy. The prevalence of lateral meniscus, medial meniscus, and MCL injuries was compared with the existence of the bone contusions.

Results.—Sixty-eight (84%) of the eighty-one knees had bone contusions on magnetic resonance imaging. The prevalence of bone contusions was 68%, 73%, 24%, and 26% in the lateral femoral condyle, lateral aspect of the tibial plateau, medial femoral condyle, and medial aspect of the tibial plateau, respectively. There were two fractures of the posterolateral aspect of the tibial plateau and two fractures of the posteromedial aspect of the tibial plateau. The overall prevalences of injury to the lateral meniscus and medial meniscus were 54% (forty-four of eighty-one) and 51% (forty-one of eighty-one), respectively. The prevalence of MCL injuries was 22% (eighteen of eighty-one). The prevalences of lateral meniscus ($p = 0.010$), medial meniscus ($p = 0.011$), and MCL ($p = 0.066$) injuries increased as the bone contusion progressed from being absent, to involving only the lateral compartment, and finally to involving both lateral and medial compartments.

Conclusions.—Bone contusions were prevalent in patients with ACL ruptures, and injuries of the menisci and the MCL tended to increase with the progression of bone contusion. The contrecoup mechanism of bone contusion on the medial compartment resulting from an ACL injury was supported. These results suggest that a higher-energy injury led to a more extensive bone contusion and a greater prevalence of associated injury of other anatomic structures in the knee.

Level of Evidence.—Diagnostic Level IV. See Instructions to Authors for a complete description of levels of evidence.

▶ This sophisticated study nicely reveals the relation of compression injuries across the knee and soft tissue injury in those with anterior cruciate ligament tears. It is surprising to see the same bone contusion pattern and prevalence for both the lateral and medial associated meniscus injury (Fig 5 in the original article). As the authors state, it does support the contrecoup theory of injury. The prevalence of medial collateral ligament injury is lower but reveals the same pattern. This study nicely highlights the complexity of the injury and undoubtedly some of the variable results with reconstruction related to less well-recognized associated injury.

B. F. Morrey, MD

Degeneration of the Knee Joint in Skeletally Immature Patients With a Diagnosis of an Anterior Cruciate Ligament Tear: Is There Harm in Delay of Treatment?

Lawrence JTR, Argawal N, Ganley TJ (Children's Hosp of Philadelphia, PA)
Am J Sports Med 39:2582-2587, 2011

Background.—In skeletally immature patients with an anterior cruciate ligament (ACL) tear and significant growth remaining, the risk of inducing a growth disturbance with early reconstruction must be balanced against the risk of further intra-articular damage by delaying treatment until closer to skeletal maturity.

Hypothesis.—Increased time from injury to ACL reconstruction in children ≤14 years of age will be associated with increased meniscal and chondral injuries at the time of reconstruction.

Study Design.—Cohort study; Level of evidence, 3.

Methods.—With institutional review board approval, the records of a consecutive series of patients 14 years of age and younger who underwent ACL reconstruction between 1991 and 2005 were reviewed. Demographic, magnetic resonance imaging (MRI), and intraoperative findings were analyzed. Meniscal and articular cartilage injuries were graded. Logistic regression models using both univariable and multivariable regression procedures were used to identify factors independently associated with intra-articular lesions. Fisher exact test and Kaplan-Meier analysis were used to test for differences in intra-articular injuries by time from injury to surgery.

Results.—Seventy patients were identified. Twenty-nine patients (41%) underwent reconstruction more than 12 weeks from the time of injury. Logistic regression analysis revealed time to surgical reconstruction (odds ratio, 4.1) and a history of a sense of knee instability (odds ratio, 11.4) to be independently associated with medial meniscal tears. Time to surgical reconstruction was also independently associated with medial and lateral compartment chondral injuries (odds ratios, 5.6 and 11.3, respectively). Testing time as a continuous variable, survivorship analysis also confirmed a significant association of time to reconstruction with medial meniscal injury as well as lateral and patellotrochlear cartilage injuries. When present, a delay in treatment of over 12 weeks (29 patients) was associated with an increase in the severity of medial meniscal tears ($P = .011$) and higher grade lateral and patellotrochlear chondral injuries ($P = .0014$ and $P = .038$, respectively).

Conclusion.—Young patients who underwent surgical reconstruction of an acute ACL tear >12 weeks after the injury were noted to have a significant increase in irreparable medial meniscal tears and lateral compartment chondral injuries at the time of reconstruction. When a subjective sense of knee instability was present, this association was even stronger (Tables 1 and 2).

▶ The issue of anterior cruciate ligament (ACL) reconstruction, in my opinion, is much more one of indication and outcome value rather than technique. The

TABLE 1.—Survivorship Analysis for Meniscal Tears[a]

	Median Time From Injury to Reconstruction (95% CI), wk		
	No Tear	Tear	*P* Value
Medial meniscus	9 (7-11)	24 (11-49)	.006
Lateral meniscus	9 (7-13)	13 (7-24)	.31

[a]Time from injury to surgical reconstruction was used as the survival time in the cohorts with and without meniscal tears noted at the time of reconstruction. CI, confidence interval.

TABLE 2.—Survivorship Analysis of Cartilage Injury[a]

	Median Time From Injury to Reconstruction (95% CI), wk		
	Grade 0 or 1	Grade 2/3 or 4	*P* Value
Medial	10 (8-12)	16 (7-30)	.33
Lateral	9 (8-11)	21 (12-50)	.009
Patellofemoral	9 (8-12)	48 (6-55)	.034

[a]Time from injury to surgical reconstruction was used as the survival time in the cohorts with and without an intact articular surface (Outerbridge 0 and 1 vs 2/3 and 4) noted at the time of reconstruction. CI, confidence interval.

central issue from this prospective is exactly that addressed here. If the ACL deficiency is not addressed, is the patient at risk for subsequent meniscus and articular cartilage injury? Virtually all the literature indicates the answer is yes to both these questions. This study further queries the data with a cohort of adolescent patients. The answer is the same. Both the meniscus (Table 1) and the articular cartilage (Table 2) are at risk if there is more than a 3-month delay of treatment. I feel these findings are relevant, especially in the symptomatic rotatory unstable knee with an ACL deficiency in the young patient.

B. F. Morrey, MD

Loss of Normal Knee Motion After Anterior Cruciate Ligament Reconstruction Is Associated With Radiographic Arthritic Changes After Surgery

Shelbourne KD, Urch SE, Gray T, et al (Shelbourne Knee Ctr, Indianapolis, IN)
Am J Sports Med 40:108-113, 2012

Background.—Meniscectomy and articular cartilage damage have been found to increase the prevalence of osteoarthritis after anterior cruciate ligament reconstruction, but the effect of knee range of motion has not been extensively studied.

Hypothesis.—The prevalence of osteoarthritis as observed on radiographs would be higher in patients who had abnormal knee range of motion compared with patients with normal knee motion, even when grouped for like meniscal or articular cartilage lesions.

Study Design.—Cohort study; Level of evidence, 3.

Methods.—We prospectively followed patients at a minimum of 5 years after surgery. The constant goal of rehabilitation was to obtain full knee range of motion as quickly as possible after surgery and maintain it in the long term. Range of motion and radiographs were evaluated at the time of initial return to full activities (early follow-up) and final follow-up according to International Knee Documentation Committee (IKDC) objective criteria. A patient was considered to have normal range of motion if extension was within 2° of the opposite knee including hyperextension and knee flexion was within 5°. Radiograph findings were rated as abnormal if any signs of joint space narrowing, sclerosis, or osteophytes were present.

Results.—Follow-up was obtained for 780 patients at a mean of 10.5 ± 4.2 years after surgery. Of these, 539 had either normal or abnormal motion at both early and final follow-up. In 479 patients who had normal extension and flexion at both early and final follow-up, 188 (39%) had radiographic evidence of osteoarthritis versus 32 of 60 (53%) patients who had less than normal extension or flexion at early and final follow-up ($P = .036$). In subgroups of patients with like meniscal status, the prevalence of normal radiograph findings was significantly higher in patients with normal motion at final follow-up versus patients with motion deficits. Multivariate logistic regression analysis of categorical variables showed that abnormal knee flexion at early follow-up, abnormal knee extension at final follow-up, abnormal knee flexion at final follow-up, partial medial meniscectomy, and articular cartilage damage were significant factors related to the presence of osteoarthritis on radiographs. Abnormal knee extension at early follow-up showed a trend toward statistical significance ($P = .0544$). Logistic regression showed the odds of having osteoarthritis were 2 times more for patients with abnormal range of motion at final follow-up; these odds were similar for those with partial medial meniscectomy and articular cartilage damage.

Conclusion.—The prevalence of osteoarthritis on radiographs in the long term after anterior cruciate ligament reconstruction is lower in patients who achieve and maintain normal knee motion, regardless of the status of the meniscus.

▶ I continue to be impressed with investigators who ask a very basic, relevant question, the answer of which will be of value to the practicing orthopedic surgeon. Such is the case here. As the authors point out in the introduction, degenerative changes are well recognized to be associated with meniscus and cartilage injury. Who would have thought to correlate subsequent arthritis with range of motion at the time of reconstruction? I did not. I credit these investigators to show this correlation. The value is clear and focused: limited flexion at the time of anterior cruciate ligament reconstruction is correlated with subsequent arthritis. The application of this information is simple: just tell the patient and proceed with the surgery.

B. F. Morrey, MD

Cartilage Injury After Acute, Isolated Anterior Cruciate Ligament Tear: Immediate and Longitudinal Effect With Clinical/MRI Follow-up

Potter HG, Jain SK, Ma Y, et al (Hosp for Special Surgery, NY)

Am J Sports Med 40:276-285, 2012

Background.—Anterior cruciate ligament (ACL) tears have been implicated in the development of osteoarthritis. Limited data exist on longitudinal follow-up of isolated ACL injury.

Hypotheses.—All isolated ACL tears are associated with some degree of cartilage injury that will deteriorate over time. There is a threshold of

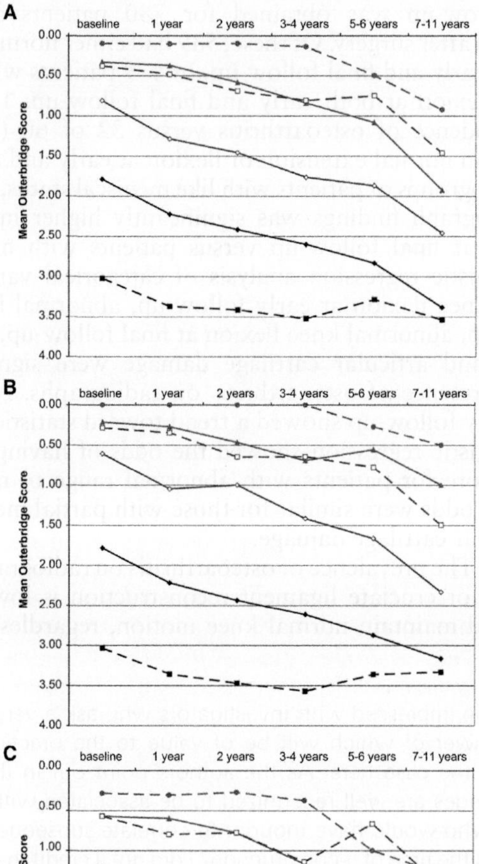

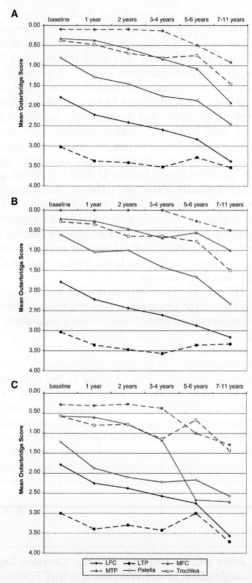

FIGURE 2.—(A) Outerbridge scores over time (all patients); (B) Outerbridge scores over time (surgical cohort); (C) Outerbridge scores over time (nonsurgical cohort). LFC, lateral femoral condyle; LTP, lateral tibial plateau; MFC, medial femoral condyle; MTP, medial tibial plateau. (Reprinted from Potter HG, Jain SK, Ma Y, et al. Cartilage injury after acute, isolated anterior cruciate ligament tear: immediate and longitudinal effect with clinical/MRI follow-up. *Am J Sports Med.* 2012;40:276-285, with permission from The Author(s).)

magnetic resonance imaging (MRI)–detectable cartilage injury that will correlate with adverse change in subjective patient-reported outcome measures.

Study Design.—Cohort study, Level of evidence, 2.

Methods.—The authors conducted a prospective, observational analysis of 42 knees in 40 patients with acute, isolated ACL injury (14 treated nonoperatively, 28 by reconstruction) with imaging at the time of injury and yearly follow-up for a maximum of 11 years. Morphologic MRI and quantitative T2 mapping was performed with validated outcome measures.

Results.—All patients sustained chondral damage at initial injury. The adjusted risk of cartilage loss doubled from year 1 for the lateral compartment and medial femoral condyle (MFC) and tripled for the patella. By years 7 to 11, the risk for the lateral femoral condyle was 50 times baseline, 30 times for the patella, and 19 times for the MFC. There was increased risk of cartilage degeneration over the medial tibial plateau (MTP) ($P = .047$; odds ratio = 6.23; 95% confidence interval [CI], 1.03-37.90) and patella ($P = .032$; odds ratio = 4.88; 95% CI, 1.14-20.80) in nonsurgical patients compared with surgically treated patients. Size of the bone-marrow edema pattern was associated with cartilage degeneration from baseline to year 3 ($P = .001$ to.039). Each increase in the MFC Outerbridge score resulted in a 13-point decrease in the International Knee Documentation Committee subjective knee score ($P = .0002$). Each increase in the MTP resulted in a 2.4-point decrease in the activity rating scale ($P = .002$).

Conclusion.—All patients with acute, traumatic ACL disruption sustained a chondral injury at the time of initial impact with subsequent longitudinal chondral degradation in compartments unaffected by the initial "bone bruise," a process that is accelerated at 5 to 7 years' follow-up (Fig 2).

► This is a great topic, addressing an essential question in sports medicine: does an anterior cruciate ligament (ACL)-deficient knee predispose to arthritis, and does ACL reconstruction protect against this tendency. While the question is an excellent one, the power and surveillance is, unfortunately, inadequate to really answer the question. With only 40 subjects and follow-up only to 5 years, in spite of the care with which the follow-up assessment was performed, this article really stimulates interest more than answering the question. Regardless, it is clearly shown the knee does deteriorate with time, even over the short term, and this is true for both the nontreated and the reconstructed patients (Fig 2) This question is begging to be answered, but with the numerous covariables, a much, much larger sample with a much longer period of surveillance will be required.

B. F. Morrey, MD

Autograft Versus Allograft: An Economic Cost Comparison of Anterior Cruciate Ligament Reconstruction

Oro FB, Sikka RS, Wolters B, et al (TRIA Orthopaedic Ctr, Minneapolis, MN)

Arthroscopy 27:1219-1225, 2011

Purpose.—The purpose of this study was to compare the costs associated with anterior cruciate ligament (ACL) reconstruction with either bone–patellar tendon–bone (BPTB) autograft or BPTB allograft.

TABLE 2.—Cost of Isolated Primary ACL Reconstruction

Procedure	n	Gender (% Male)	Age (yr)	Supply Cost ($)	Case Time (min)	Personnel Cost ($)	Facility Cost ($)	Total Expense ($)	Reimbursement ($)	Margin ($)
Autograft	60	62%	25.4 ± 9.8	1,715 ± 487	91 ± 23	237 ± 59	1,030 ± 258	2,983 ± 508	2,774 ± 1,285	−208 ± 1,419
Allograft	27	59%	39.5 ± 12.3	3,132 ± 794	83 ± 32	215 ± 84	936 ± 365	4,283 ± 852	3,640 ± 2,298	−644 ± 2,015
P value		*P* =.980	*P* < .001	*P* < .001	*P* =.170	*P* =.170	*P* =.170	*P* < .001	*P* =.027	*P* =.251

Methods.—Surgical costs are reported, including supply costs, based on invoice costs per item used per procedure, and personnel costs calculated as cost per minute. All operations were performed at an ambulatory surgery center between March 2005 and March 2006. A total of 160 patients underwent primary ACL reconstruction with either BPTB autograft (n = 106) or BPTB allograft (n = 54). Procedure cost data were retrieved from a financial management database and divided into various categories for comparison of the 2 groups. Payment data were provided by the surgery center's billing office.

Results.—The total mean cost per case was \$4,147 ± \$943 in the allograft group compared with \$3,154 ± \$704 in the autograft group; this was statistically significant ($P < .001$). The mean operating room time was 12 minutes greater in autograft cases ($P = .006$). Supply costs comprised a mean of 58.7% of total expenses in the autograft group and 72.2% in the allograft group.

Conclusions.—Allograft reconstruction of the ACL was significantly more expensive than autograft reconstruction.

Level of Evidence.—Level II, economic analysis (Table 2).

▶ I truly commend the authors for undertaking this study. They face an age-old question as to whether the savings in operating room (OR) time associated with the allograft is justified by the cost incurred. The answer, at least based on their procurement costs and OR costs, are clear. It is cheaper to use the patients own tissue. The study does not completely answer the issue of morbidity or subsequent management of patella tendon complication, but it does offer a strong basis to use the autograft. I use allografts for my elbow reconstructions. Whether this is a more or less cost-effective approach deserves to be studied.

B. F. Morrey, MD

A Surgical Technique Using Presoaked Vancomycin Hamstring Grafts to Decrease the Risk of Infection After Anterior Cruciate Ligament Reconstruction

Vertullo CJ, Quick M, Jones A, et al (Pindara Hosp & Griffith Univ, Gold Coast, Australia; Mater Adults and Mothers Hosp, South Brisbane, Australia; Pindara Private Hosp, Southport, Australia; et al)

Arthroscopy 28:337-342, 2012

Purpose.—The purpose of this study was to investigate whether presoaking hamstring graft with a dilute antibiotic solution provides a potential new tool to improve measures to prevent joint infection.

Methods.—This is a retrospective analysis of data that were prospectively collected for 1,135 consecutive patients who underwent anterior cruciate ligament reconstruction (ACLR) during a 7-year period. In the initial 3-year period, 285 patients (group 1) underwent ACLR with a hamstring autograft with preoperative intravenous (IV) antibiotics. In the subsequent 4-year period, 870 patients underwent ACLR with a vancomycin-presoaked

TABLE 1.—Patients Reviewed for Infection After ACLR

	Period of Study (yr)	No. of Patients	No. of Male Patients	No. of Female Patients	Mean Age at Surgery (yr)
Group 1	3	285	195	90	30
Group 2	4	870	599	271	31

hamstring autograft (group 2) with preoperative IV antibiotics. Presoaking involved wrapping hamstring tendon autografts in a sterile gauze swab, which had been previously saturated with 5-mg/mL vancomycin solution.

Results.—In group 1 a total of 4 postoperative joint infections were documented (1.4%). Each case showed increasing pain and effusion, as well as a high intra-articular white blood cell count and increased C-reactive protein level. Of the 4 infected cases, 3 cultured coagulase-negative *Staphylococcus (Staphylococcus epidermidis)*. The fourth case was treated as a postoperative infection despite a negative culture and responded to arthroscopic washout and IV antibiotics. In group 2 no infections (0%) were recorded, and no investigatory washouts occurred. The difference was statistically significant. Known failures were similar in each group.

Conclusions.—Prophylactic vancomycin presoaking of hamstring autografts statistically reduced the infection rate in this series compared with IV antibiotics alone.

Level of Evidence.—Level IV, therapeutic case series (Table 1).

▶ Like total joints, the infection rate with anterior cruciate ligament (ACL) reconstruction is very low. But, also like joint replacement sepsis, the consequences are often devastating. This is actually a technique article, but it does convey a valuable insight. It is difficult to ignore a sample of more than 800 ACL reconstructions without an infection after introducing the presoak technique (Table 1). One must be concerned about a possible synovial allergic or irritative reaction to the presence of vancomycin in the joint, but this did not appear to be a problem. Hence, for those who have had some concern about their specific infection rate, this technique might be considered.

B. F. Morrey, MD

Factors Used to Determine Return to Unrestricted Sports Activities After Anterior Cruciate Ligament Reconstruction

Barber-Westin SD, Noyes FR (Cincinnati Sportsmedicine Res and Education Foundation, OH)

Arthroscopy 27:1697-1705, 2011

Purpose.—Anterior cruciate ligament (ACL) reconstruction is commonly performed in athletes, with the goal of return to sports activities. Unfortunately, this operation may fail, and the rates of either reinjuring an

ACL-reconstructed knee or sustaining an ACL rupture to the contralateral knee range from 3% to 49%. One problem that exists is a lack of information and consensus regarding the appropriate criteria for releasing patients to unrestricted sports activities postoperatively. The purpose of this study was to determine the published criteria used to allow athletes to return to unrestricted sports activities after ACL reconstruction.

Methods.—A systematic search was performed to identify the factors investigators used to determine when return to athletics was allowed after primary ACL reconstruction. Inclusion criteria were English language, publication within the last 10 years, clinical trial, all adult patients, primary ACL reconstruction, original research investigation, and minimum 12 months' follow-up.

Results.—Of 716 studies identified, 264 met the inclusion criteria. Of these, 105 (40%) failed to provide any criteria for return to sports after ACL reconstruction. In 84 studies (32%) the amount of time postoperatively was the only criterion provided. In 40 studies (15%) the amount of time along with subjective criteria were given. Only 35 studies (13%) noted objective criteria required for return to athletics. These criteria included muscle strength or thigh circumference (28 studies), general knee examination (15 studies), single-leg hop tests (10 studies), Lachman rating (1 study), and validated questionnaires (1 study).

Conclusions.—The results of this systematic review show noteworthy problems and a lack of objective assessment before release to unrestricted

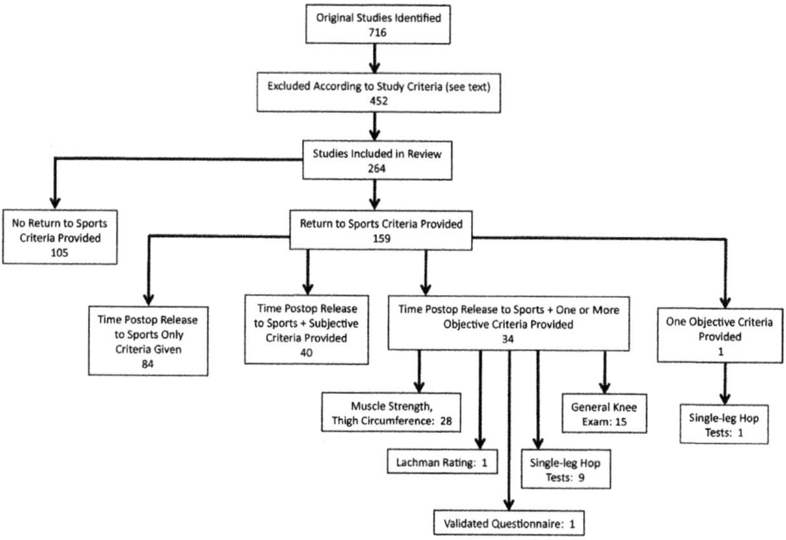

FIGURE 1.—Flowchart of ACL reconstruction studies with criteria for return to athletics. (Reprinted from Arthroscopy: The Journal of Arthroscopic and Related Surgery. Barber-Westin SD, Noyes FR. Factors used to determine return to unrestricted sports activities after anterior cruciate ligament reconstruction. *Arthroscopy.* 2011;27:1697-1705, Copyright 2011, with permission from the Arthroscopy Association of North America.)

TABLE 3.—Subjective Criteria Provided for Release to Sports Activities

Criteria	No. of Studies
Good firm anterior tibial stop	1
Good firm point on clinical evaluation	1
Knee stability confirmed on clinical examination	3
Stable knee	1
Good stability	1
Normal laxity of knee	1
Satisfactory stability	1
Ability to pass sports-specific tests such as cutting, squatting, and jumping	1
Knee function normal or nearly normal on clinical examination	1
Satisfactory clinical examination	1
Confirmation of recovery of quadriceps strength	2
Functional quadriceps control	1
Sufficient muscle recovery after specified athletic training accomplished	1
Depending on functional capacity	2
Good recovery of ROM, muscle strength, and stability	1
Regained full subjective functional stability	5
Regained full functional stability	9
Regained full functional strength and stability	2
Full functional stability in terms of strength, coordination, and balance	3
No significant side-to-side deficits If all parameters met	1
Depending on individual progress	1
After ACL accelerated rehabilitation program	1
No problematic symptoms in knee joint	1
Only after rehabilitation goals met	1
Controlled functional training had been performed without difficulty	2
Good muscle coordination in agility training and balance equal to opposite side	1
If patient's rehabilitation of limb and stability warrant	1
Satisfactory performance on agility drills	1
Depending on functional ability, including run-to-sprint intervals, sidestep cutting, and timed recreational drills	1
Close to full ROM and muscle strength	1

NOTE. Multiple subjective criteria were given in 10 of the 40 studies included.

sports activities. General recommendations are made for quantification of muscle strength, stability, neuromuscular control, and function in patients who desire to return to athletics after ACL reconstruction, with acknowledgment of the need for continued research in this area.

Level of Evidence.—Level IV, systematic review of Level I to IV studies (Fig 1, Tables 3 and 4).

► I find it interesting that with time my interests change. I am currently ever drawn into analytical interpretations of the literature. The reason is that this is the most efficient way to understand what has been studied and concluded. Most involve controversial or poorly understood issues, such as this study. What is the basis for return to sport, really? Ideally, it is based on evidence. But, as is documented here, in spite of numerous studies and comments, evidence is lacking (Fig 1). A massive review of more than 700 studies found only just greater than 250 met inclusion criteria. It is worthwhile to note the subjective (Table 3) and the objective variables (Table 4) used to make the decision. But even within these groups, opinions

TABLE 4.—Objective Criteria Provided for Release to Sports Activities

Criteria Categories	No. of Studies
Time postoperatively, muscle strength	16
Time postoperatively, muscle strength, ROM/effusion	3
Time postoperatively, thigh circumference, single-leg hop test	3
Time postoperatively, ROM/effusion	4
Time postoperatively, muscle strength, single-leg hop test	2
Time postoperatively, muscle strength, ROM	2
Time postoperatively, Lachman rating, effusion	1
Time postoperatively, muscle strength/thigh circumference, single-leg hop test	1
Time postoperatively, muscle strength, single-leg hop test, ROM/effusion	1
Time postoperatively, muscle strength, 4 single-leg hop tests, ROM/effusion, validated questionnaires	1
Single-leg hop test	1

NOTE. Data are presented for 35 studies that provided objective criteria for return to sports.

vary. At the end of the day, one must conclude the basis for answering the question raised by this study is personal opinion, not science.

B. F. Morrey, MD

Accelerated Versus Nonaccelerated Rehabilitation After Anterior Cruciate Ligament Reconstruction: A Prospective, Randomized, Double-Blind Investigation Evaluating Knee Joint Laxity Using Roentgen Stereophotogrammetric Analysis

Beynnon BD, Johnson RJ, Naud S, et al (Univ of Vermont College of Medicine, Burlington; et al)

Am J Sports Med 39:2536-2548, 2011

Background.—The relationship between the biomechanical dose of rehabilitation exercises administered after anterior cruciate ligament (ACL) reconstruction and the healing response of the graft and knee is not well understood.

Hypothesis.—After ACL reconstruction, rehabilitation administered with either accelerated or nonaccelerated programs produces the same change in the knees' 6 degrees of freedom, or envelope, laxity values.

Study Design.—Randomized controlled trial; Level of evidence, 1.

Methods.—Patients who underwent ACL reconstruction with a bone–patellar tendon–bone autograft were randomized to rehabilitation with either accelerated (19 week) or nonaccelerated (32 week) programs. At the time of surgery, and then 3, 6, 12, and 24 months later, the 6 degrees of freedom knee laxity values were measured using roentgen stereophotogrammetric analysis and clinical, functional, and patient-oriented outcome measures.

Results.—Eighty-five percent of those enrolled were followed through 2 years. Laxity of the reconstructed knee was restored to within the limits

TABLE 1.—Patient Data for Participants in Accelerated and Nonaccelerated Rehabilitation Programs[a]

	Accelerated	Nonaccelerated	Comparison (*P* Value)
Number of patients enrolled in investigation	24	18	
Number of dropouts	5	1	
Number of patients studied >2 years and retained for analyses	19	17	
Suspected ACL graft failure, n (%)	0 (0)	1 (6)	.47
Age in years, mean (range; SD)	29.7 (16-48; 10.1)	30.2 (16-46; 9.9)	.89
Weight in kg, mean (range)	75.3 (49-98)	71.8 (55-97)	
Gender			
Males, no. (%)	13 (68)	9 (53)	
Females, no. (%)	6 (32)	8 (47)	.34
Days between index injury and surgery, mean (range; SD)	56 (13-102; 23.5)	66 (29-134; 31.6)	.30
Meniscal lesion identified at surgery			
Medial	7 (37)	7 (41)	.79
Lateral	5 (26)	6 (35)	.56
Meniscal debridement/resection			
Medial	3 (16)	3 (18)	.88
Lateral	5 (26)	3 (18)	.53

[a]ACL, anterior cruciate ligament; SD, standard deviation.

of the contralateral, normal side at the time of surgery (baseline) in all participants. Patients in both programs underwent a similar increase in the envelope of knee laxity over the 2-year follow-up interval (anterior-posterior translation 3.2 vs 4.5 mm, and coupled internal-external rotations 2.6° vs 1.9° for participants in the accelerated and nonaccelerated programs, respectively). Those who underwent accelerated rehabilitation experienced a significant improvement in thigh muscle strength at the 3-month follow-up ($P < .05$) compared with those who participated in nonaccelerated rehabilitation, but no differences between the programs were seen after this time interval. At the 2-year follow-up, the groups were similar in terms of clinical assessment, patient satisfaction, function, proprioception, and isokinetic thigh muscle strength.

Conclusion.—Rehabilitation with the accelerated and nonaccelerated programs administered in this study produced the same increase in the envelope of knee laxity. A majority of the increase in the envelope of knee laxity occurred during healing when exercises were advanced and activity level increased. Patients in both programs had the same clinical assessment, functional performance, proprioception, and thigh muscle strength, which returned to normal levels after healing was complete. For participants in both treatment programs, the Knee Injury and Osteoarthritis Outcome Score (KOOS) assessment of quality of life did not return to preinjury levels (Table 1).

▶ Once again I am drawn to a very well-done prospective, randomized study. The value of this contribution rests in the clinically relevant question and a study design that did answer the question definitively. With the limitations that this trial studied only bone-patella-bone grafts, and with only a single rehabilitation protocol for each group, there were no differences in the long-term outcomes of the 2 programs (Table 1). It should be noted that both groups did suffer from postoperative laxity. Their conclusion that is obvious is at least there is no measurable downside from the early rehabilitation program. The short-term morbidity is less, however, and this might be the most important implication in selecting between the 2 programs.

B. F. Morrey, MD

9 Foot and Ankle

Introduction

I was fortunate early in my career to have been mentored by Ken Johnson, one of the early pioneers of foot and ankle surgery in the United States. I practiced as a surgeon in the Mayo Foot Clinic for 7 years before becoming more focused in hip, knee, sports and elbow. This background has provided an ongoing interest in the area, and it is for this reason that I continue to review the foot and ankle articles. In this year's volume, articles that are felt to be most relevant to the general practice of orthopedic surgery have been selected. We feel as though this is the most useful information for the majority of orthopedic surgeons, particularly those who do not specifically specialize in foot and ankle surgery. The quality of the clinical research, as well as the specific topic and its relevance, were the primary basis for this year's selections. It is hoped that this section will be of value to the majority of those who have interest in this area.

Bernard F. Morrey, MD

Incidence of venous thromboembolism in elective foot and ankle surgery with and without aspirin prophylaxis

Griffiths JT, Matthews L, Pearce CJ, et al (Basingstoke and North Hampshire NHS Foundation Trust, Basingstoke, UK)
J Bone Joint Surg Br 94-B:210-214, 2012

The incidence of deep-vein thrombosis (DVT) and pulmonary embolism (PE) is thought to be low following foot and ankle surgery, but the routine use of chemoprophylaxis remains controversial. This retrospective study assessed the incidence of symptomatic venous thromboembolic (VTE) complications following a consecutive series of 2654 patients undergoing elective foot and ankle surgery. A total of 1078 patients received 75 mg aspirin as routine thromboprophylaxis between 2003 and 2006 and 1576 patients received no form of chemical thromboprophylaxis between 2007 and 2010. The overall incidence of VTE was 0.42% (DVT, 0.27%; PE, 0.15%) with 27 patients lost to follow-up. If these were included to create a worst case scenario, the overall VTE rate was 1.43%. There was no apparent protective effect against VTE by using aspirin.

TABLE 1.—The Incidence of a Venous Thromboembolic Event (VTE; Either Deep-Vein Thrombosis (DVT) or Pulmonary Embolism (PE)) in the Aspirin, no Thromboprophylaxis and Combined Study Groups, Excluding the Patients Lost to Follow-up

	Number of Patients	DVT Number	DVT Incidence (%)	PE Number	PE Incidence (%)	Total Number of VTEs	Overall Incidence (%)
Aspirin	1068	4	*0.37*	1	*0.09*	5	*0.47*
No thromboprophylaxis	1559	3	*0.19*	3	*0.19*	6	*0.39*
Combined	2627	7	*0.27*	4	*0.15*	11	*0.42*

We conclude that the incidence of VTE following foot and ankle surgery is very low and routine use of chemoprophylaxis does not appear necessary for patients who are not in the high risk group for VTE (Table 1).

▶ Concern about thromboembolic complications after foot surgery is not very high in most surgeons' minds, yet it does exist. This study was included to provide "scientific basis for clinical practice." In other words, with this large sample of patients, the conclusion that aspirin prophylaxis is not indicated appears to be documented. The incidence of about 1 in 1000 is the same, roughly, as spontaneous development in the general population. So, even with aspirin being as inexpensive and safe as it is, it is probably still unnecessary, unless there is a documented underlying risk present.

B. F. Morrey, MD

Formulated collagen gel accelerates healing rate immediately after application in patients with diabetic neuropathic foot ulcers

Blume P, Driver VR, Tallis AJ, et al (Affiliated Foot Surgeons, New Haven, CT; Boston Univ Med Ctr and School of Medicine, MA; Associated Foot and Ankle Specialists, Phoenix, AZ; et al)

Wound Repair Regen 19:302-308, 2011

We assessed the safety and efficacy of Formulated Collagen Gel (FCG) alone and with Ad5PDGF-B (GAM501) compared with Standard of Care (SOC) in patients with 1.5–10.0 cm^2 chronic diabetic neuropathic foot ulcers that healed <30% during Run-in. Wound size was assessed by planimetry of acetate tracings and photographs in 124 patients. Comparison of data sets revealed that acetate tracings frequently overestimated areas at some sites. For per-protocol analysis, 113 patients qualified using acetate tracings but only 82 qualified using photographs. Prior animal studies suggested that collagen alone would have little effect on healing and would serve as a negative control. Surprisingly trends for increased incidence of complete closure were observed for both GAM501 (41%) and FCG (45%) vs. Standard of Care (31%). By photographic data, Standard of Care had no significant effect on change in wound radius (mm/week) from during Run-in to Week

1 (-0.06 ± 0.32 to 0.78 ± 1.53, $p =$ ns) but both FCG (-0.08 ± 0.61 to 1.97 ± 1.77, $p < 0.002$) and GAM501 (-0.02 ± 0.58 to 1.46 ± 1.37, $p < 0.002$) significantly increased healing rates that gradually declined over subsequent weeks. Both GAM501 and FCG appeared to be safe and well tolerated, and alternate dosing schedules hold promise to improve overall complete wound closure in adequately powered trials.

▶ As the authors point out, the problem of diabetic ulcers increases as does the prevalence of the disease. Because this is one of the most problematic diseases in all of medicine, any improvement in management is welcome. This industry-supported study clearly supports the value of growth factor applied to the neurotrophic ulcer. The variability in the data, however, also emphasizes the long road ahead to optimize the formulation, frequency, and concentration of the application. I was also not clear as to the exact location or the means of supportive management during the study. Regardless, collagen gel as a carrier of growth factors does appear to be a promising adjunct to the management of this difficult problem.

B. F. Morrey, MD

Ankle Tourniquet Pain Control in Forefoot Surgery: A Randomized Study

Burg A, Tytiun Y, Velkes S, et al (Rabin Med Ctr, Petach-Tikva, Israel)
Foot Ankle Int 32:595-598, 2011

Background.—Forefoot surgery is often performed under regional anesthesia in awake patients, using tourniquet or Esmarch bandage to obtain a bloodless field. The purpose of this study was to examine the value and need for local tourniquet pain control using local subcutaneous analgesic mixture in patients undergoing forefoot surgery under ankle block anesthesia.

Materials and Methods.—We prospectively randomized 56 patients who underwent forefoot surgery under ankle block to receive either subcutaneous local anesthetic mixture under the tourniquet or no additional anesthetic. We checked for local tourniquet pain score (VAS 0 to 100) and skin condition during and after the procedure.

Results.—The tourniquet was quite tolerable in both groups, with an average VAS score of 7 to 21. No difference was observed between groups throughout most of the procedure. No correlation between VAS scores and procedure length or patient's age or gender was found.

Conclusion.—An ankle tourniquet was well-tolerated by patients without need for local anesthetic beneath the cuff.

Level of Evidence.—II, Prospective Comparative Study (Fig 1).

▶ I am attracted to simple studies that address clinically relevant issues. This straightforward study simply asks whether local anesthesia is of value to enhance tolerance for an ankle or calf tourniquet. Using the visual analogue pain score the

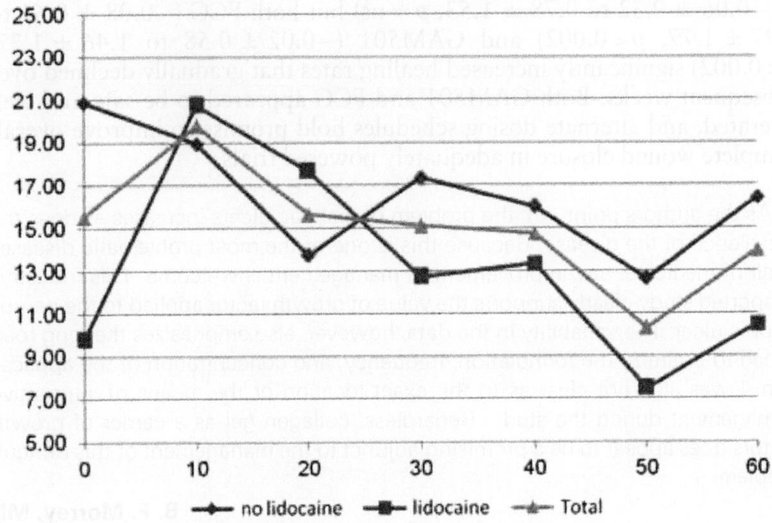

FIGURE 1.—Mean VAS scores. (Reprinted from Burg A, Tytiun Y, Velkes S, et al. Ankle tourniquet pain control in forefoot surgery: a randomized study. *Foot Ankle Int*. 2011;32:595-598, Copyright © 2011 by the American Orthopaedic Foot and Ankle Society, Inc., originally published in Foot & Ankle International 32:595-598 and reproduced here with permission.)

answer is clear (Fig 1). Local anesthesia is of no added value. My one question is that if, in fact, patients tolerate this type tourniquet so well, which Fig 1 would suggest, why was the study performed?

B. F. Morrey, MD

Accuracy of MRI findings in chronic lateral ankle ligament injury: Comparison with surgical findings

Park H-J, Cha S-D, Kim SS, et al (Sungkyunkwan Univ School of Medicine, Seoul, Republic of Korea; Kwandong Univ, Koyang, Republic of Korea; Kangwon Natl Univ, Chuncheon, Republic of Korea)
Clin Radiol 67:313-318, 2012

Aim.—To evaluate the accuracy of magnetic resonance imaging (MRI) findings in chronic lateral ankle ligament injury in comparison with that of surgical findings.

Materials and Methods.—Forty-eight cases (25 men, 23 women, mean age 36 years) of clinically suspected chronic ankle ligament injury underwent MRI studies and surgery. Sagittal, coronal, and axial, T1-weighted, spin-echo, proton density and T2-weighted, fast spin-echo images with fat saturation were obtained in all patients. MRI examinations were read in consensus by two fellowship-trained academic musculoskeletal radiologists who evaluated the lateral ankle ligaments, including the anterior talofibular

TABLE 3.—Validity of MRI (%) in the Diagnosis of Anterior Talofibular Ligament (ATFL) and Calcaneofibular Ligament (CFL) Lesions

MRI	Location	Sensitivity	Specificity	PPV	NPV	Accuracy	*p*-Value
Normal	ATFL	75	88	38	98	88	<0.001
	CFL	97	79	88	94	90	
Sprain	ATFL	44	88	88	44	58	0.120
	CFL	55	100	100	88	90	
Partial tear	ATFL	75	78	40	94	77	0.165
	CFL	83	93	63	98	92	
Complete tear	ATFL	75	86	33	97	85	<0.001
	CFL	50	98	50	98	96	

PPV, positive predictive value; NPV, negative predictive value.

ligament (ATFL) and calcaneofibular ligament (CFL) without clinical information. The results of the MRI studies were then compared with the surgical findings.

Results.—The MRI findings of ATFL injury showed a sensitivity of detection of complete tears of 75% and specificity of 86%. The sensitivity of detection of partial tears was 75% and the specificity was 78%. The sensitivity of detection of sprains was 44% and the specificity was 88%. Regarding the MRI findings of CFL injury, the sensitivity of detection of complete tears was 50% and the specificity was 98%. The sensitivity of detection of partial tear was 83% and the specificity was 93%. The sensitivity of detection of sprains was 100% and the specificity was 90%. Regarding the ATFL, the accuracies of detection were 88, 58, 77, and 85% for no injury, sprain, partial tear, and complete tear, respectively, and for the CFL the accuracies of detection were 90, 90, 92, and 96% for no injury, sprain, partial tear, and complete tear, respectively.

Conclusions.—The diagnosis of a complete tear of the ATFL on MRI is more sensitive than the diagnosis of a complete tear of the CFL. MRI findings of CFL injury are diagnostically specific but are not sensitive. However, only normal findings and complete tears were statistically significant between ATFL and CFL ($p < 0.001$) (Table 3).

► In general, I feel studies such as this one are quite useful. We are constantly faced with the dilemma of knowing whether or to what extent the shadows observed by the imagers correlate to true pathology. Hence, the burden of such a study is an adequate sample size of patients with surgical observation of the documented image. In this particular instance, the authors were able to show better specificity than sensitivity for both anatomic sites of injury. The overall accuracy was better for calcaneofibular than for anterior talofibular ligament injury. These findings have clinical relevance when deciding the true extent of the injury and hence the need for surgical intervention.

B. F. Morrey, MD

A 5-year follow-up study of Alfredson's heel-drop exercise programme in chronic midportion Achilles tendinopathy

van der Plas A, de Jonge S, de Vos RJ, et al (The Hague Med Centre, Leidschendam, The Netherlands; et al)

Br J Sports Med 46:214-218, 2012

Background.—Eccentric exercises have the most evidence in conservative treatment of midportion Achilles tendinopathy. Although short-term studies show significant improvement, little is known of the long-term (>3 years) results.

Aim.—To evaluate the 5-year outcome of patients with chronic midportion Achilles tendinopathy treated with the classical Alfredson's heel-drop exercise programme.

Study Design.—Part of a 5-year follow-up of a previously conducted randomised controlled trial.

Methods.—58 patients (70 tendons) were approached 5 years after the start of the heel-drop exercise programme according to Alfredson. At baseline and at 5-year follow-up, the validated Victorian Institute of Sports Assessment–Achilles (VISA-A) questionnaire score, pain status, alternative treatments received and ultrasonographic neovascularisation score were recorded.

Results.—In 46 patients (58 tendons), the VISA-A score significantly increased from 49.2 at baseline to 83.6 after 5 years ($p<0.001$) and from the 1-year to 5-year follow-up from 75.0 to 83.4 ($p<0.01$). 39.7% of the patients were completely pain-free at follow-up and 48.3% had received one or more alternative treatments. The sagittal tendon thickness decreased

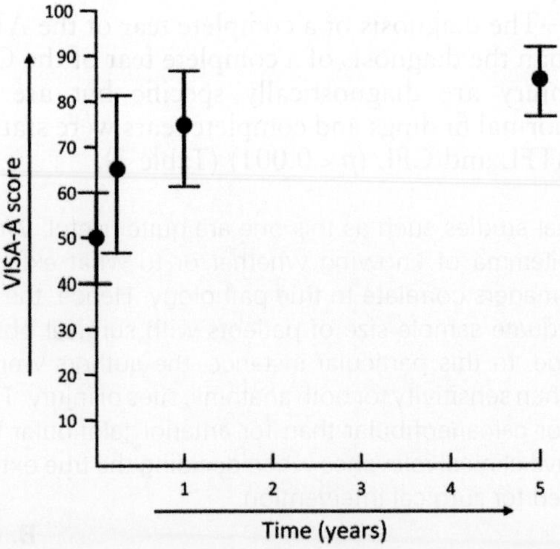

FIGURE 2.—The VISA-A score in time. (Reprinted from van der Plas A, de Jonge S, de Vos RJ, et al. A 5-year follow-up study of Alfredson's heel-drop exercise programme in chronic midportion Achilles tendinopathy. *Br J Sports Med.* 2012;46:214-218.)

from 8.05 mm (SD 2.1) at baseline to 7.50 mm (SD 1.6) at the 5-year follow-up (p=0.051).

Conclusion.—At 5-year follow-up, a significant increase of VISA-A score can be expected. After the 3-month Alfredson's heel-drop exercise programme, almost half of the patients had received other therapies. Although improvement of symptoms can be expected at long term, mild pain may remain (Fig 2).

▶ Controversy continues, and probably always will, regarding the optimum management of mid-substance Achilles tendinopathy. The merits of this study are obviously as much in the design as in the findings. A prospective, randomized study was continued for a longer period (5 years) assessing the effectiveness of a basic exercise program. The findings are quite straightforward: improvement up to a year can be anticipated. After that, there is little improvement, but importantly, there is not a deterioration either (Fig 2). The reader should note, that even with the long-term, sustained benefit, most patients still had pain. Why? The tendon is still degenerated.

B. F. Morrey, MD

Ankle and Hindfoot Fusions: Comparison of Outcomes in Patients With and Without Diabetes

Myers TG, Lowery NJ, Frykberg RG, et al (Univ of Pittsburgh Med Ctr, PA; Carl T Hayden VA Med Ctr, Phoenix, AZ)

Foot Ankle Int 33:20-28, 2012

Background.—Patients with diabetes mellitus (DM) are believed to have higher complication rates when undergoing ankle and hindfoot fusions, but data is lacking. The purpose of this study was to compare the postoperative outcomes of major foot and ankle arthrodeses in patients with and without DM. Another goal was to evaluate what effect glycemic control had on the outcomes of patients with diabetes.

Methods.—A retrospective review of charts from operative years 2005 to 2010 was performed. Inclusion criteria encompassed patients requiring major hindfoot and/or ankle fusion. Exclusion criteria included any patient who did not have at least 6-month followup. Seventy four patients with DM were matched with 74 non-DM patients based on age, gender, and length of surgery. Significance was set at $p < 0.05$ with associated 95% confidence intervals.

Results.—The overall complication rate was found to be significantly higher in patients with DM, a history of tobacco use, and peripheral neuropathy. The postoperative infection rate was found to be significantly higher in patients with DM, poor long-term glucose control (Hgb A1c levels greater than or equal to 7%), a history of tobacco use, peripheral artery disease, and peripheral neuropathy. Our rate of noninfectious complications was found to be significantly higher in patients with DM, poor short-term glucose control (a preoperative glucose greater than 200 mg/dL), a history

TABLE 2.—Results

Patient Characteristics	Number of Patients	Any Complication (%) ($n = 49$)	OR (95% CI)	p Value
Diabetes	74	33 (44.6%)	**2.9 (1.42–5.96)**	$p < 0.005$
No Diabetes	74	16 (21.6%)		
Age ≥65 years	33	7 (21.2%)	**0.35 (0.13–0.99)**	$p < 0.05$
Obesity (BMI >30)	93	30 (32.2%)		$p > 0.05$
Preoperative Glucose >140 mg/dL	39	16 (41.0%)		$p > 0.05$
Preoperative Glucose >200 mg/dL	13	8 (61.5%)		$p > 0.05$
Hemoglobin AIC ≥7%	44	20 (45.5%)		$p > 0.05$
Length of surgery ≥156 minutes	63	25 (39.7%)		$p > 0.05$
History of tobacco use	36	20 (55.5%)	**3.58 (1.64–7.82)**	$p < 0.001$
ASA ≥3	94	35 (37.2%)		$p > 0.05$
History of previous ulcer	22	10 (45.5%)		$p > 0.05$
Peripheral artery disease	16	5 (31.5%)		$p > 0.05$
Peripheral neuropathy	67	30 (44.7%)	**2.64 (1.31–5.35)**	$p < 0.01$
Transplant	5	4 (80%)		$p > 0.05$
		Infection (%) ($n = 15$)		
Diabetes	74	14 (18.9%)	**17 (2.18–133.28)**	$p < 0.01$
No Diabetes	74	1 (1.4%)		
Age ≥65 years	33	0		*$p < 0.05$
Obesity (BMI >30)	93	12 (10.7%)		$p > 0.05$
Preoperative Glucose >140 mg/dL	39	7 (17.9%)		$p > 0.05$
Preoperative Glucose >200 mg/dL	13	3 (23.1%)		$p > 0.05$
Hemoglobin AIC ≤7%	44	12 (27.3%)	**5.06 (1.04–24.03)**	$p < 0.05$
Length of surgery ≥156 minutes	63	11 (17.5%)		$p > 0.05$
History of tobacco use	36	8 (22.2%)	**4.29 (1.43–12.83)**	$p < 0.01$
ASA ≥3	94	13 (13.8%)		$p > 0.05$
History of previous ulcer	22	4 (18.2%)		$p > 0.05$
Peripheral artery disease	16	5 (31.3%)	**5.54 (1.61–19.13)**	$p < 0.01$
Peripheral neuropathy	67	13 (19.4%)	**21.13 (2.70–165.51)**	$p < 0.005$
Transplant	5	0		$p > 0.05$
		Noninfectious Complication (%) ($n = 49$)		
Diabetes	74	25 (33.8%)	**2.19 (1.03–4.65)**	$p < 0.05$
No Diabetes	74	14 (18.9%)		
Age ≥65 years	33	7 (21.2%)		$p > 0.05$
Obesity (BMI >30)	93	23 (27.7%)		$p > 0.05$
Preoperative Glucose >140 mg/dL	39	12 (30.8%)		$p > 0.05$
Preoperative Glucose >200 mg/dL	13	7 (53.8%)	**3.19 (1.04–9.77)**	$p < 0.05$
Hemoglobin AIC ≥7%	44	15 (34.1%)		$p > 0.05$
Length of surgery ≥156 minutes	63	19 (30.2%)		$p > 0.05$
History of tobacco use	36	15 (41.7%)	**2.62 (1.17–5.83)**	$p < 0.05$
ASA ≥3	94	27 (28.7%)		$p > 0.05$
History of previous ulcer	22	8 (36.4%)		$p > 0.05$
Peripheral artery disease	16	2 (12.5%)		$p > 0.05$
Peripheral neuropathy	67	22 (32.8%)		$p > 0.05$
Transplant	5	4 (80%)	**12.34 (1.33–114.13)**	$p < 0.05$

R, Odds ratio; CI, 95% Confidence interval; n/a = Not applicable because these are continuous variables.
*Unable to determine CI because no infections occurred in patients who were 65 years or older.

of tobacco use, and previous solid organ transplantation. Patients greater than or equal to 65 years of age were significantly associated with fewer overall complications and postoperative infections.

Conclusion.—This study confirmed our hypothesis that patients with DM were at increased risk for postoperative complications after foot and/or ankle arthrodesis when compared to patients without DM. A secondary finding of this study demonstrated patients with poor short- and long-term glucose control experienced more complications (Table 2).

► Pathology associated with the diabetic foot is increasing in incidence, and the problems it poses continue to be challenging. Although this is a retrospective, this descriptive case-controlled study offers findings that are of value. The entire essence of the study is summarized in Table 2. The true importance is to glean the issues that are amenable to intervention or prevention. Once again this points to control of the underlying diagnosis. Today this means not using just the blood sugar level as an indicator of control, but also, and possibly more sensitive, is the hemoglobin A1c levels. This is especially true as the incidence of infection is significantly greater when the A1c is in excess of 7%.

B. F. Morrey, MD

Medium- to Long-Term Outcome of Ankle Arthrodesis

Hendrickx RPM, Stufkens SAS, de Bruijn EE, et al (Academic Med Ctr, Amsterdam, The Netherlands)

Foot Ankle Int 32:940-947, 2011

Background.—Despite improvement in outcome after ankle arthroplasty, fusion of the ankle joint is still considered the gold standard. A matter of concern is deterioration of clinical outcome as a result of loss of motion and advancing degeneration of adjacent joints. We performed a long-term study to address these topics.

Methods.—Between 1990 and 2005 a total of 121 ankle arthrodeses were performed at our institute. Thirty-five cases were excluded because of simultaneous subtalar arthrodesis. Ten had died and ten were lost to followup. Six had a bilateral ankle arthrodeses, leaving 60 patients (66 ankles) eligible for followup. There were 40 males and 26 females with a mean age at surgery of 47 years. In 60 ankles, fusion was obtained using a two-incision, three-screw technique. All patients were assessed using validated questionnaires and clinical rating systems: Short Form 36 (SF-36), American Orthopaedic Foot and Ankle Society (AOFAS) Ankle and Hindfoot scale, Foot and Ankle Ability Measure (FAAM) and a subjective satisfaction rating. Radiological progression of osteoarthritis of the adjacent joints was assessed.

Results.—Fusion was achieved in 91% after primary surgery. In six patients rearthrodesis was needed to obtain fusion. The mean SF-36 score was 63 (SD, 22) for the physical component scale and 81 (SD, 15) for the mental component scale. The mean FAAM score was 69 (SD, 17) and the mean AOFAS Ankle Hindfoot score was 67 (SD, 12). Ninety-one percent were satisfied with their clinical result. Infection occurred once. No other serious adverse events were encountered. In all contiguous joints significant progression of arthritis was appreciated.

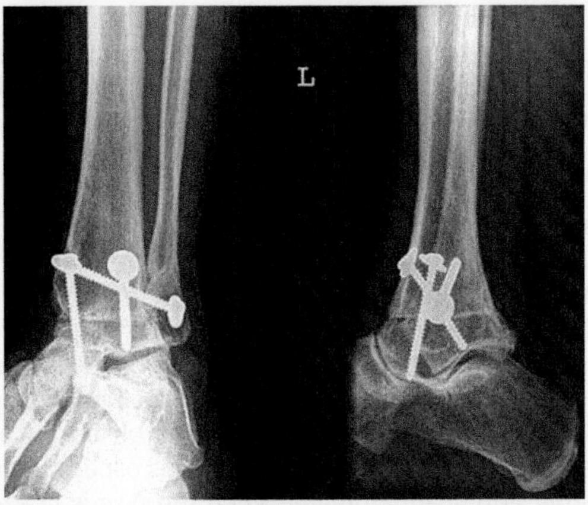

FIGURE 1.—X-ray illustrating the screw placement and postoperative result. (Reprinted from Hendrickx RPM, Stufkens SAS, de Bruijn EE, et al. Medium- to long-term outcome of ankle arthrodesis. *Foot Ankle Int.* 2011;32:940-947, with permission from American Orthopaedic Foot & Ankle Society.)

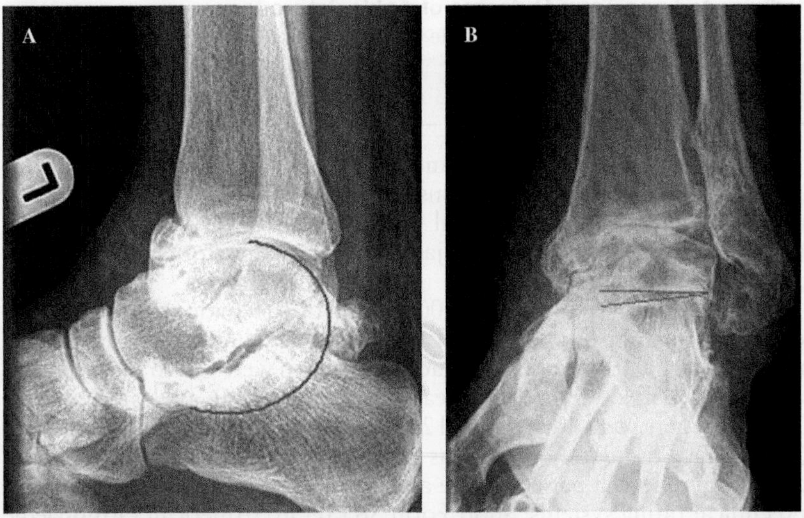

FIGURE 3.—A, The "C-sign": a curved continuous line visible on lateral images as indicated by the gray line. When this line is visible it indicates marked cartilage loss of the subtalar joint. B, Asymmetric subtalar joint. The gray line shows the lateral joint space narrowing of the subtalar joint, as visible on an anteroposterior X-ray. (Reprinted from Hendrickx RPM, Stufkens SAS, de Bruijn EE, et al. Medium- to long-term outcome of ankle arthrodesis. *Foot Ankle Int.* 2011;32:940-947. Copyright © 2011 by the American Orthopaedic Foot and Ankle Society, Inc., originally published in Foot & Ankle International, 32:940-947, and reproduced here with permission.)

Conclusion.—Ankle arthrodesis using a two-incision, three-screw technique was a reliable and safe technique for the treatment of end-stage osteoarthritis of the ankle. It resulted in a good functional outcome at a mean followup of 9 years. Progressive osteoarthritis of the contiguous joints was clearly appreciated but the functional and clinical importance of these findings remains unclear (Figs 1 and 3).

▶ I will readily confess I am drawn to studies and reports that I personally find interesting, and they are often on topics I have also studied. Such is the case here. But there are some legitimate reasons to consider this article. The study is of a relatively large sample, with good follow-up and objective study data. Further, as the authors note, ankle replacement is still emerging as a reliable option, so the alternative salvage procedure is worthy of study to serve as a baseline comparison. Note, therefore, the 91% patient satisfaction at less than 10 years. Also note the tendency to less invasive procedures (Fig 1). The main concern, other than initial fusion, is the tendency for development of arthritis in the adjacent joints—Chopart's and subtalar. The authors do a nice job of pointing out that often the arthritis already exists before the fusion (Fig 3). So it is not necessarily caused by the fusion, but may be aggravated by the procedure. Regardless, with modest, not long-term follow-up, ankle fusion remains a viable salvage option for end-stage ankle arthritis.

B. F. Morrey, MD

Combined Medial and Lateral Anatomic Ligament Reconstruction for Chronic Rotational Instability of the Ankle

Buchhorn T, Sabeti-Aschraf M, Dlaska CE, et al (Sporthopaedicum Straubing, Germany; Med Univ of Vienna, Austria)

Foot Ankle Int 32:1122-1126, 2011

Background.—This study aimed to extend knowledge on the arthroscopic evaluation of the unstable ankle joint and the outcome of ligament reconstruction on rotational instability. In contrast to previous studies, we investigated the combined repair of lateral and medial ligaments.

Methods.—Ninety-six patients underwent medial and lateral ligament reconstruction between 2006 and 2008, 81 of whom, with a mean age of 31.9 (range, 14 to 44) years, completed the 12-month followup and were therefore included in this study (Table 1). Clinical, radiographic, and concomitant arthroscopic examination was performed prior to the ligament stabilization. Postoperative followup included clinical and radiographic evaluation after 3, 6, and 12 months.

Results.—Arthroscopy showed a lesion of the anterior fibulotalar ligament (AFTL), calcaneofibular ligament (CFL), and tibiocalcanear ligament (TCL) (Deep part of deltoid ligament complex) in 67 patients. An avulsion of the proximal insertion point of the ATTL was additionally found in 14 cases. Clinical results 3 months after surgery showed a significant increase in the AOFAS-Hindfoot Score as well as a significant decrease of the Visual Analogue-Scale for pain (VAS) ($p < 0.0001$). This outcome persisted at the 12-month examination.

Conclusion.—Rotational instability of the ankle joint in most cases has an injury of the lateral ligaments and a component of the deltoid, the TCL,

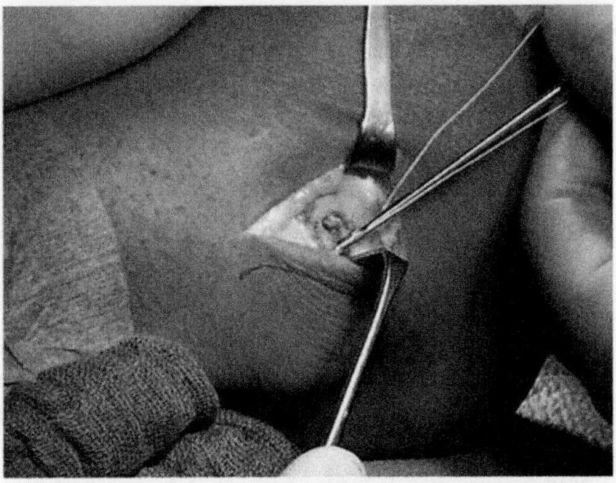

FIGURE 3.—Anchor placed with a press fit technique. (Reprinted from Buchhorn T, Sabeti-Aschraf M, Dlaska CE, et al. Combined medial and lateral anatomic ligament reconstruction for chronic rotational instability of the ankle. *Foot Ankle Int.* 2011;32:1122-1126, Copyright © 2011 by the American Orthopaedic Foot and Ankle Society, Inc., originally published in Foot & Ankle International 32:1122-1126 and reproduced here with permission.)

but rarely with a combined lesion of the TCL and the anterior tibiotalar ligament (ATTL) (Superficial part of deltoid ligament complex). The combined lateral and medial ligament reconstruction with an anchor technique had a good clinical outcome with high patient satisfaction with few complications (Fig 3).

▶ I was struck by the clinical practice of medial and lateral ligament reconstruction, as this is not typically felt to be indicated. I was possibly even more impressed that the authors performed almost 100 of these procedures in the 2006–2008 study period. The documentation of the pathology is descriptive and largely gleaned from arthroscopic interpretation. The technique uses suture anchors and is performed in a less-invasive manner. The authors conclude the technique is of value and produce comparative data to substantiate their claim (Fig 3).

I do not get a good feel for the degree of instability before and after the procedure nor the precise indications for a medial and lateral reconstructive technique. Interesting.

B. F. Morrey, MD

Critical Review of Self-Reported Functional Ankle Instability Measures
Donahue M, Simon J, Docherty CL
Foot Ankle Int 32:1140-1146, 2011

Background.—Since functional ankle instability (FAI) lacks a "gold standard" measure, a variety of self-reported ankle instability measures have been created. The purpose of this study was to determine which ankle instability measure identifies individuals who meet a minimum acceptable criterion for FAI.

TABLE 3.—Sensitivity and Specificity of Significant Predictor Variables From the Reduced Model

	Sensitivity (95% CI)	Specificity (95% CI)	Odds-Ratio (95% CI)	Risk (95% CI)
AII	0.73 (0.59-0.83)	0.85 (0.79-0.83)	16.10 (7.84-33.02)	6.99 (4.15-11.77)
CAIT	0.56 (0.45-0.67)	0.86 (0.79-0.90)	7.88 (4.18-14.89)	3.20 (2.33-4.65)
AII&CAIT	0.82 (0.66-0.92)	0.82 (0.76-0.87)	21.21 (8.68-51.83)	11.70 (5.4-25.22)

Methods.—Participants volunteered from a large university population which included 242 participants (104 males, 138 females; 21.4 ± 1.4 years). The predictor variables were seven ankle instability questionnaires: Ankle Instability Instrument (AII), Ankle Joint Functional Assessment Tool (AJFAT), Chronic Ankle Instability Scale (CAIS), Cumberland Ankle Instability Tool (CAIT), Foot and Ankle Ability Measure (FAAM), Foot and Ankle Instability Questionnaire (FAIQ), and Foot and Ankle Outcome Score (FAOS). The outcome variable (MC_FAI) was created based on the minimum acceptable criteria for FAI. This was established as at least one ankle sprain and an episode of giving way. Data were modeled using chi-square and multinomial logistic regression.

Results.—The regression model revealed all of the questionnaires were more useful at identifying participants who did not meet the minimum criteria for FAI (No MC_FAI = 95.7%, MC_FAI = 55.6%, overall = 84.6%). Based on the Wald criterion, the full model was reduced to the CAIT, AII, and FAAM. The reduced model revealed the CAIT ($X^2 = 8.756$, $p = 0.003$) and AII ($X^2 = 31.992$, $p = 0.001$) as the only variables that had a significant relationship with the outcome variable.

Conclusion.—The model illustrates no single measure was able to predict if individuals met the minimally accepted criteria for FAI. However, a significantly accurate prediction of ankle stability status was produced by combining the CAIT and AII.

Clinical Relevance.—Based on the results we recommend that researchers and clinicians use both the CAIT and AII to determine ankle stability status (Table 3).

▶ As mentioned in the past, I am intentionally presenting clinical studies that I hope can shape our thinking in a manner that will be required in the future. This might in general be referred to as *evidence-based medicine*. In this instance, the hypothesis investigates the reliability of self-reported function of the ankle as a means of accurately determining clinically relevant ankle instability. Of interest is that no single measure was adequate, but the specificity and sensitivity of the combination of the Cumberland Ankle Instability Tool and the Ankle Instability Index were both greater than 80. In addition to the obvious value of the specific findings, this study also reveals the potential complexity of the entire subject.

B. F. Morrey, MD

Functional Treatment After Surgical Repair for Acute Lateral Ligament Disruption of the Ankle in Athletes

Takao M, Miyamoto W, Matsui K, et al (Teikyo Univ, Tokyo, Japan)

Am J Sports Med 40:447-451, 2012

Background.—There have been several reports showing 20% to 40% failure after nonoperative functional treatment for acute lateral ligament disruption of the ankle.

Hypothesis.—Functional treatment after primary surgical repair has the advantage of decreasing the failure rate in comparison with functional treatment alone.

Study Design.—Cohort study; Level of evidence, 3.

Methods.—A total of 132 feet of 132 patients were included in this study. Of these, 78 patients were treated with functional treatment alone (group F), and the remaining 54 patients were treated with functional treatment after primary surgical repair (group RF). The clinical results were evaluated using the Japanese Society for Surgery of the Foot Ankle-Hindfoot scale (JSSF) score, measuring the talar tilt angle and the anterior displacement of the talus in stress radiography, and noting the elapsed time between the injury and the return to the full athletic activity with no external supports.

Results.—The mean JSSF scores at 2 years after injury were 95.6 ± 5.0 points in group F and 97.5 ± 2.6 points in group RF ($P = .0669$). The differences of the talar tilt angles compared with the contralateral side and displacement of the talus on stress radiography at 2 years after injury were 1.1° ± 1.5° and 3.6 ± 1.6 mm in group F, and 0.8° ± 0.9° and 3.2 ± 0.8 mm in group RF, respectively ($P = .4093$, .1883). In group F, 8 cases showed fair to poor results, with JSSF scores below 80 points and instability at 2 years after injury. In group RF, 9 cases (9.4%) showed dorsum foot pain along the superficial peroneal nerve, which disappeared within a month. The time elapsed between the injury and the patient's return to full athletic activity without any external supports was 16.0 ± 5.6 weeks in group F and 10.1 ± 1.8 weeks in group RF ($P < .0001$).

Conclusion.—Nonoperative functional treatment alone and functional treatment after primary surgical repair showed similar overall results after acute lateral ankle sprain, but functional treatment alone had an approximately 10% failure rate and a slower return to full athletic activity. The authors recommend that treatment be tailored to suit each individual athlete (Table 1).

▶ Ankle sprain remains a major issue for the competitive and recreational athlete alike. This large series again revisits the difference between surgical and nonsurgical intervention, but in this instance, it is assessed in the acute stage. Although the randomized process was by even or odd numbers, the difference in nonoperative (78) and operative (54) patients suggests some selection bias. The study is rather comprehensive with clinical, radiographic, and subjective parameters being assessed. Although the data at 2 years do not reveal dramatic differences (Table 1), careful assessment would suggest a slightly better result in virtually

TABLE 1.—Treatment Outcomes[a]

	Group F	Group RF	*P* Value
JSSF score 2 years after surgery	67-100 (95.6 ± 5.0)	90-100 (97.5 ± 2.6)	.0669
Stress radiography			
Talar tilt angle compared with the contralateral side, deg			
Before surgery	7-15 (11.7 ± 1.8)	7-15 (12.1 ± 1.6)	.4587
2 years after surgery	0-13 (1.1 ± 1.5)	0-3 (0.8 ± 0.9)	.4093
Anterior displacement of the talus, mm			
Before surgery	6-12 (8.6 ± 1.7)	7-12 (8.9 ± 1.6)	.4319
2 years after surgery	2-10 (3.6 ± 1.6)	2-5 (3.2 ± 0.8)	.1883
Duration between the injury and their returning to full athletic activity, wk			
With external support	3-12 (6.3 ± 1.3)	3-8 (5.7 ± 1.3)	.0498[b]
Without external support	8-48 (16.0 ± 5.6)	8-15 (10.1 ± 1.8)	<.0001[b]

[a]Data are expressed as range (mean ± standard deviation). Group F, functional treatment alone; group RF, functional treatment after primary surgical repair; JSSF, Japanese Society for Surgery of the Foot Ankle-Hindfoot scale.
[b]p-value < .05.

every parameter in the operated group. The study leaves one to consider possibly being more aggressive, especially with the more severe, acute ankle sprain.

B. F. Morrey, MD

Comparison of Magnetic Resonance Imaging to Physical Examination for Syndesmotic Injury After Lateral Ankle Sprain

de César PC, Avila EM, de Abreu MR (Hospital Mãe de Deus de Porto Alegre, RS, Brazil)
Foot Ankle Int 32:1110-1114, 2011

Background.—Clinical assessment of syndesmotic injury usually consists of two tests: the ankle external rotation test and squeeze test. This study sought to determine the sensitivity and specificity of both for syndesmotic injury secondary to lateral ankle sprain.

Methods.—Fifty-six patients with sprained ankles underwent clinical examination for syndesmotic injury with the aforementioned tests. Clinical findings were compared against magnetic resonance imaging (MRI) of the ankle. Sprains were graded on anatomical and functional classification scales, and correlation and agreement between both scales were assessed.

Results.—The MRI prevalence of syndesmotic injury in patients with lateral ankle sprains was 17.8%. Sensitivity and specificity were 30% and 93.5% for the squeeze test, and 20% and 84.8% for the external rotation test, respectively. Using the anatomical scale for sprain grading, 40% of syndesmotic injuries occurred in Grade I, 40% in Grade II, and 20% in Grade III sprains. Ten percent of patients with syndesmotic injury had no lateral ligament injury on MRI, 70% had injury of the anterior talofibular (ATFL) ligament, and 20% had injury to the ATFL and calcaneofibular (CFL).

Conclusion.—The sensitivity of the squeeze test and external rotation test was low, suggesting that physical examination often fails to diagnose syndesmotic injury. Conversely, specificity was very high; nearly all patients with a positive test actually had syndesmotic injury. Severity of ankle sprain was not associated with prevalence of syndesmotic injury.

▶ This clean, straightforward study addresses a clinical problem: accurate diagnosis of syndesmotic injuries. Using MRI as the gold standard, the 2 most commonly used clinical tests—the squeeze test and the external rotation test—were evaluated. The study allows one to conclude that if the tests are negative, the patient may still have a syndesmotic injury. However, if the test is positive, one can be quite sure this documents ligament injury. What was unexpected was the lack of correlation between the severity of the lateral ankle ligament injury and the associated injury of the syndesmosis.

B. F. Morrey, MD

Clinical and Computed Tomography Evaluation of Surgical Outcomes in Tarsal Navicular Stress Fractures

McCormick JJ, Bray CC, Davis WH, et al (Washington Univ Orthopaedics, Chesterfield, MO; Carolinas Med Ctr, Charlotte, NC; et al)

Am J Sports Med 39:1741-1748, 2011

Background.—As clinical suspicion increases and radiographic evaluation improves, navicular stress fractures are becoming a more recognized injury. To date, there is a small volume of literature examining these stress fractures, particularly as it pertains to outcomes of surgical management.

Purpose.—To evaluate the clinical and computed tomography (CT) outcomes of surgically treated navicular stress fractures.

Study Design.—Case series; Level of evidence, 4.

Methods.—Ten navicular stress fractures in 10 patients were available for follow-up at an average of 42.4 months postoperatively (range, 16.8-79.9). These patients underwent a clinical examination and a CT scan of their operatively treated foot. The American Orthopaedic Foot & Ankle Society (AOFAS) and SF-36 scores were completed for each fracture at the time of examination. The CT scans were blindly evaluated for bony union.

Results.—According to the CT scan evaluation, 8 of 10 navicula (80%) had gone on to union. Clinical outcome scores on all patients were an average AOFAS hindfoot score of 88.5 and an average SF-36 score of 88.3. The feet with united fractures had an average AOFAS score of 92.1 (range, 83-100) and an average SF-36 score of 91.9 (range, 79-98). The 2 patients with nonunions had AOFAS scores of 74 and 74 and SF-36 scores of 70 and 78, respectively. Both nonunions were complete, displaced fractures on preoperative imaging.

Conclusion.—In our series of operatively treated navicular stress fractures, 80% went on to union, as verified by CT scan. Patients with united fractures had a clinically significant improvement in outcome, with higher AOFAS and SF-36 scores as compared with the 2 patients with nonunions.

Patients with complete, displaced navicular stress fractures may be more likely to develop nonunions.

► As the authors indicate, navicular stress fracture is not common, but it can be a sinister and disabling injury. Surgery is uncommonly required, occurring in less than 20% in this experience. That 2 of 10 did not initially unite is of note and concern. Unfortunately, the precise indications for surgery are not clear, and it should be noted that 4 surgeons contributed to the series. In my experience, it is of concern that not all stress fractures heal spontaneously, that protected weight bearing is required, and the healing process may be prolonged. Hence the need for fixation in selected cases.

B. F. Morrey, MD

Functional Outcome of Endoscopic Plantar Fasciotomy

Bader L, Park K, Gu Y, et al (Hosp for Special Surgery, NY)

Foot Ankle Int 33:37-43, 2012

Background.—The majority of cases of plantar fasciitis can be treated nonoperatively; however, a small number of patients remain refractory to nonoperative treatment and operative intervention is indicated. Historically, open treatment has been recommended, but more recently endoscopic plantar fasciotomy (EPF) has produced promising results.

Methods.—Forty-eight patients (56 feet) were identified who underwent endoscopic plantar fasciotomy. Forty-one patients (49 feet) were available for followup. There were 15 men and 26 women, with an average age of 53.8 (range, 42 to 68) years. The mean followup time was 49.5 (range, 6 to 142) months. An AOFAS Hind foot Scale was used for analysis. The influence of gender, duration of symptoms, severity of symptoms, and bilateral verses unilateral release were examined.

Results.—Pain resolved completely in 37 feet, decreased in 11 feet, and increased in one foot. The mean postoperative AOFAS Hindfoot score improved 39 points (54 to 93, $p < 0.001$). Patients with severe symptoms achieved higher mean improvement than the moderate symptom group ($p < 0.0001$). Patients with symptoms greater than 24 months trended towards lower mean improvement and lower post operative AOFAS Hindfoot scores. Both gender and laterality did not significantly influence outcome. There was one superficial infection, one third and fourth metatarsal stress fracture in the same patient, and transient lateral hindfoot pain in five patients.

Conclusion.—EPF was an effective operation with reproducible results, low complication rate, and little risk of iatrogenic nerve injury with proper technique (Fig 2).

► Plantar fasciitis remains an enigma. The condition frequently becomes chronic, and the impact is debilitating. As noted, there are few if any reliable interventions.

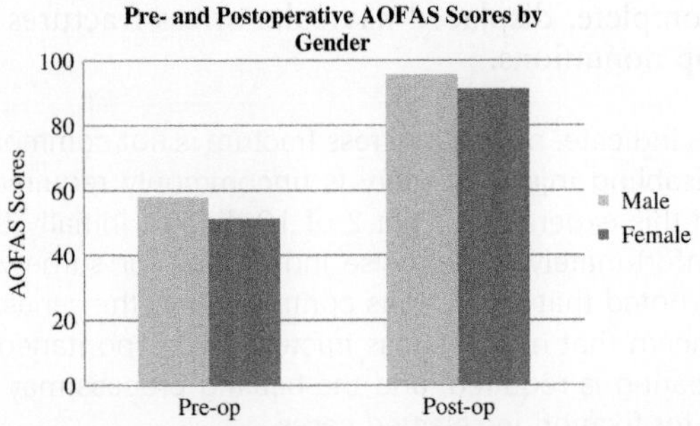

FIGURE 2.—Pre- and postoperative scores for 15 men and 26 women. In men, there was a 37-point improvement from 58 to 95. In women, there was a 40-point improvement, from 51 to 91. No statistical difference was found between men and women postoperative scores. (Reprinted from Bader L, Park K, Gu Y, et al. Functional outcome of endoscopic plantar fasciotomy. *Foot Ankle Int*. 2012;33:37-43. Copyright © 2012 by the American Orthopaedic Foot and Ankle Society, Inc., originally published in Foot & Ankle International, 33:37-43 and reproduced here with permission.)

Any intervention that is reliable and effective and has minimal morbidity is superior to any current option. The minimally invasive endoscopic adjunct is, therefore, a useful advance in the management of this condition. The data in this report suggest this technique is consistently reliable, regardless of gender (Fig 2). We have been involved in yet another technology using ultrasonic energy to address this problem. The results are very encouraging.

B. F. Morrey, MD

10 Spine

Introduction

The articles chosen for the Spine section of the YEAR BOOK OF ORTHOPEDICS 2012 represent the very best in quality and design and are sure to be both provocative and informative to the YEAR BOOK's readership. The reference articles span both the basic science and clinical realms and provide insight into health policy, basic science and the economics of spinal practice. Readers will be briefed on the latest knowledge learned form treating spinal injuries from the conflicts in Afghanistan and Iraq as well as controversies related to spinal wound infections after surgery and the use of prophylactic antibiotics in the wound to prevent infection. Articles on the significance and basic science of the epidemic of obesity and its impact on back pain, the surprising biomechanical significance of vertebral body osteophytes along with a treatise questioning the usefulness of the Lenke classification for scoliosis surgery, and scoliosis surgery in adults are included. Complications related to spinal surgery spotlight the frequency of facet violation with percutaneous pedicle screw insertion and dysphagia after anterior cervical surgery as well as continued controversies involving the use of infuse for lumbar fusion. We have reviewed articles concerning the changing payer policies and clinical guidelines for fusion for chronic low back pain and the effects of intraoperative waste in spine surgery. Some sobering information of the survival analysis after the diagnosis of spinal metastatics disease will be informative to clinicians as well as a wonderful review on the use of growing rods to treat scoliosis. There was certainly no shortage of enlightening and controversial articles to select for this year's YEAR BOOK, and I hope you enjoy these selections and commentaries as a succinct and useful reference for the best of last year's publications and a useful reference for the year to come!

Paul M. Huddleston, MD

Risk-Benefit Assessment of Surgery for Adult Scoliosis: An Analysis Based on Patient Age

Smith JS, the Spinal Deformity Study Group (Univ of Virginia, Charlottesville; et al)

Spine 36:817-824, 2011

Study Design.—Retrospective review of a prospective, multicenter database.

Objective.—The purpose of this study was to assess whether elderly patients undergoing scoliosis surgery had an incidence of complications and improvement in outcome measures comparable with younger patients.

Summary of Background Data.—Complications increase with age for adults undergoing scoliosis surgery, but whether this impacts the outcomes of older patients is largely unknown.

Methods.—This is a retrospective review of a prospective, multicenter spinal deformity database. Patients complete the Oswestry Disability Index (ODI), SF-12, Scoliosis Research Society-22 (SRS-22), and numerical rating scale (NRS; 0–10) for back and leg pain. Inclusion criteria included age 25 to 85 years, scoliosis (Cobb ≥ 30°), plan for scoliosis surgery, and 2-year follow-up.

Results.—Two hundred six of 453 patients (45%) completed 2-year follow-up, which is distributed among age groups as follows: 25 to 44 (n = 47), 45 to 64 (n = 121), and 65 to 85 (n = 38) years. The percentages of patients with 2-year follow-up by age group were as follows: 25 to 44 (45%), 45 to 64 (48%), and 65 to 85 (40%) years. These groups had perioperative complication rates of 17%, 42%, and 71%, respectively ($P < 0.001$). At baseline, elderly patients (65–85 years) had greater disability (ODI, $P = 0.001$), worse health status (SF-12 physical component score (PCS), $P < 0.001$), and more severe back and leg pain (NRS, $P = 0.04$ and $P = 0.01$, respectively) than younger patients. Mean SRS-22 did not differ significantly at baseline. Within each age group, at 2-year follow-up there were significant improvements in ODI ($P \leq 0.004$), SRS-22 ($P \leq 0.001$), back pain ($P < 0.001$), and leg pain ($P \leq 0.04$). SF-12 PCS did not improve significantly for patients aged 25 to 44 years but did among those aged 45 to 64 ($P < 0.001$) and 65 to 85 years ($P = 0.001$). Improvement in ODI and leg pain NRS were significantly greater among elderly patients ($P = 0.003$, $P = 0.02$, respectively), and there were trends for greater improvements in SF-12 PCS ($P = 0.07$), SRS-22 ($P = 0.048$), and back pain NRS ($P = 0.06$) among elderly patients, when compared with younger patients.

Conclusion.—Collectively, these data demonstrate the potential benefits of surgical treatment for adult scoliosis and suggest that the elderly, despite facing the greatest risk of complications, may stand to gain a disproportionately greater improvement in disability and pain with surgery.

▶ It would be tempting to see this publication by the Spinal Deformity study group as nothing more than an organized corporate-funded cheerleading effort for complex spine surgery in the elderly. The massive amounts of money flowing throughout the instrumented spinal fusion for deformity business line is staggering.[1] Health care expenditures related to disorders of the spine have grown 65% between 1997 and 2005, totaling $86 billion in 2005.[2] Many recent efforts have admirably tried to make an argument to justify the expense by calculating quality-adjusted life-years for these complex spinal interventions and have, as a result, suggested increasing benefit with time.[3] Methodology notwithstanding, the correct question is not whether funding these interventions is financially beneficial, but whether funding them at all is indicated. With numerous other chronic diseases such as obesity, diabetes, tobacco abuse, and heart disease causing an avalanche of death disability, is it worth supporting operations for pain and deformity when they are not life-threatening? Should highly morbid and expensive surgeries be funded when adult scoliosis has always been present in the human form and until recent history was treated without surgery in this patient population? These are the important questions that society, and their elected policy makers, will need to decide in the near future.

P. Huddleston, MD

References

1. Martin BI, Deyo RA, Mirza SK, et al. Expenditures and health status among adults with back and neck problems. *JAMA*. 2008;299:656-664.
2. Babu MA, Coumans JV, Carter BS, et al. A review of lumbar spinal instrumentation: evidence and controversy. *J Neurol Neurosurg Psychiatry*. 2011;82:948-951.
3. Tosteson AN, Tosteson TD, Lurie JD, et al. Comparative effectiveness evidence from the spine patient outcomes research trial: surgical versus nonoperative care for spinal stenosis, degenerative spondylolisthesis, and intervertebral disc herniation. *Spine (Phila Pa 1976)*. 2011;36:2061-2068.

2011 Young Investigator Award Winner: Increased Fat Mass Is Associated With High Levels of Low Back Pain Intensity and Disability

Urquhart DM, Berry P, Wluka AE, et al (Monash Univ, Melbourne, Victoria, Australia; et al)
Spine 36:1320-1325, 2011

Study Design.—A cross-sectional study.

Objective.—To determine whether body composition is associated with low back pain intensity and/or disability.

Summary of Background Data.—The relationship between obesity and low back pain and disability is unclear. No study has examined the role of body composition in low back pain and disability.

Methods.—A total of 135 participants (25–62 years), with a range of body mass indices (18–55 kg/m^2), were recruited for a study examining the relationship between obesity and musculoskeletal disease. Participants completed the Chronic Back Pain Grade Questionnaire, which examines individuals' levels of low back pain intensity and disability. Body composition was assessed using dual radiograph absorptiometry.

Results.—Body mass index was associated with higher levels of back pain intensity (Odds ratio [OR] = 1.35; 95% confidence interval [CI] = 1.09, 1.67) and disability (OR = 1.66; 95% CI = 1.31, 2.09). Higher levels of pain intensity were positively associated with total body (OR = 1.19; 95% CI = 1.04, 1.38) and lower limb fat mass (OR = 1.51; 95% CI = 1.04, 2.20), independent of lean tissue mass. There were also positive associations between higher levels of low back disability and total body (OR = 1.41; 95% CI = 1.20, 1.67) and upper (OR = 1.67; 95% CI = 1.27, 2.19) and lower (OR = 2.29; 95% CI = 1.51, 3.49) limbs fat mass. Similar relationships were observed with trunk, android, and gynoid fat mass. After adjusting for confounders, no measures of lean tissue mass were associated with higher pain intensity or disability ($P > 0.10$).

Conclusion.—Greater fat, but not lean tissue mass, was associated with high levels of low back pain intensity and disability. Longitudinal investigation is needed to determine whether fat mass is predictive of low back pain and disability, as this may have important implications for further prevention strategies. Understanding the mechanism for these relationships may provide novel approaches to managing low back pain.

▶ This very interesting cross-sectional study from authors in Australia adds to the growing literature describing the deleterious musculoskeletal effects of obesity, specifically in the spine. One of the more interesting points discussed in the study describes a strong association between higher levels of pain intensity and total body and lower limb fat mass, independent of lean tissue mass. This research improves on the work of others in that the study recorded body mass percentages and not just weight, body mass index, and waist/hip ratio as measures of obesity. These measurements can be unrepresentative of an individual's actual healthy weight, especially in heavily muscled or stocky individuals. The authors speculate a fascinating hypothesis, that in addition to the pure weight effect of excess adipose tissue, the metabolic activity of fat could exacerbate low back pain by releasing a multitude of proinflammatory cytokines and key mediators of metabolism termed the *adipokines*. The results of the study were strongly significant, and while the authors correctly predict that "future longitudinal studies, in larger populations with a wide spectrum of back pain and disability, will be needed to determine the predictive nature of our findings," common sense would dictate we share this information with our patients and colleagues as 1 more weapon in the fight against obesity.

P. Huddleston, MD

Intrawound Application of Vancomycin for Prophylaxis in Instrumented Thoracolumbar Fusions: Efficacy, Drug Levels, and Patient Outcomes

Sweet FA, Roh M, Sliva C (Rockford Spine Ctr, IL)

Spine 36:2084-2088, 2011

Study Design.—A retrospective cohort study from a single institution of a consecutive series of spine surgery patients.

Objective.—To evaluate the safety and efficacy of adjunctive local application of vancomycin for infection prophylaxis in posterior instrumented thoracic and lumbar spine wounds compared to IV cephalexin alone.

Summary of Background Data.—Cephalosporin resistant strains of staphylococcus (MRSA and coagulase negative staph) have diminished the efficacy of intravenous antibiotic prophylaxis for instrumented spine fusion. Intravenous vancomycin prophylaxis has not been shown to decrease wound infection rates compared to IV cephalosporins. Adjunctive application of vancomycin powder in wounds for instrumented spinal fusion surgery may decrease infection rates.

Methods.—Since 2000, 1732 consecutive thoracic and lumbar posterior instrumented spinal fusions have been performed with routine 24 hours of perioperative intravenous antibiotic prophylaxis with cephalexin. Since 2006, 911 of these instrumented thoracic and lumbar cases had 2 g of vancomycin powder applied to the wound before closure in addition to intravenous antibiotics. A retrospective review for infection rates and complications was performed. Oswestry and SF-36 outcomes instruments were completed before surgery, immediately after surgery, and at latest follow-up. The average follow-up is 2.5 years, range 1 to 7 years.

Results.—Eight hundred twenty-one posterior instrumented thoracic and lumbar fusions were preformed using intravenous cephalexin prophylaxis with a total of 21 deep wound infections (2.6%). Coag negative staph was the most commonly isolated organism. Nine hundred eleven posterior instrumented thoracic and lumbar fusions have been performed with IV cephalexin plus adjunctive local vancomycin powder with two deep wound infections (0.2%). The reduction in wound infections was statistically significant ($P < 0.0001$). There were no adverse clinical outcomes or wound complications related to the local application of vancomycin.

Conclusion.—Adjunctive local application of vancomycin powder decreases the postsurgical wound infection rate with statistical significance in posterior instrumented thoracolumbar spine fusions.

▶ I would like to commend the authors of this retrospective case-control study for their interest and discipline in studying one of the more catastrophic complications of spine surgery—wound infection. Deep wound infection, especially those associated with implants, can lead to both short-term and long-term pain and disability. In their larger review, Kowalski et al[1] reported that of implant-associated spine infractions occurring at a referral spine center, even at 2-year follow-up after appropriate treatment, the estimated rate of 2-year survival free of treatment failure was only 71% (95% confidence interval, 51%–85%) for all patients with early-onset infection. Faced with such a difficult diagnostic dilemma, it is easy to understand why surgeons would try to mitigate the risk with an untried and developed intervention. The ends do not justify the means in this case, and until some very basic questions are answered, the practice should be condemned. The authors fail to describe whether there was any attempt to implement best infection practices to combat their 2% infection rate. It is not clear what methicillin-resistant *Staphylococcus aureus* (MRSA) was the prevalent organism in their infection population preintervention and whether a *Staphylococcus* bacteria screening program existed at their institution to attempt to identify populations at risk. It would be very short-sighted and metaphorically "kicks the can down the road" to take the conclusions of this report and apply them to large groups of patients as standard practice. Issues about the proper dosing of the drug, the method and manner of tissue absorption, and the eventual increased antibiotic resistance from a singular dose of the antibiotic should be the research focus. As an alternative, practitioners should concentrate on other, less-invasive interventions such as preoperative optimization of the patients' known health conditions, reduction of operative time, strict glucose preoperative control, and MRSA screening. A multidisciplinary work group led by a neutral third party such as the Centers for Disease Control and Prevention or the Infectious Diseases Research Society should take up the mantle on this topic and provide evidence-based recommendations as soon as possible.

P. Huddleston, MD

Reference

1. Kowalski TJ, Berbari EF, Huddleston PM, Steckelberg JM, Mandrekar JN, Osmon DR. The management and outcome of spinal implant infections: contemporary retrospective cohort study. *Clin Infect Dis*. 2007;44:913-920.

Survival Analysis of 254 Patients After Manifestation of Spinal Metastases: Evaluation of Seven Preoperative Scoring Systems

Wibmer C, Leithner A, Hofmann G, et al (Med Univ of Graz, Austria; et al)
Spine 36:1977-1986, 2011

Study Design.—Retrospective study.

Objective.—This study analyzed the predictive value of the scoring systems of Bauer, Bauer modified, Tokuhashi, Tokuhashi revised, Tomita, van der Linden, and Sioutos as well as the parameters included in these systems.

Summary of Background Data.—Metastases of the spinal column are a common manifestation of advanced cancer. Severe pain, pathologic fracture, and neurologic deficit due to spinal metastases need adequate treatment. Besides oncologic aspects and quality of life, treatment decisions should also include the survival prognosis.

Methods.—Two hundred fifty-four patients with confirmed spinal metastases were investigated retrospectively (treatment 1998–2006; 62 underwent surgery and 192 had conservative treatment only). Factors related to survival, such as primary tumor, general condition (Karnofsky Performance Status Scale), neurologic deficit, number of spinal and extra-spinal bone metastases, visceral metastases, and pathologic fracture, were analyzed. The survival period was calculated from date of diagnosis of the spinal metastases to date of death or last follow-up (minimum follow-up: 12 months). For statistical analysis, univariate and stepwise multivariate Cox regression analyses were performed.

Results.—Median overall survival for all patients was 10.6 months. The following factors showed significant influence on survival in multivariate analysis: primary tumor ($P < 0.0001$), status of visceral metastases ($P < 0.0001$), and systemic therapy ($P < 0.0001$). Using the recommended group assignment for each system, only Bauer and Bauer modified showed significant results for the distinction between good, moderate, and poor prognosis. The other systems failed to distinguish significantly between good and moderate prognosis. The hazard ratio of the absolute score of all analyzed systems was, however, statistically significant, with a better score leading to lower risk of death.

Conclusion.—According to this analysis, the Bauer and the Bauer modified scores are the most reliable systems for predicting survival. Since the Bauer modified score furthermore consists of only four positive prognostic factors, we emphasize its impact and simplicity.

▶ This retrospective study performed by researchers in Austria strongly suggests and independently confirms that the Bauer modified[1] scoring system for assisting in planning surgical care of patients with spinal metastases is superior to 6 other proposed systems. The strength of this statement comes out in the statistical analysis of the article but confirms the conventional wisdom summarized by Albert Einstein: "Everything should be as simple as it can be, but not simpler." With the proliferation of the electronic medical record, a superabundance of information, images, and data points have allowed researchers the power to create more progressively complex analyses of patient outcomes. I think in all of this progress the wisdom of Einstein should still apply. It is not clear to me that the classification exercise provides value, however, and the Austrian authors clearly advocate for the simple, yet predictive, Bauer modified scoring system. They do allow, and I agree, that the decision to proceed with a spinal operation should additionally take into account the presence of spinal instability, spinal cord progression, and all other possible treatment options, not life expectancy alone. A perfect treatment algorithm would incorporate all these issues and additionally insert a way to value the patient's needs, concerns, and beliefs into an all-encompassing patient-centered solution. So, there is still much to do!

P. Huddleston, MD

Reference

1. Bauer H, Tomita K, Kawahara N, Abdel-Wanis ME, Murakami H. Surgical strategy for spinal metastases. *Spine*. 2002;27:1124-1126.

Outcomes for Single-Level Lumbar Fusion: The Role of Bone Morphogenetic Protein

Cahill KS, Chi JH, Groff MW, et al (Brigham and Women's Hosp, Boston, MA; Beth Israel Med Ctr, Boston, MA; et al)
Spine 36:2354-2362, 2011

Study Design.—Retrospective analysis of a population-based insurance claims data set.

Objective.—To determine the risk of repeat fusion and total costs associated with bone morphogenetic protein (BMP) use in single-level lumbar fusion for degenerative spinal disease.

Summary of Background Data.—The use of BMP has been proposed to reduce overall costs of spinal fusion through prevention of repeat fusion procedures. Although radiographic fusion rates associated with BMP use have been examined in clinical trials, few data exist regarding outcomes associated with BMP use in the general population.

Methods.—Using the MarketScan claims data set, 15,862 patients that underwent single-level lumbar fusion from 2003 to 2007 for degenerative disease were identified. Propensity scores were used to match 2372 patients who underwent fusion with BMP to patients who underwent fusion without BMP. Logistic regression models, Kaplan-Meier estimates, and Cox proportional hazards models were used to examine risk of repeat fusion, length of stay, and 30-day readmission by BMP use. Cost comparisons were evaluated with linear regression models using logarithmic transformed data.

Results.—At 1 year from surgery, BMP was associated with a 1.1% absolute decrease in the risk of repeat fusion (2.3% with BMP vs. 3.4% without BMP, $P = 0.03$) and an odds ratio for repeat fusion of 0.66 (95% confidence interval [CI] = 0.47–0.94) after multivariate adjustment. BMP was also associated with a decreased hazard ratio for long-term repeat fusion (adjusted hazards ratio = 0.74, 95% CI = 0.58–0.93). Cost analysis indicated that BMP was associated with initial increased costs for the surgical procedure (13.9% adjusted increase, 95% CI = 9.9%–17.9%) as well as total 1-year costs (10.1% adjusted increase, 95% CI = 6.2%–14.0%).

Conclusion.—At 1 year, BMP use was associated with a decreased risk of repeat fusion but also increased health care costs.

► The very small decreased risk of repeat fusion (1.1%) in this retrospective, large, matched case-control study may at first glance seem to justify the increased cost of the drug, but in a large dataset such as this, it would have been more meaningful to define a probability value of 0.01 as the mark for significance. I did find it interesting but not surprising that specific populations with the analysis had higher rates of refusion, as those patients with the diagnosis of degenerative disc disease (DDD) had a higher rate than those with the diagnosis of degenerative spondylolisthesis. In my practice, DDD can be a difficult diagnosis, with the clinician often attempting to make decisions about including or excluding spinal levels based on a complex and often confusing mix of patient symptoms, radiographs, magnetic resonance, and discography. Patients with degenerative spondylolisthesis rarely present the same diagnostic dilemma and subsequently may not be at the same level of risk for subsequent arthrodesis. For the use of recombinant human BMP-2 (INFUSE; Medtronic, Inc, Minneapolis, MN) to make economic sense from a societal perspective, the additional cost of INFUSE at the point of use and at 1 year should offset the subsequent need for further spinal fusion. Cost savings could of course be accomplished by other methods, such as restricting payment for fusion for the diagnosis of DDD whether INFUSE is used or not. The metric of interest could be changed and large payers could find patient-reported pain from radiculitis meaningful; the outcome of such an analysis might be very different with a higher reported incidence of that complication being present with INFUSE. It would be even more interesting to see the results at even longer follow-ups, such as 2 and 5 years. The final decision, it seems, is increasingly going to be taken out of the individual surgeon's prevue as more private payers and hospitals place increasingly higher restrictions on the drug's use and reimbursement.

P. Huddleston, MD

Dysphagia Following Cervical Spine Surgery With Anterior Instrumentation: Evidence From Fluoroscopic Swallow Studies

Leonard R, Belafsky P (Univ of California, Davis)

Spine 36:2217-2223, 2011

Study Design.—Retrospective review.

Objective.—The purpose of this study was to evaluate alterations in objective swallowing parameters in patients reporting dysphagia after anterior cervial-spine surgery.

Summary of Background Data.—Dysphagia is increasingly recognized as a potential complication of anterior surgical approaches to the cervical spine. Retraction pressure on the esophagus that alters blood flow, edema of the pharynx, and laryngeal nerve injury are among factors implicated. There has been little investigation of the biomechanics of swallowing in a large cohort of patients reporting postoperative dysphagia.

Methods.—The fluoroscopic swallow studies of all persons reporting dysphagia after anterior c-spine surgery between January 1, 2000, and December 31, 2008, were retrospectively reviewed. The dysphagic cohort was divided into early (<2 months postsurgery) and late (>2 months) groups. Aspiration and completeness of epiglottic inversion were noted. Objective measures of pharyngeal wall thickness, upper esophageal sphincter opening, hyoid displacement, pharyngeal constriction, and pharyngeal transit time were abstracted and compared to the same parameters in age and sex-matched normal control subjects. Analysis of variance was used for statistical comparison of objective measures across groups.

Results.—Sixty-seven patients were identified. Significant differences were identified between control subjects and both patient groups, as well as between the 2 patient groups, for most objective measures considered. Instances of aspiration were identified in 50% of patients in the early post-operative group, reduced to 18% in the later group. Significantly increased pharyngeal wall thickness and poor epiglottic inversion were characteristic of both c-spine groups.

Conclusion.—Significant alterations in swallowing mechanics can accompany c-spine surgery with anterior plating. A number of these changes improve over time, leaving patients with relatively minor impairment;

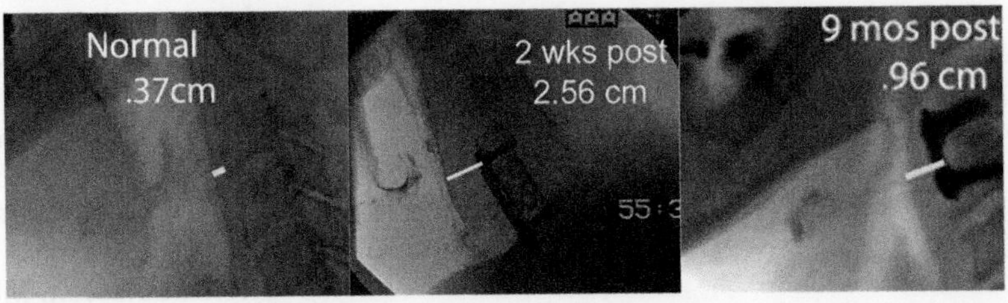

FIGURE 6.—Examples of pharyngeal wall thickness (PPWthk) measured posterior to the epiglottis. Examples represent normal subject, and patients from early and later postoperative groups. (Reprinted from Leonard R, Belafsky P, Dysphagia following cervical spine surgery with anterior instrumentation: evidence from fluoroscopic swallow studies. *Spine*. 2011;36:2217-2223, with permission from Lippincott Williams & Wilkins.)

however, some appear to be long-lasting. Education and dysphagia therapy can be useful treatment adjuncts (Fig 6).

▶ The authors, both otorhinolaryngologists from the Department of Otolaryngology/HNS, University of California–Davis, have reported on another disappointing complication of spinal surgery, specifically dysphagia after anterior cervical spine surgery. Although the study does not describe an incidence for this complication, it does provide some very interesting objective swallowing study data from patients with postoperative swallowing complaints versus an asymptomatic comparison control group. The most striking and impressive portions of the article are the images demonstrating changes of esophageal thickening, both acutely and chronically, after surgery (Fig 6). Postoperative dysphagia is most certainly underreported, as is retrograde ejaculation after anterior lumbar spine surgery, and with the resultant chronic difficulties and disability possible, physicians should regularly ask their patients if they experience this complication. Practitioners whose practice includes a large portion of anterior cervical surgery should consider the authors' experience and recommendations for evaluation of postoperative dysphagia and incorporate a suitable protocol to address any issues discovered.

P. Huddleston, MD

Did the Lenke Classification Change Scoliosis Treatment?

Clements DH, Harms Study Group (Shriners' Hosp for Children, Philadelphia, PA; et al)
Spine 36:1142-1145, 2011

Study Design.—A retrospective review of data prospectively entered into a multicenter database.

Objective.—To evaluate the adherence to classification-specific surgical treatment recommendations for adolescent idiopathic scoliosis (AIS) before and after the Lenke classification system introduction in 2001.

Summary of Background Data.—The Lenke classification system of AIS was developed in 2001 to provide a comprehensive and reliable means to categorize and guide treatment. The treatment recommendations of the system state that major and structural minor curves are included in the instrumentation and fusion and the nonstructural minor curves are excluded.

Methods.—Surgical AIS cases for each Lenke classification (curve types 1–6) were queried for "Rule-breakers," in which the treatment performed *did not* follow the recommendations of the Lenke classification system. Each "Rule-breaker" case was individually evaluated to ensure correct Lenke classification and radiographic image verification was performed. "Rule-breaker" patients were expressed as a percentage of the total number of patients for each curve type. The presence of "Rule-breakers" before and after the introduction of the Lenke classification system in 2001 was evaluated for statistical difference using a chi-square analysis.

Results.—The data for 1310 AIS patients who underwent surgical correction for their deformity were included in this analysis. Overall, treatment of 191 patients did not follow the classification recommendations; the rules are broken 15% of the time. The proportion of "Rule-breakers" (18%) was significantly greater prior to the introduction of the Lenke classification system than it was after (12%) ($P = 0.001$).

Conclusion.—The introduction of this system has led to a reduction in the variation of treatment approaches; however, our data suggest that 6%

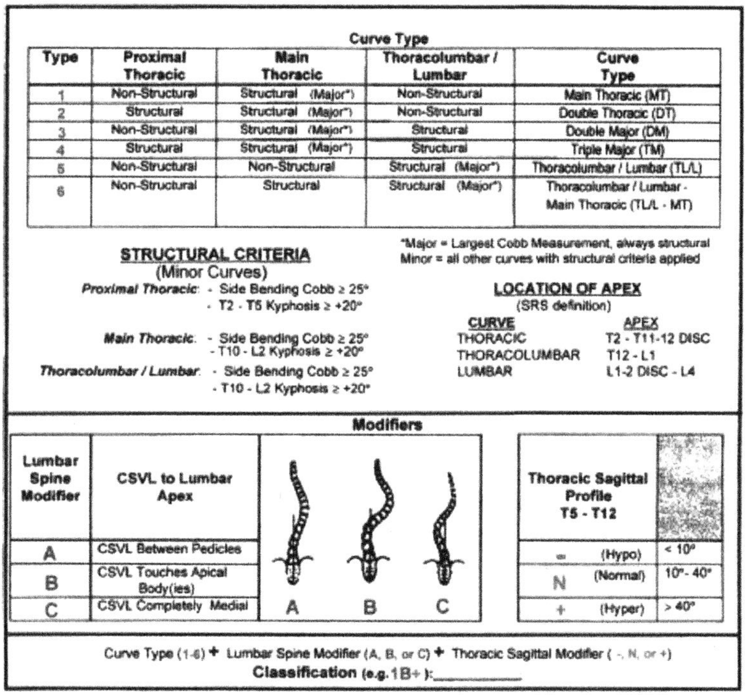

FIGURE 1.—Lenke classification: synopsis of all necessary criteria for curve classification. (Reprinted from Clements DH, Harms Study Group. Did the Lenke classification change scoliosis treatment? *Spine.* 2011;36:1142-1145, with permission from Lippincott Williams & Wilkins.)

to 29% of the time, depending on the curve pattern, there are other aspects of the clinical and radiographic deformity that suggest deviation from the recommendations of the classification system. The outcome of adherence to this system remains yet to be evaluated (Fig 1).

▶ When I was completing my spine surgery fellowship at the turn of the century, I can tell you confidently that I believed the last thing orthopedics or spine surgery needed was another classification system (Fig 1). Wasn't the AO trauma system proof that detailed orthopedic classification could be very useful from a research standpoint but yet fall down when used by clinicians to guide clinical care? How could you use something that nobody could remember because of the complexity? Didn't Drs. King and Moe get it right the first time? While many freely acknowledged the importance of sagittal balance and the need to fuse structural curves and not fuse flexible nonstructural curves, I had many questions about the Scoliosis Research Society (SRS) Lenke classification then and continue to do so. The good news is that over the past 10 years or so, the Lenke classification system has shown wide adoption and use and appears to additionally provide clinical value in guiding surgeons with a surgical recommendation and strategy. It has been shown in peer-reviewed studies to be reliable and reproducible and clearly addresses the deficiencies inherent in the King/Moe classification toward lumbar curves, sagittal balance, and lower reproducibility. The question remains, however, if the system will improve scoliosis surgical care over the long-term and whether issues regarding the definition of the curves themselves (structural vs nonstructural) can be resolved. An unanswered question is how to capture, in the authors' words, the fact that in a select group of power-users, "6% to 29% of the time, there are other aspects of the clinical and radiographic deformity that suggest deviation from the recommendations of the Lenke classification system."

P. Huddleston, MD

Artificial Cervical Disc Arthroplasty: A Systematic Review

Cepoiu-Martin M, Faris P, Lorenzetti D, et al (Univ of Calgary, Alberta, Canada)
Spine 36:E1623-E1633, 2011

Study Design.—Systematic Review.

Objective.—(1) To qualitatively analyze the literature on the efficacy and effectiveness of artificial cervical disc arthroplasty (ACDA). (2) To highlight methodological and reporting issues of randomized controlled trials (RCT) reports on effectiveness of ACDA compared to cervical fusion.

Summary of Background Data.—ACDA is an alternate surgical procedure that may replace cervical fusion in selected patients suffering from cervical degenerative disc disease.

Methods.—We searched seven electronic databases, including MEDLINE, Cochrane Library, and EMBASE, unpublished sources, and reference lists for studies on the efficacy and effectiveness of ACDA compared to cervical fusion—the surgical standard of care for patients with cervical degenerative disc disease.

Results.—A total of 622 studies were retrieved, of which 18 (13 case series, four RCT reports, one nonrandomized comparative study) met the inclusion criteria for this review. The four RCTs and the nonrandomized comparative study concluded that the effectiveness of ACDA is not inferior to that of cervical fusion in the short term (up to 2-yr follow-up). The safety profile of both procedures appears similar. The case series reviewed noted improved clinical outcomes at 1 or 2 years after one or multiple-level ACDA.

Conclusion.—ACDA is a surgical procedure that may replace cervical fusion in selected patients suffering from cervical degenerative disc disease. Within 2 years of follow-up, the effectiveness of ACDA appears similar to that of cervical fusion. Weak evidence exists that ACDA may be superior to fusion for treating neck and arm pain. Future studies should report change scores and change score variance in accordance with RCT guidelines, in order to strengthen credibility of conclusions and to facilitate meta-analyses of studies (Table 4).

► The authors from the Department of Community Health Sciences, University of Calgary, Alberta, Canada have published an excellent systemic review of the use and outcomes of artificial cervical disc arthroplasty (ACDA) that supports the conclusion that the procedure is not inferior to anterior discectomy and fusion (ACDF) at outcomes of 2 years. The study also reveals the scarcity of stringent studies on this topic and suggests longer follow-up is needed. In my spine practice I have seen continued excitement and interest by patients and clinicians with this procedure and its larger relative, artificial lumbar disc arthroplasty. Only the

TABLE 4.—Summary of the Methodological Quality Assessment of the RCT Reports (Cochrane Musculoskeletal Injuries Group)

	Mummaneni et al 2007[6]	Murrey et al 2009[27]	Nabhan et al 2007[28]	Sasso et al 2007[29]
Concealment	2	2	2	2
ITT analysis	0	0	1	0
Blinding of assessors	0	0	0	0
Baseline	2	2	0	2
Blinding of patients	0	0	2	0
Blinding of treatment provider	0	0	0	0
Care programs	2	2	0	2
Inclusionexclusion criteria	2	2	2	2
Intervention	2	2	2	2
Outcomes	2	2	2	2
Diagnostic test	2	2	2	2
Follow-up	2	2	2	2
TOTAL	16	16	15	16

Cochrane Musculoskeletal Injuries Group Methodological Assessment Tool includes aspects of internal and external validity of RCTs. Individual scores for each item are assigned (2, 1, or 0), and a total score is optional and may be obtained by summing the scores of individual items. The scores for the last three items used in the total score are those for the primary measure of the systematic review. In cases where the items remain unknown, all items are designated the lowest score except for allocation concealment where the middle score is given. The higher the total score, the higher quality of the RCT is. The maximum possible total score is 24.

Editor's Note: Please refer to original journal article for full references.

truly jaded would say that this procedure is only gliding down the gilded path of similar past spine technological "advances," such as stand-alone cylindrical interbody cages. The well-known parabolic curve of excitement travels upward with the new technology until the inevitable accumulation of patient follow-up either sustains the arc or, more commonly, leads to its predictable decline. Dissatisfaction with the latest new toy will not always be related to a suboptimal clinical result but can be associated with a prohibitive cost, poor logistics in obtaining the device, or something as granular as poor handling characteristics in vivo. On the topic of ACDA, the authors suggest, and I agree, that the perfunctory 2-year follow-up that is culturally required to satisfy the Food and Drug Agency and editors for peer-reviewed journals may be wholly inadequate to determine the 2 most important questions concerning potential benefits of the devices: How long will it last, and will the Holy Grail of arthroplasty benefits actually come to fruition? That is, will continued motion at the operated level alter the natural history of the adjacent unoperated spine? As a specialty, I believe we should be cautious before abandoning ACDF for ADCA, as nothing ruins good results like follow-up, and none of the randomized, controlled trials (RCTs) to date have definitively proven that ACDA is more effective or superior to an ACDF. Lastly, the quality of future RCTs will need to improve as the authors identified several basic methodologic flaws in each of the 4 RCTs that had been performed to evaluate ACDA (Table 4).

P. Huddleston, MD

Growing Rods for Scoliosis in Spinal Muscular Atrophy: Structural Effects, Complications, and Hospital Stays

McElroy MJ, Shaner AC, Crawford TO, et al (Johns Hopkins Med Institutions, Baltimore, MD; et al)
Spine 36:1305-1311, 2011

Study Design.—Retrospective analysis of patients with spinal muscular atrophy (SMA) treated with growing rod (GR) instrumentation for scoliosis.

Objective.—To evaluate structural effectiveness, complications, and length of hospital stay associated with GRs for scoliosis in SMA and to compare values with those of infantile and juvenile idiopathic scoliosis (IIS/JIS).

Summary of Background Data.—Most studies evaluate GR effectiveness in all patients. We specifically examined SMA and IIS/JIS.

Methods.—We searched a multicenter database and found 15 patients with SMA and scoliosis treated with GRs for 54 ± 33 months. Radiographic measurements, complications, and hospital stay durations were compared with those of 80 GR patients with IIS/JIS observed for 43 ± 31 months. Measures of rib collapse, including T6: T10 mean rib-vertebral angle and T6: T12 thoracic width, were compared. Student t test was used to compare SMA and IIS/JIS values (significance level, $P = 0.05$).

Results.—Primary radiographic measurements in patients with SMA improved from preoperative to latest follow-up as follows: curve,

89° ± 19° to 55° ± 17°; pelvic obliquity, 31° ± 14° to 11° ± 10°; space-available-for-lung ratio, 0.86 ± 0.15 to 0.94 ± 0.21; and T1–S1 length grew 8.7 ± 3.2 cm. Rib collapse continued despite GR treatment in SMA but not in IIS/JIS. Hospital stays were longer for SMA than for IIS/JIS for lengthening procedures ($P = 0.01$) and trended to be longer for initial surgery ($P = 0.08$) and final fusion ($P = 0.06$). Patients with SMA and IIS/JIS experienced, respectively, 0.5 and 1.1 major complications per patient ($P = 0.02$).

Conclusion.—GRs improve trunk height and the space-available-for-lung ratio while controlling curve and pelvic obliquity in young patients with SMA with severe scoliosis, but they do not halt rib collapse. For patients with SMA, hospital stays were longer than those for patients with IIS/JIS, whereas the rate of major complications was lower.

▶ Patients with spinal muscular atrophy (SMA) are a particular challenge for any spine surgeon to manage. Although there are many tools to help address their care, 3 main challenges remain: progression of scoliosis, compensating for moderate to severe muscle weakness, and management of complications related to surgical treatment. The authors of this multicenter study have put together a well-done, case-control study that also serves as an insightful review on the characteristics of patients with the condition of SMA and the patients' expected hospital course after surgery and latest outcomes with growing rod (GR) surgery. I was surprised that the SMA patients had statistically fewer major inpatient complications than a matched cohort of infantile and juvenile idiopathic scoliosis patients but believe their increased length of stay compared to controls is consistent with their baseline weakness and resultant vulnerability. At the very minimum, having a safe alternative to ineffectual bracing or spinal fusion with possible resultant "crankshaft" phenomenon is attractive. With the surprisingly good outlook for patients with SMA being treated with GRs, it once again brings to the fore the lengthy, flawed, and frustrating regulations put in place by the Food and Drug Administration to develop, study, and distribute new technology for children. We can only hope that studies on GRs and other devices for children will provide focus on this flawed process and help facilitate, not deter, future technological breakthroughs and treatments for children with difficult to manage clinical diseases or injuries.

P. Huddleston, MD

Facet Violation With the Placement of Percutaneous Pedicle Screws

Patel RD, Graziano GP, Vanderhave KL, et al (Univ of Michigan, Ann Arbor; et al)

Spine 36:E1749-E1752, 2011

Study Design.—Independent review and classification of therapeutic procedures performed on cadavers by surgeons blinded to purpose of study.

Objective.—The objective of this study is to determine the rate of facet violation with the placement of percutaneous pedicle screws.

Summary of Background Data.—Improvements in percutaneous instrumentation and fluoroscopic imaging have led to a resurgence of percutaneous pedicle screw insertion in lumbar spine surgery in an attempt to minimize many of the complications associated with open techniques of pedicle screw placement. Rates of pedicle breech and neurologic injury resulting from percutaneous insertion are reportedly similar to those of open techniques. Postoperative pain because of impingement and instability is believed to result from violation of the facet capsule or facet joint. To the authors' knowledge, however, the rate of facet injury associated with the placement of percutaneous pedicle screws is unreported in the literature.

Methods.—Percutaneous pedicle screw placement was performed on 4 cadaveric specimens by 4 certified orthopedic surgeons who had clinical experience in the procedure and who were blinded to the study's purpose. The surgeons were instructed to place pedicle screws from L1–S1 using their preferred clinical techniques and a 5.5-mm screw system with which they were all familiar. All surgeons utilized 1 OEC C-arm for fluoroscopic imaging. After insertion, 2 independent spine surgeons each reviewed and classified the placement of all facet screws.

Results.—A total of 48 screws were inserted and classified. The placement of 28 screws (58%) resulted in violation of facet articulation, with 8 of these screws being intra-articular. Interobserver reliability of the classification system was 100%.

Conclusion.—Percutaneous pedicle screw placement may result in a high rate of facet violation. Facet injury can be reliability classified and therefore, perhaps, easily prevented.

▶ One of the challenges when adopting any new technique is proving to yourself it is at least not inferior to the old technique. The authors of this cadaver study address this very challenge by confronting one of the "dirty little secrets" of minimal access spine surgery—accurate placement of the implants. One of the most common reasons I will see a patient in consultation for continuing pain after a minimal access surgery is for symptoms or signs of implant misplacement or impingement at the cranial or caudal end of the implant construct. This research publication, performed at the University of Michigan–Ann Arbor, demonstrates this very point by identifying a 58% facet violation with fluoroscopy-guided, percutaneous-placed lumbosacral implants. A full 16% of the screws placed by board-certified, experienced spine surgeons familiar with the percutaneous technique were identified to be intra-articular by postplacement anatomic dissection. I applaud the authors' recognition of a significant risk with minimal access surgery and encourage other surgeons to adjust their techniques to accommodate facet morphology, especially when instrumenting the upper lumbar vertebra.

P. Huddleston, MD

Intraoperative Waste in Spine Surgery: Incidence, Cost, and Effectiveness of an Educational Program

Soroceanu A, Canacari E, Brown E, et al (Dalhousie Univ, Halifax (NS), Canada; Beth Israel Deaconess Med Ctr, Boston, MA)

Spine 36:E1270-E1273, 2011

Study Design.—Prospective observational study.

Objective.—This study aims to quantify the incidence of intraoperative waste in spine surgery and to examine the efficacy of an educational program directed at surgeons to induce a reduction in the intraoperative waste.

Summary of Background Data.—Spine procedures are associated with high costs. Implants are a main contributor of these costs. Intraoperative waste further exacerbates the high cost of surgery.

Methods.—Data were collected during a 25-month period from one academic medical center (15-month observational period, 10-month post–awareness program). The total number of spine procedures and the incidence of intraoperative waste were recorded prospectively. Other variables recorded included the type of product wasted, cost associated with the product or implant wasted, and reason for the waste.

Results.—Intraoperative waste occurred in 20.2% of the procedures prior to the educational program and in 10.3% of the procedures after the implementation of the program ($P < 0.0001$). Monthly costs associated with surgical waste were, on average, $17680 prior to the awareness intervention and $5876 afterwards ($P = 0.0006$). Prior to the intervention, surgical waste represented 4.3% of total operative spine budget. After the awareness program this proportion decrease to an average of 1.2% ($P = 0.003$).

Conclusion.—Intraoperative waste in spine surgery exacerbates the already costly procedures. Extrapolation of this data to the national level leads to an annual estimate of $126,722,000 attributable to intraoperative spine waste. A simple educational program proved to be and continues to be effective in making surgeons aware of the import of their choices and the costs related to surgical waste (Fig 2).

▶ This wonderful article from Dr Soroceanu and colleagues is a demonstration on what a large dose of awareness and a small bit of education can have on reducing operative waste in spine surgery. Medical costs are increasing and payment cuts are being implemented almost across the board for the surgical specialties, especially in government-funded patients. As referenced by the authors, Medicare spending for inpatient back surgery more than doubled over the last decade, as the spending for lumbar fusion increased more than 500%.[1] This, coupled with an avalanche of migrations from private practice into large single and multispecialty groups by orthopedic surgeons[2] in the coming years, will bring cost awareness into the forefront of clinicians and surgeons minds and practices. When the surgeon was functioning as a private contractor to the hospital, with surgical privileges and admitting costs, the hospital bore the brunt of the expenses performed

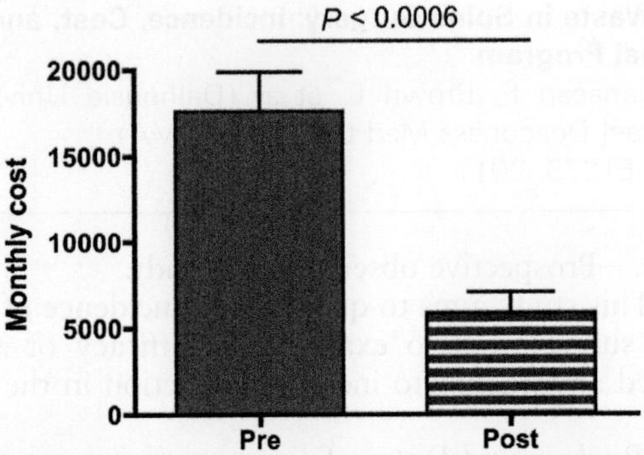

FIGURE 2.—The difference in mean monthly cost related to waste before and after the awareness program. (Reprinted from Soroceanu A, Canacari E, Brown E, et al. Intraoperative waste in spine surgery: incidence, cost, and effectiveness of an educational program. *Spine*. 2011;36:E1270-E1273, with permission from Lippincott Williams & Wilkins.)

in surgery. For example, if a surgeon wished to use the most expensive spinal implants and off-label or physician-directed use of Infuse without clinical data to support it, this was often allowed. Unless the hospital administrator approached the surgeon about the financial losses the hospital was taking on the nonreimbursed implants and biologics on their Medicare patients, the surgeon was immune to the cost of medicine, as they still received their surgeon's fee for performing the procedure. Now, if the surgeon works as an employee of the hospital, the "tables turn," and the effects of cost and waste related to the surgeon's style of practice directly affect their employer and indirectly themselves. The authors from Boston Massachusetts and Halifax, Canada will describe to the readers a simple yet very effective program that could potentially reduce equipment in the operating room related to spine surgery. Most interesting was the finding that the education program proposed by the authors also decreased the frequency of how often the surgeons themselves consciously chose to waste an implant from 42.20% to 24.10%.

This change was also statistically significant ($P < .0001$).

P. Huddleston, MD

References

1. Weinstein JN, Lurie JD, Olson PR, Bronner KK, Fisher ES. United States' trends and regional variations in lumbar spine surgery: 1992-2003. *Spine*. 2006;31:2707-2714.
2. Kocher R, Sahni NR. Hospitals' race to employ physicians—the logic behind a money-losing proposition. *N Engl J Med*. 2011;364:1790-1793.

On total disc replacement

Berg S (Löwenströmska Hosp, Upplands Väsby, Sweden)

Acta Orthop Suppl 82:1-29, 2011

Low back pain consumes a large part of the community's resources dedicated to health care and sick leave. Back disorders also negatively affect the individual leading to pain suffering, decreased quality-of-life and disability. Chronic low back pain (CLBP) due to degenerative disc disease (DDD) is today often treated with fusion when conservative treatment has failed and symptoms are severe. This treatment is as successful as arthroplasty is for hip arthritis in restoring the patient's quality of life and reducing disability. Even so, there are some problems with this treatment, one of these being recurrent CLBP from an adjacent segment (ASD) after primarily successful surgery. This has led to the development of alternative surgical treatments and devices that maintain or restore mobility, in order to reduce the risk for ASD. Of these new devices, the most frequently used are the disc prostheses used in Total Disc Replacement (TDR).

This thesis is based on four studies comparing total disc replacement with posterior fusion. The studies are all based on a material of 152 patients with DDD in one or two segments, aged 20-55 years that were randomly treated with either posterior fusion or TDR.

The first study concerned clinical outcome and complications. Follow-up was 100% at both one and two years. It revealed that both treatment groups had a clear benefit from treatment and that patients with TDR were better in almost all outcome scores at one-year follow-up. Fusion patients continued to improve during the second year. At two-year follow-up there was a remaining difference in favour of TDR for back pain. 73% in the TDR group and 63% in the fusion group were much better or totally pain-free (n.s.), while twice as many patients in the TDR group were totally pain free (30%) compared to the fusion group (15%).

Time of surgery and total time in hospital were shorter in the TDR group.

There was no difference in complications and reoperations, except that seventeen of the patients in the fusion group were re-operated for removal of their implants.

The second study concerned sex life and sexual function. TDR is performed via an anterior approach, an approach that has been used for a long time for various procedures on the lumbar spine. A frequent complication reported in males when this approach is used is persistent retrograde ejaculation. The TDR group in this material was operated via an extraperitoneal approach to the retroperitoneal space, and there were no cases of persistent retrograde ejaculation. There was a surprisingly high frequency of men in the fusion group reporting deterioration in ability to have an orgasm postoperatively. Preoperative sex life was severely hampered in the majority of patients in the entire material, but sex life underwent a marked improvement in both treatment groups by the two-year follow-up that correlated with reduction in back pain.

The third study was on mobility in the lumbar spinal segments, where X-rays were taken in full extension and flexion prior to surgery and at two-year follow-up. Analysis of the films showed that 78% of the patients in the fusion group reached the surgical goal (non-mobility) and that 89% of the TDR patients maintained mobility.

Preoperative disc height was lower than in a normative database in both groups, and remained lower in the fusion group, while it became higher in the TDR group. Mobility in the operated segment increased in the TDR group postoperatively. Mobility at the rest of the lumbar spine increased in both treatment groups. Mobility in adjacent segments was within the norm postoperatively, but slightly larger in the fusion group.

In the fourth study the health economics of TDR vs Fusion was analysed. The hospital costs for the procedure were higher for patients in the fusion group compared to the TDR group, and the TDR patients were on sick-leave two months less.

In all, these studies showed that the results in the TDR group were as good as in the fusion group. Patients are more likely to be totally pain-free when treated with TDR compared to fusion. Treatment with this new procedure seems justified in selected patients at least in the short-term perspective. Long-term follow-up is underway and results will be published in due course.

▶ This article is a comprehensive study of patients seen and treated for chronic low back pain within the Swedish health system. Written in a thesis format, it is a nice complement to the many short-form publications available on this topic to date. It is worth reading as a primary source for the thorough nature of the research, its 100% clinical follow-up, its novel reporting of sexual function both before and after lumbar fusion, and its analysis of the EQ-5D to report cost-effectiveness. I was surprised to note the author's discovery of a preoperative incidence of retrograde ejaculation almost equal to postoperative incidence. Reported sexual satisfaction was increased in both fusion and total disc replacement (TDR) groups inversely to their reduction in pain scores. The author's conclusions are sound in that I believe that TDR can be a beneficial treatment for patients with "definable" discogenic chronic low back pain, but then "therein lies the rub!"

P. Huddleston, MD

Patients' Perspective on Full Disclosure and Informed Consent Regarding Postoperative Visual Loss Associated With Spinal Surgery in the Prone Position

Corda DM, Dexter F, Pasternak JJ, et al (Mayo Clinic, Jacksonville, FL; Univ of Iowa, Iowa City; Mayo Clinic, Rochester, MN; et al)
Mayo Clin Proc 86:865-868, 2011

Objective.—To determine patients' opinions regarding the person, method, and timing for disclosure of postoperative visual loss (POVL) associated with high-risk surgery.

Patients and Methods.—On the basis of findings of a pilot study involving 219 patients at Mayo Clinic in Florida, we hypothesized that at least 80% of patients would prefer disclosure of POVL by the surgeon, during a face-to-face discussion, before the day of scheduled surgery. To test the hypothesis, we sent a questionnaire to 437 patients who underwent prolonged prone spinal surgical procedures at Mayo Clinic in Rochester, MN, or Mayo Clinic in Arizona from December 1, 2008, to December 31, 2009.

Results.—Among the 184 respondents, 158 patients gave responses supporting the hypothesis vs 26 with at least 1 response not supporting it, for an observed incidence of 86%. The 2-sided 95% confidence interval is 80% to 91%.

Conclusion.—At least 80% of patients prefer full disclosure of the risk of POVL, by the surgeon, during a face-to-face discussion before the day of scheduled surgery. This finding supports development of a national patient-driven guideline for disclosing the risk of POVL before prone spinal surgery.

▶ Although not a lethal event, there may be no more devastating complication for the patient than to suffer permanent postoperative visual loss (POVL) in the perioperative period. The result is final, tragic, and leaves a sense of grief and loss in the survivors. Paralysis, another uncommon but dreadfully feared complication, may lead to great disability but can be accommodated with training and adaptive devices, and survivors can still lead meaningful lives. It is the unfortunate patients who suffer the unexpected but permanent POVL from ischemic optic neuropathy. This infrequent but controversial complication can occur in prone as well as supine patients and has been most commonly reported in coronary bypass surgery prior to the explosion of complex spine surgery. With such an infrequent occurrence, determining etiology has been difficult and may well prove impossible, so efforts about disclosure have gained prominence. Regardless how the surgeon, team, or institution chooses to characterize the visual loss, the more important point is to disclose it. In my practice, I have never once had a single patient who refused spine surgery after hearing about POVL; the most the surgeon can expect is a lengthy discussion about how much the profession does not know about the etiology. A standard protocol of disclosure is most effective, and in my experience, I see no downside to having the message repeated by numerous caregivers such as the surgeon and the anesthesiologist. Because there is no effective treatment for the problem once it occurs, the professional, medical-legal, and moral imperative is that the patient be fully advised of all the risks that a reasonable person would wish to know and that they might personally find important. These can be difficult conversations, and I agree with the authors that they should ideally be discussed on at least one other day than that of the surgical procedure to maximize understanding and minimize stress.

P. Huddleston, MD

Risk Factors for Surgical Site Infections Following Spinal Fusion Procedures: A Case-Control Study

Rao SB, Vasquez G, Harrop J, et al (Thomas Jefferson Univ, Philadelphia, PA)
Clin Infect Dis 53:686-692, 2011

Background.—Spinal fusion procedures are associated with a significant rate of surgical site infection (SSI) (1%–12%). The goal of this study was to identify modifiable risk factors for spinal fusion SSIs at a large tertiary care center.

Methods.—A retrospective, case-control (1:3 ratio) analysis of SSIs following posterior spine fusion procedures was performed over a 1-year period. Clinical and surgical data were collected through electronic database and chart review. Variables were evaluated by univariate analysis and multivariable logistic regression.

Results.—In total, 57 deep SSIs were identified out of 1587 procedures (3.6%). Infections were diagnosed a mean of 13.5 ± 8 days postprocedure. *Staphylococcus aureus* was the predominant pathogen (63%); 1/3 of these isolates were methicillin resistant. Significant patient risk factors for infection by univariate analysis included ASA score >2 and male gender. Among surgical variables, infected cases had significantly higher proportions of staged procedures and thoracic level surgeries and had a greater number of vertebrae fused. Notably, infected fusion procedures had a longer duration of closed suction drains than controls (5.1 ± 2 days vs 3.4 ± 1 day, respectively; $P < .001$). Drain duration (unit odds ratio [OR], 1.6 per day drain present; 95% confidence interval [CI], 1.3–1.9), body mass index (OR, 1.1; 95% CI, 1.0–1.1), and male gender (OR, 2.7; 95% CI, 1.4–5.6) were significant risk factors in the multivariate analysis.

Conclusions.—Prolonged duration of closed suction drains is a strong independent risk factor for SSI following instrumented spinal fusion procedures. Therefore, removing drains as early as possible may lower infection rates.

▶ This article describes the extended use of closed suction drains as a strongly significant independent risk factor ($P < .001$) for surgical site infection (SSI). Previous studies in spine surgery have questioned the effectiveness of drains at all in routine postoperative wound care.[1] In clinical practice, it is common for clinicians to leave the suction drain in place until the drainage falls below some historically significant level. This level can vary from practice to practice, but the constant is that if the wound drainage continues to be above the level of comfort, the surgeon will leave it in. It is likely that within this study some of the patients who had developed a postoperative wound infection initially manifest this as an increased wound drainage and that the infection was therefore an "inside-out" infection and not "outside-in." I personally routinely use postoperative suction drains unless I encounter a dural leak that cannot be repaired watertight, in the case of an operation to address a known infection, or to manage large dead space issues relating to oncology surgery. Eliminating the drain eliminates the risk of accidentally sewing it into the wound and having it retained and the question of an outside-in drain-related infection. This article supports eliminating the closed suction drain as soon as possible and the need to study this clinical question in a prospective randomized fashion.

P. Huddleston, MD

Reference

1. Brown MD, Brookfield KF. A randomized study of closed wound suction drainage for extensive lumbar spine surgery. *Spine (Phila Pa 1976)*. 2004;29:1066-1068.

Fusion *Versus* Nonoperative Management for Chronic Low Back Pain: Do Comorbid Diseases or General Health Factors Affect Outcome?

Choma TJ, Schuster JM, Norvell DC, et al (Univ of Missouri, Columbia; Univ of Pennsylvania, Philadelphia; Spectrum Res, Inc, Tacoma, WA; et al)
Spine 36:S87-S95, 2011

Study Design.—Systematic review of literature focused on heterogeneity of treatment effect analysis.

Objective.—The objectives of this systematic review were to determine if comorbid disease and general health factors modify the effect of fusion *versus* nonoperative management in chronic low back pain (CLBP) patients?

Summary of Background Data.—Surgical fusion as a treatment of back pain continues to be controversial due to inconsistent responses to treatment. The reasons for this are multifactorial but may include heterogeneity in the patient population and in surgeon's attitudes and approaches to this complex problem. There is a relative paucity of high quality publications from which to draw conclusions. We were interested in investigating the possibility of detecting treatment response differences comparing fusion to conservative management for CLBP among subpopulations with different disease specific and general health risk factors.

Methods.—A systematic search was conducted in MEDLINE and the Cochrane Collaboration Library for literature published from 1990 through December 2010. To evaluate whether the effects of CLBP treatment varied by disease or general health subgroups, we sought randomized controlled trials or nonrandomized observational studies with concurrent controls evaluating surgical fusion *versus* nonoperative management for CLBP. Of the original 127 citations identified, only 5 reported treatment effects (fusion *vs.* conservative management) separately by disease and general health subgroups of interest. Of those, only two focused on patients who had primarily back pain without spinal stenosis or spondylolisthesis.

Results.—Few studies comparing fusion to nonoperative management reported differences in outcome by specific disease or general health subpopulations. Among those that did, we observed the effect of fusion compared to nonoperative management was slightly more favorable in patients with no additional comorbidities compared with those with additional comorbidities and more marked in nonsmokers compared with smokers.

Conclusion.—It is unclear from the literature which patients are the best candidates for fusion *versus* conservative management when experiencing CLBP without significant neurological impairment. Nonsmokers may be more likely to have a favorable surgical fusion outcome in CLBP patients. Comorbid disease presence has not been shown to definitively modify the effect of fusion. Further prospective studies that are designed to evaluate these and other subgroup effects are encouraged to confirm these findings.

Clinical Recommendations.—We recommend optimizing the management of medical co-morbidities and smoking cessation before considering surgical fusion in CLBP patients. Strength of recommendation: Weak.

▶ This impressive literature review from the University of Missouri suggests that there are large gaps in the literature prospectively analyzing the outcomes of lumbar fusion for chronic low back pain (CLBP). This is not surprising, but what readers may find interesting is that in their analysis, the presence of medical morbidities was only weakly associated with decreased outcome in patients undergoing fusion for CLBP without significant neurologic impairment. Smoking was more strongly associated, but not conclusively. Will this change our preoperative counseling for patients prior to surgery? Probably not, as I believe that as a physician and not just a surgeon, there are plenty of other great reasons to counsel your patients to discontinue smoking and lose weight while participating in meaningful exercise, such as preventing cardiovascular disease and reducing the risk of adult onset diabetes and cancer. But it is curious that many surgeons will refuse to perform the most elementary of spinal surgeries on patients if they are still smoking. Numerous reports exist describing comparable outcomes for smokers and nonsmokers, even with complex spine surgery.[1] That seems to be a very strong statement based on such weak evidence. Other interesting research questions would help define whether the use of nicotine gum or patches definitively hinders both spinal fusion and outcomes after spinal fusion surgery.

P. Huddleston, MD

Reference

1. Bertagnoli R, Yue JJ, Kershaw T, et al. Lumbar total disc arthroplasty utilizing the ProDisc prosthesis in smokers versus nonsmokers: a prospective study with 2-year minimum follow-up. *Spine (Phila Pa 1976)*. 2006;31:992-997.

Clinical Guidelines and Payer Policies on Fusion for the Treatment of Chronic Low Back Pain

Cheng JS, Lee MJ, Massicotte E, et al (Vanderbilt Univ Med Ctr, Nashville, TN; Univ of Washington Med Ctr, Seattle; Univ of Toronto, Ontario, Canada; et al)
Spine 36:S144-S163, 2011

Study Design.—Systematic review.

Objective.—The purpose of this review is to provide a critical appraisal of general and fusion–specific clinical practice guidelines on the treatment of chronic nonradicular low back pain and compare the quality and evidence base of fusion guidelines and select payer policies.

Summary of Background Data.—The treatment of lumbar spondylosis associated with low back pain with lumbar arthrodesis, or fusion, has risen fourfold in the past two decades. Given the significant associated health care costs, there is an increase in clinical guidelines and payer policies influencing patient treatment options. Assessment of the medical necessity of a treatment, such as lumbar fusions, based on medical literature will frequently supersede the determination of the physician in the care of their patient. Concerns regarding the effectiveness and costs of the surgical treatment of spinal disorders presenting with low back pain has placed enormous scrutiny on the value of surgical treatments to our patients. As both clinical guidelines and payer policies have a major impact on the perceived effectiveness, or medical necessity, of lumbar fusions for the treatment of chronic nonradicular low back pain, a review of this topic was undertaken.

Methods.—An electronic literature search of PubMed, the National Guideline Clearinghouse and the International Network of Agencies for Health Technology Assessment was performed to identify clinical practice guidelines on assessment and treatment of chronic nonradicular low back pain, including those on use of lumbar fusion, as well as relevant technology assessments. A Google search for publicly available private and public payer policies related to fusion was also performed. A hand search was used to identify specific studies cited for support of the recommendations made. A modified Appraisal of Guidelines Research and Evaluation instrument was used to provide a standardized assessment method for evaluating the quality of development of the evidence base and recommendations in guidelines and selected health policies. This was combined with appraisal of the evidence base supporting the recommendations.

Results.—Three systematic reviews of general guidelines from a PubMed search yielding 94 citations were included. A convenience sample of five guidelines with recommendations on fusion was taken from 182 citations identified by the National Guideline Clearinghouse and the International Network of Agencies for Health Technology Assessment searches. Two guidelines were developed by US professional societies, (neurosurgery and pain management), and three were European-based guidelines (Belgium, United Kingdom, and the European Cooperation in Science and Technology). The general guidelines were consistent with their recommendations for diagnosis, but inconsistent regarding recommendations for treatment. All guidelines and payer policies with recommendations on fusion included some set of the primary randomized controlled trials comparing fusion to other treatment options with the exception of one policy. However, no clear pattern with regard to the quality of development was identified based on the modified Appraisal of Guidelines Research and Evaluation tool. There were differences in specialty society recommendations.

Conclusion.—Three systematic reviews of evidence-based guidelines that provide general guidance for the assessment and treatment of chronic low back pain described consistent recommendations and guidance for the evaluation of chronic low back pain but inconsistent recommendations and guidance for treatment. Five evidence-based guidelines with recommendations on the use of fusion for the treatment of chronic low back pain were evaluated. There is some consistency across guidelines and policies that are government sponsored with regard to development process and critical evaluation of index studies as well as overall recommendations. There were differences in specialty society recommendations. There is heterogeneity in the medical payer policies reviewed possibly due to variations in the literature cited and transparency of the development process. A description of how recommendations are formulated and disclosure of any potential bias in policy development is important. Three—medical payer policies reviewed are of poor quality with one rated as good with respect to their development based on the modified Appraisal of Guidelines Research and Evaluation tool. Medical payer policies influence patient care by defining medical necessity for approving treatments, and should be held to the same standards for transparency and development as guidelines.

Clinical Recommendations.—The spine care community needs to develop (or update) high—quality treatment guidelines. The process should be transparent, methodologically rigorous, and consistent with the Appraisal of Guidelines Research and Evaluation and Institute of Medicine recommendations. This effort should be collaborative across specialty/society groups and would benefit from patient and public input.

Payer policies and treatment guidelines need to be transparent and based on the highest quality evidence available. Clinicians from specialty/society groups, guideline developers and policy makers should collaborate on their development. This process would also benefit from public and patient input.

▶ This very thorough review of medical payer clinical practice guidelines touches on one of the most controversial and contested issues in spinal surgery in my region. It is tempting to believe that the entire process would be improved with more transparency to guideline development and more involvement of the stakeholders, especially patients. But this misses the point. We then assume that the only goal is to facilitate the easier evaluation, approval, and reimbursement of patients thought to benefit from spinal fusion. I would ask the simple question: Who has defined the patient population for the procedure, and, just as importantly, the best technique and follow-up care? In an era of decreasing medical resources, I believe that medical payers should themselves fund the clinical research to improve the care of these cost-intensive procedures and the patients they are inflicted upon. The best balance would be a compromise between a large health system determining internally the best practice and refusing to publicize it for internal political reasons and the government funding a large unwieldy effort through the National Institutes of Health that is too ungainly and awkward to be applicable to the real world. We can only hope. I will say that any large-scale guideline development that does not involve the patient from the start of its creation is, by definition, fatally flawed. Efforts like the Minnesota Community Measurement have shown that it is possible to tackle difficult and complex problems with patient stakeholders as active participants in guideline development and could serve as a model for others to emulate.

P. Huddleston, MD

Primary Vertebral Tumors: A Review of Epidemiologic, Histological, and Imaging Findings, Part I: Benign Tumors

Ropper AE, Cahill KS, Hanna JW, et al (Brigham and Women's Hosp, Boston, MA; et al)
Neurosurgery 69:1171-1180, 2011

Primary vertebral tumors, although less common than metastases to the spine, make up a heterogeneous group of neoplasms that can pose diagnostic and treatment challenges. They affect both the adult and the pediatric population and may be benign, locally aggressive, or malignant. An understanding of typical imaging findings will aid in accurate diagnosis and help neurosurgeons appreciate anatomic subtleties that may increase their effective resection. An understanding of the histological similarities and differences between these tumors is imperative for all members of the clinical team caring for these patients. In this first review of 2 parts, we discuss the epidemiological, histological, and imaging features of the most common benign primary vertebral tumors—aneurysmal bone cyst, chondroma and enchondroma, hemangioma, osteoid osteoma, and osteoblastoma—and lesions related to eosinophilic granuloma and fibrous dysplasia. In addition, we discuss the basic management paradigms for each of these diagnoses. In combination with part II of the review, which focuses on locally aggressive and malignant tumors, this article provides a comprehensive review of primary vertebral tumors.

▶ This fantastic article from researchers at the Brigham and Women's Hospital, Dana-Farber Cancer Institute, and Harvard Medical School is my favorite contribution to the Year Book from *Spine* this year. This one-stop article, complete with color photographs of tumor pathology and beautiful diagnostic imaging, would be the only article I would recommend to the private practice orthopedic surgeon if he or she were contemplating a review of benign spinal tumors this year. Although the article suffers from a slight neurosurgical tilt to its perspective, it more than makes up for this small shortcoming with good organization and content. Any improvement to the article would include some more atypical examples to complement the more straightforward clinical presentations. Adding this to your article folder, whether in paper format or electronic, and pairing it with the classic atlas by Wold et al[1] will be all that most orthopedists will ever need to satisfy (or overwhelm) their desire to maintain their knowledge base for spine pathology!

P. Huddleston, MD

Reference

1. Wold LE, McLeod RA, Sim FH, Unni KK. *Atlas of Orthopedic Pathology.* WB Saunders Company; 1990.

Spinal Injuries After Improvised Explosive Device Incidents: Implications for Tactical Combat Casualty Care

Comstock S, Pannell D, Talbot M, et al (Canadian Forces Health Services, Toronto, Ontario, Canada)

J Trauma 71:S413-S417, 2011

Background.—Tactical Combat Casualty Care aims to treat preventable causes of death on the battlefield but deemphasizes the importance of spinal immobilization in the prehospital tactical setting. However, improvised explosive devices (IEDs) now cause the majority of injuries to Canadian Forces (CF) members serving in Afghanistan. We hypothesize that IEDs are more frequently associated with spinal injuries than non-IED injuries and that spinal precautions are not being routinely employed on the battlefield.

Methods.—We examined retrospectively a database of all CF soldiers who were wounded and arrived alive at the Role 3 Multinational Medical Unit in Kandahar, Afghanistan, from February 7, 2006, to October 14, 2009. We collected data on demographics, injury mechanism, anatomic injury descriptions, physiologic data on presentation, and prehospital interventions performed. Outcomes were incidence of any spinal injuries.

Results.—Three hundred seventy-two CF soldiers were injured during the study period and met study criteria. Twenty-nine (8%) had spinal fractures identified. Of these, 41% (n = 12) were unstable, 31% (n = 9) stable, and 28% indeterminate. Most patients were injured by IEDs (n = 212, 57%). Patients injured by IEDs were more likely to have spinal injuries than those injured by non—IED-related mechanisms (10.4% vs. 2.3%; $p < 0.01$). IED victims were even more likely to have spinal injuries than patients suffering blunt trauma (10.4% vs. 6.7%; $p = 0.02$). Prehospital providers were less likely to immobilize the spine in IED victims compared with blunt trauma patients (10% [22 of 212] vs. 23.0% [17 of 74]; $p < 0.05$).

Conclusions.—IEDs are a common cause of stable and unstable spinal injuries in the Afghanistan conflict. Spinal immobilization is an underutilized intervention in the battlefield care of casualties in the conflict in Afghanistan. This may be a result of tactical limitations; however, current protocols should continue to emphasize the judicious use of immobilization in these patients.

▶ It seems that conflict has been the driver of many inventions over the millennia with regard to the study of medical injuries. Whether studying the effects of blast injuries on the lower extremity, rationales for whole-blood transfusion, or the epidemiology of military casualty injuries, many of the developments in military medical care will, or already have, directly impacted civilian care. Even when an injury mechanism like improvised explosive devices (IEDs) might not seem to have a civilian equivalent, it is still worth understanding in an effort to improve knowledge and training for future conflicts. These authors from the Canadian Forces Health Services have made an important observation: current doctrinal military medical training has not emphasized that the spinal immobilization of combatants injured by penetrating trauma as lessons learned in Vietnam "suggests that stabilization in penetrating missile injuries is not necessary, as patients either have complete, irreversible neurologic injury or no significant injury." They cite statistics from the current Afghanistan conflict in which only 11% of Canadian troops brought injured to the military hospital in Kandahar Airfield Base were delivered with spinal immobilization in place, even when 8% of all injured Canadian Forces members had at least 1 spinal fracture, of which 41% were unstable fractures. In my experience as an Army Reserve Orthopedic Surgeon serving in the Army Medical Corp in both the Afghanistan and Iraq theaters, I can confirm similar statistics on my rotations. I agree with the authors that the evolution of current combat with the increasing frequency of the use of IEDs should force specific training of medical personnel to recognize the increased risk of spinal injury with these violent injury mechanisms and adjust the training treatment and hopefully the outcome of these wounded warriors.

P. Huddleston, MD

Mortality in the Vertebroplasty Population

McDonald RJ, Achenbach SJ, Atkinson EJ, et al (Mayo Clinic, Rochester, MN)
AJNR Am J Neuroradiol 32:1818-1823, 2011

Background and Purpose.—Vertebroplasty is an effective treatment for painful compression fractures refractory to conservative management. Because there are limited data regarding the survival characteristics of this patient population, we compared the survival of a treated with an untreated vertebral fracture cohort to determine whether vertebroplasty affects mortality rates.

Materials and Methods.—The survival of a treated cohort, comprising 524 vertebroplasty recipients with refractory osteoporotic vertebral compression fractures, was compared with a separate historical cohort of 589 subjects with fractures not treated by vertebroplasty who were identified from the Rochester Epidemiology Project. Mortality was compared between cohorts by using Cox proportional hazards models adjusting for age, sex, and Charlson indices of comorbidity. Mortality was also correlated with pre-, peri-, and postprocedural clinical metrics (eg, cement volume use, RDQ score, analog pain scales, frequency of narcotic use, and improvement in mobility) within the treated cohort.

Results.—Vertebroplasty recipients demonstrated 77% of the survival expected for individuals of similar age, ethnicity, and sex within the US population. Compared with individuals with both symptomatic and asymptomatic untreated vertebral fractures, vertebroplasty recipients retained a 17% greater mortality risk. However, compared with symptomatic untreated vertebral fractures, vertebroplasty recipients had no increased mortality following adjustment for differences in age, sex, and comorbidity (HR, 1.02; 95% CI, 0.82–1.25). In addition, no clinical metrics used to assess the efficacy of vertebroplasty were predictive of survival.

Conclusions.—Vertebroplasty recipients have mortality rates similar to those of individuals with untreated symptomatic fractures but have worse mortality compared with those with asymptomatic vertebral fractures.

▶ This article once again impresses upon me the terrible morbidity and mortality associated with osteoporotic or "fragility" fractures. It would be hard to find other common nononcologic disease entities in the surgical field that are associated with such a high 1-year mortality or, by association, decrease the 77% survival expected for individuals of similar age, ethnicity, and sex within the U.S. population. Although it is recognized that in many cases the fragility fracture is simply a surrogate for a general physical and mental decline, the authors additionally suggest that performing vertebroplasty does not alter the natural history of this decline. Many advocates of the procedure have argued that the symptomatic pain relief will minimize the possible deleterious effects of pain medications and immobility that can occur. Although prospective studies have failed to identify the pain generator and called into question the effectiveness of vertebroplasty or kyphoplasty as an intervention, I was still surprised by the study results suggesting that vertebroplasty recipients have worse mortality compared with those with asymptomatic vertebral fractures. The differences defy easy explanation, but the authors suggest that patients with a higher risk of mortality are possibly being selected for cement vertebral augmentation, or restated, "the increased mortality risk seen among vertebroplasty recipients compared with the general US population or among the asymptomatic fracture population simply represents a selection bias because the medical community is treating with vertebroplasty the patients with the most severe vertebral fractures." On a historical note, this research publication joins the several hundred publications related to osteoporosis supported by the Rochester Epidemiology Project and authored, either directly or indirectly, by the always impressive, and newly retired, physician epidemiologist, Larry Joe Melton III.[1]

P. Huddleston, MD

Reference

1. Melton LJ III. History of the Rochester epidemiology project. *Mayo Clin Proc.* 1996;71:266-274.

Mechanical Function of Vertebral Body Osteophytes, as Revealed by Experiments on Cadaveric Spines

Al-Rawahi M, Luo J, Pollintine P, et al (Sultan Qaboos Univ Hosp, Sultanate of Oman; Univ of Bristol, UK; Univ of Bath, UK)

Spine 36:770-777, 2011

Study Design.—Mechanical testing of cadaveric spines.

Objective.—To determine whether vertebral body osteophytes act primarily to reduce compressive stress on the intervertebral discs, or to stabilize the spine in bending.

Summary of Background Data.—The mechanical significance of vertebral osteophytes is unclear.

Methods.—Thoracolumbar spines were obtained from cadavers, aged 51 to 92 years, with vertebral body osteophytes, mostly anterolateral. Twenty motion segments, from T5–T6 to L3–L4, were loaded in compression to 1.5 kN, and then in flexion, extension, and lateral bending to 10 to 25 Nm (depending on specimen size) with a compressive preload. Vertebral movements were tracked using an optical 2-dimensional MacReflex system. Tests were performed in random order, and were repeated after excision of all osteophytes. Osteophyte function was inferred from (a) changes in the force or moment resisted and (b) changes in tangent stiffness, measured at maximum displacement or rotation angle. Volumetric bone mineral density (BMD) was measured using dual photon x-ray absorptiometry and water immersion. Results were analyzed using repeated measures analysis of variance.

Results.—Resistance to compression was reduced by an average of 17% after osteophyte removal ($P < 0.05$), and resistance to bending moment in flexion, extension, and left and right lateral bending was reduced by 49%, 36%, 36%, and 35%, respectively (all $P < 0.01$). Changes in tangent stiffness were similar. Osteophyte removal increased the neutral zone in bending ($P < 0.05$) and, on average, reduced motion segment BMD by 7% to 9%. Results were insensitive to applied loads and moments, but several changes were proportional to osteophyte size.

Conclusion.—Vertebral body osteophytes resist bending movements more than compression. Because they reverse the instability in bending that can stimulate their formation, these osteophytes seem to be adaptive rather than degenerative. Results suggest that osteophytes could cause clinical BMD measurements to underestimate vertebral compressive strength.

► Adaptive not degenerative. The authors from the University of Bristol, United Kingdom, have put forth a very provocative hypothesis that questions more than just the terminology we use to describe the spine. The idea that the morphological changes seen as osteophytes but that patients, radiologists, and spine surgeons have labeled as signs of wearing out, aging, or deteriorating could instead be a sign that the spine is adapting, responding, and minimizing forces that could be potentially painful or destructive on the spine is revolutionary at best and heretical at worst. It is easier to see the condition of a painful, arthritic stiff low back as a hopelessly lost state with no chance of improvement that needs to be "fixed" than to accept that this is the natural history for the condition and that the deterioration manifesting as osteophytes is just Mother Nature's own way of stiffening or fusing the spine, but without the risk and uncertainty of surgery. I could see a profound difference in the mental picture of the disorder if I as a patient or physician read the x-ray report as "adaptive lumbar disc changes" instead of "degenerative disc disease." The authors rightly recommend further longitudinal studies to determine that motion segment instability is a stimulus for osteophyte formation. Similarly, studies that demonstrated a reduction in osteophyte size with improved motion segment stability as a result of fibrosis would be supportive to the hypothesis. A very useful conclusion is that the increased bony density of osteophytes in the osteoporotic spine may well falsely increase the measured bone density and lead to misguided conclusions regarding indicated care for those patients being considered for osteoporosis therapy.

P. Huddleston, MD

11 Orthopedic Oncology

Introduction

We continue to be the benefactors of wide ranging literature in orthopedic oncology; I have selected articles for this YEAR BOOK to represent the diversity of the field.

The issue of biopsy is a continuing theme in oncology, and two articles dealing with this subject are summarized below. In addition to the disease-oriented articles that form the backbone of our field (eg osteosarcoma and soft tissue sarcomas), I have included articles on the treatment of benign bone tumors that are commonly seen in practice. Several outcome-related papers for oncologic limb salvage are discussed. In an expansion of the scope of this section of the YEAR BOOK, I have also included papers dealing with metastatic spine disease, a common problem our patients face.

The paper selection is intended to be of interest to the general orthopedic surgeon and of use for those specializing in oncology. I hope it is an enjoyable section of the YEAR BOOK.

Peter S. Rose, MD

Tumor General

Bisphosphonate Use and the Risk of Subtrochanteric or Femoral Shaft Fractures in Older Women

Park-Wyllie LY, Mamdani MM, Juurlink DN, et al (Inst for Clinical Evaluative Sciences, Toronto, Ontario, Canada; et al)
JAMA 305:783-789, 2011

Context.—Osteoporosis is associated with significant morbidity and mortality. Oral bisphosphonates have become a mainstay of treatment, but concerns have emerged that long-term use of these drugs may suppress bone remodeling, leading to unusual fractures.

Objective.—To determine whether prolonged bisphosphonate therapy is associated with an increased risk of subtrochanteric or femoral shaft fracture.

Design, Setting, and Patients.—A population-based, nested case-control study to explore the association between bisphosphonate use and fractures in a cohort of women aged 68 years or older from Ontario, Canada, who initiated therapy with an oral bisphosphonate between April 1, 2002, and

March 31, 2008. Cases were those hospitalized with a subtrochanteric or femoral shaft fracture and were matched to up to 5 controls with no such fracture. Study participants were followed up until March 31, 2009.

Main Outcome Measures.—The primary analysis examined the association between hospitalization for a subtrochanteric or femoral shaft fracture and duration of bisphosphonate exposure. To test the specificity of the findings, the association between bisphosphonate use and fractures of the femoral neck or intertrochanteric region, which are characteristic of osteoporotic fractures, was also examined.

Results.—We identified 716 women who sustained a subtrochanteric or femoral shaft fracture following initiation of bisphosphonate therapy and 9723 women who sustained a typical osteoporotic fracture of the intertrochanteric region or femoral neck. Compared with transient bisphosphonate use, treatment for 5 years or longer was associated with an increased risk of subtrochanteric or femoral shaft fracture (adjusted odds ratio, 2.74; 95% confidence interval, 1.25-6.02). A reduced risk of typical osteoporotic fractures occurred among women with more than 5 years of bisphosphonate therapy (adjusted odds ratio, 0.76; 95% confidence interval, 0.63-0.93). Among 52 595 women with at least 5 years of bisphosphonate therapy, a subtrochanteric or femoral shaft fracture occurred in 71 (0.13%) during the subsequent year and 117 (0.22%) within 2 years.

Conclusion.—Among older women, treatment with a bisphosphonate for more than 5 years was associated with an increased risk of subtrochanteric or femoral shaft fractures; however, the absolute risk of these fractures is low (Table 2).

▶ There has been increasing concern in the orthopedic literature as clinical experience accumulates of patients treated with long-term bisphosphonates presenting with atypical subtrochanteric fractures. Evidence in the literature to date has been conflicting, and 3 recent bisphosphonate trials did not find a clear association between bisphosphonate use and these fractures; however, in this large population-based study (the largest to date on the subject), these authors found that bisphosphonate treatment for greater than 5 years in older women

TABLE 2.—Risk of Subtrochanteric or Femoral Shaft Fractures Among Women Taking Bisphosphonate Therapy

	Duration of Bisphosphonate Therapy			
	Transient, <100 Days	Short-term Use, 100 Days to 3 Years	Intermediate Use, 3 to 5 Years	Long-Term Use, ≥5 Years
No. (%) of patients				
Case (n = 716)	42 (5.9)	349 (48.7)	204 (28.5)	121 (16.9)
Control (n = 3580)	218 (6.1)	1832 (51.2)	1070 (29.9)	460 (12.9)
Odds Ratio (95% CI)				
Crude	1.0 [Reference]	1.00 (0.70-1.43)	1.08 (0.73-1.59)	1.74 (1.11-2.73)
Adjusted[a]	1.0 [Reference]	0.90 (0.48-1.68)	1.59 (0.80-3.15)	2.74 (1.25-6.02)

Abbreviation: CI, confidence interval.
[a]The full list of covariates for the adjusted model are given in eAppendix 2 (available at http://www.jama.com).

clearly increased the risk of atypical subtrochanteric fractures. The study population included only women who are age 68 or older, but clinical experience has shown that younger patients treated with high-dose and prolonged bisphosphonate therapy either for osteoporosis or as a part of chemotherapy protocols for multiple myeloma or other tumors appear to be at similar risk.

The study was drawn from an administrative database, which limits its ability to control for direct issues of patients' activities and some risk factors. As shown in Table 2 reproduced below, short- and intermediate-term use (less than 5 years) did not confer a significantly increased odds ratio of fracture but use greater than 5 years did.

It is important to remember that the absolute risk of these atypical fractures is quite low (0.13% in the year after 5 years of treatment) and that typical osteoporotic hip fractures outnumbered these subtrochanteric fractures by greater than 12 to 1 during the study period. As such, this article confirms the strong clinical impression that many surgeons have, as they see and treat these patients, of a relationship between prolonged bisphosphonate therapy and atypical fractures. It also gives us a greater understanding of the risk factors and the duration of treatment that appears necessary to confer a significant risk of atypical fracture on this population. It should not, however, discourage us from the use of bisphosphonate therapy in patients with osteoporosis, as a benefit in osteoporotic fractures is clearly present. Rather, studies of this nature inform our selection of bisphosphonate therapy duration as we proceed with clinical care.

P. S. Rose, MD

The Current Practice of Orthopaedic Oncology in North America

White J, Toy P, Gibbs P, et al (Univ of Oklahoma Health Sciences Ctr; Univ of Tennessee, Memphis; Univ of Florida, Gainesville)

Clin Orthop Relat Res 468:2840-2853, 2010

Background.—The field of orthopaedic oncology in North America has been formalized over the past 30 years with the development of the Musculoskeletal Tumor Society (MSTS) and fellowship education opportunities.

Questions/Purposes.—To characterize current practices we assessed the fellowship education, practice setting, constitution of clinical practice, bone and soft tissue sarcoma treatment volume, perceived challenges and rewards of the career, and the nonclinical activities of orthopaedic oncologists.

Methods.—Members of the MSTS and attendees of the 2009 AAOS–MSTS Specialty Day meeting were invited to participate in a twenty-three question online survey. One hundred and four surgeons including 99 of the 192 (52%) MSTS members completed the online survey.

Results.—Sixty-nine of the 104 (66%) responding surgeons completed a 1-year musculoskeletal oncology fellowship. Thirty-eight (37%) completed an additional orthopaedic subspecialty fellowship. Seventy-four (79%) work in an academic practice and 70 (+/− 16) % of clinical time is spent practicing musculoskeletal oncology. An average of 20 (+/− 16) bone and 40 (+/− 36) soft tissue sarcomas were treated annually. Insufficient institutional support,

TABLE 3.—Results of the Survey: Career Challenges and Rewards

Importance of Factors in Providing Significant Career Challenges

Factor	Percent Reporting as "Not Important" or "Somewhat Important"	Percent Reporting as "Important" or "Very Important"
Reimbursement	44	56
Emotional stress	57	43
Insufficient institutional support	58	42
Insufficient case volume	72	28
Time commitment for research	72	28
Time commitment for administrative efforts	81	19
Change of interest	88	12

Importance of Factors in Providing Significant Career Satisfaction

Factor	Percent Reporting as "Not Important" or "Somewhat Important"	Percent Reporting as "Important" or "Very Important"
Case variety	3	97
Complex and challenging surgery	4	96
Challenge of diagnosis	9	91
Multidisciplinary care aspect	16	84
Furthers academic career	36	64
Research interest	46	54
Reimbursement	66	34

reimbursement, and emotional stresses were perceived as the most important challenges in a musculoskeletal oncology practice. Sixty-seven (64%) of the surgeons reported serving in a leadership position at the departmental or national level.

Conclusions.—Professional time distribution is similar to other academic orthopaedists. The members of the MSTS are responsible for the treatment of more than two-thirds of bone and soft tissue sarcomas in the United States.

Clinical Relevance.—This information can assist the fellowship directors and related professional societies in tailoring their educational programs and the interested orthopaedic resident to make a more informed career choice (Table 3).

▶ Orthopedic oncology is a new subspecialty of orthopedics dedicated to the management of complex bone and soft tissue disorders usually resulting in large musculoskeletal defects requiring unique reconstructive surgery. This subspecialty was born in the 1970s and has since grown into a group that has a huge impact on diseases that otherwise were poorly managed. This article is a must read for those interested in entering the challenging field of orthopedic oncology. Insufficient institutional support, relatively poor reimbursement, and the overall stresses of dealing with life- and limb-threatening illnesses are some of the remaining challenges to overcome in this subspecialty. The rewards of caring for this group of patients, however, are immense.

C. P. Beauchamp, MD

Outcomes and Prognostic Factors for a Consecutive Case Series of 115 Patients with Somatic Leiomyosarcoma

Abraham JA, Weaver MJ, Hornick JL, et al (Rothman Inst of Orthopedic Surgery, Philadelphia, PA; Brigham and Women's Hosp, Boston, MA; et al)
J Bone Joint Surg Am 94:736-744, 2012

Background.—Leiomyosarcoma is an uncommon tumor that affects 500 to 1000 patients in the United States annually. The purpose of our study was to further define survival rates as well as to identify multivariable predictors of disease-specific mortality, local recurrence, and development of distant metastasis following surgical resection.

Methods.—We studied a consecutive series of patients treated for leiomyosarcoma at our institution (a tertiary-care referral center) over a ten-year period. Only patients with leiomyosarcoma of soft tissues, vasculature, or bone were included. Those with uterine, gastrointestinal, or cutaneous forms of the disease were excluded. This yielded a cohort of 115 patients with complete follow-up data on which statistical analysis was performed.

Results.—One-year, five-year, and ten-year disease-specific survival rates were 87%, 57%, and 19%, respectively. Tumor depth ($p < 0.01$), histological grade ($p < 0.01$), and metastasis at presentation ($p = 0.03$) were found to be multivariable predictors of mortality. Both retroperitoneal location ($p = 0.01$) and mitotic rate ($p < 0.001$) were predictive of distant metastasis. Resection margin was the only multivariable significant predictor of local recurrence in the group treated with surgical resection ($p < 0.001$).

Conclusions.—Leiomyosarcoma is an aggressive disease, with a generally poor prognosis. Depth of tumor and high histological grade are indicators of a poor prognosis. Retroperitoneal tumors have a particularly high potential to metastasize.

Level of Evidence.—Prognostic Level II. See Instructions for Authors for a complete description of levels of evidence.

▶ The Harvard Brigham and Women's Hospital group brings us this consecutive series of patients treated for somatic leiomyosarcoma, the largest series reported to date. This article highlights the poor oncologic outcome of this tumor and the importance of wide surgical margins in dealing with it. This is a recurring theme in soft tissue sarcoma oncology that bears emphasis given the trends toward closer and closer resections.

The article suffers from the usual limitations of a retrospective analysis of a rare tumor. Nongastrointestinal and gynecologic retroperitoneal tumors were included in this cohort and faired especially poorly. This point is brought out but not fully emphasized in the article; most orthopedic oncologists do not directly manage retroperitoneal tumors, and as Fig 1D in the original article shows, the metastasis-free survival of truncal and extremity tumors approximates that of other high-grade soft tissue sarcomas. Thus, the treatment of this tumor in the trunk or extremities remains one of aggressive orthopedic surgical oncology with appropriate adjuvant treatments. Readers need not be put off by the poor statistics quoted in the abstract that are biased by the retroperitoneal portion of the cohort.

P. S. Rose, MD

Epithelioid Hemangioma of Bone and Soft Tissue: A Reappraisal of a Controversial Entity

Errani C, Zhang L, Panicek DM, et al (Memorial Sloan-Kettering Cancer Ctr, NY)

Clin Orthop Relat Res 470:1498-1506, 2012

Background.—The controversy surrounding diagnosis of an epithelioid hemangioma (EH), particularly when arising in skeletal locations, stems not only from its overlapping features with other malignant vascular neoplasms, but also from its somewhat aggressive clinical characteristics, including multifocal presentation and occasional lymph node involvement. Specifically, the distinction from epithelioid hemangioendothelioma (EHE) has been controversial. The recurrent t(1;3)(p36;q25) chromosomal translocation, resulting in WWTR1-CAMTA1 fusion, recently identified in EHE of various anatomic sites, but not in EH or other epithelioid vascular neoplasms, suggests distinct pathogeneses.

Question/Purposes.—We investigated the clinicopathologic and radiologic characteristics of bone and soft tissue EHs in patients treated at our institution with available tissue for molecular testing.

Patients and Methods.—Seventeen patients were selected after confirming the pathologic diagnosis and fluorescence in situ hybridization analysis for the WWTR1 and/or CAMTA1 rearrangements. Four patients had multifocal presentation. Most patients with EH of bone were treated by intralesional curettage. None of the patients died of disease and only four patients had a local recurrence.

Results.—Our results, using molecular testing to support the pathologic diagnosis of EH, reinforce prior data that EH is a benign lesion characterized by an indolent clinical course with an occasional multifocal presentation and rare metastatic potential to locoregional lymph nodes.

Conclusion.—These findings highlight the importance of distinguishing EH from other malignant epithelioid vascular tumors as a result of differences in their management and clinical outcome.

Level of Evidence.—Level IV, prognostic study. See Guidelines for Authors for a complete description of levels of evidence.

▶ Vascular tumors exist along a spectrum of benign, aggressive benign, and malignant tumors or bone and soft tissue. Additionally, their nomenclature is distinct and can often lead to confusion, particularly for epithelioid variants.

This article presents data from the Memorial Sloan-Kettering group on 17 patients with epithelioid hemangioma with molecular confirmation of disease (2 being recharacterized from hemangioendotheliomas). The article provides a clinicopathologic description of this disease process and will be a lasting reference for epithelioid hemangioma. The only patient who died succumbed to complications of radiotherapy, and the disease had a generally benign course.

However, at least as valuable to the orthopedic oncologist is the discussion of other similar vascular tumors (eg, the malignant epithelioid hemangioendothelioma) and how they are distinguished from epithelioid hemangioma. The first hurdle in the treatment of these patients is establishing the correct diagnosis and recognizing the treatment implications; in this manner, this article informs the care of patients with other vascular neoplasms as well.

P. S. Rose, MD

Systemic Therapy for Advanced Soft Tissue Sarcoma: Highlighting Novel Therapies and Treatment Approaches

Riedel RF (Duke Univ Med Ctr, Durham, NC)

Cancer 118:1474-1485, 2012

Soft tissue sarcomas (STS) are a rare, heterogeneous group of solid tumors in need of improved therapeutic options. First-line chemotherapy is considered the current standard of care for patients with advanced, symptomatic STS, but the median survival is only 8 to 12 months. Efforts to increase response rates by using combination or dose-dense regimens have largely failed to improve patient outcomes. However, increasing evidence supports the use of specific treatments for certain histological subtypes of STS, and novel therapies, including tyrosine kinase and mammalian target of rapamycin inhibitors, are currently under active investigation. In addition, novel treatment approaches (such as maintenance therapy) designed to prolong the duration of response to chemotherapy and delay disease progression are being explored. This article provides an overview of current systemic therapies for patients with advanced STS and discusses ongoing efforts designed to improve patient outcomes through the use of novel therapeutic agents and treatment strategies.

▶ This article deals with chemotherapeutic management of patients with unresectable or metastatic soft tissue sarcoma; why, then, select it for inclusion in the Oncology section of the YEAR BOOK OF ORTHOPEDICS?

As oncologic surgeons, we are often faced with making or delivering the diagnosis of advanced soft tissue sarcoma. Although the management of these patients is then transferred to our colleagues in medical oncology, it is important for us as surgeons to understand the treatment options and paradigms to which we send our patients. In this article, Dr Riedel provides a readable and practical summary of treatment options for such patients. The article includes treatment considerations that are evolving for specific sarcoma subtypes and the use of new targeted and maintenance therapies. It is worthwhile reading for anybody who cares for these patients.

P. S. Rose, MD

Outcome of Lower-Limb Preservation with an Expandable Endoprosthesis After Bone Tumor Resection in Children

Henderson ER, Pepper AM, Marulanda G, et al (H. Lee Moffitt Cancer Ctr & Res Inst, Tampa, FL; All Children's Hosp, St Petersburg, FL)
J Bone Joint Surg Am 94:537-547, 2012

Background.—The optimal treatment of malignant pediatric lower-extremity bone tumors is controversial. Expandable endoprostheses allow limb preservation, but the revision rate and limited function are considered barriers to their use. This study investigated the functional, emotional, and oncologic outcomes of thirty-eight patients treated with an expandable endoprosthesis.

Methods.—A retrospective chart review was performed, and surviving patients were asked to complete the Musculoskeletal Tumor Society (MSTS) outcomes instrument and the Pediatric Outcomes Data Collection Instrument (PODCI). Additional data including the range of hip and knee motion, limb-length discrepancy, and total lengthening were also obtained.

Results.—Thirty-eight patients were treated with an expandable endoprosthesis, and twenty-six of these patients were alive at the time of the study. The mean global MSTS score was 26.1, and the mean global PODCI score was 85.8. The mean emotional acceptance and happiness subscores were high. The mean sagittal-plane hip motion in patients who had undergone replacement of the proximal aspect of the femur was 103°. The mean knee motion in patients who had undergone replacement of the proximal aspect of the femur, the distal aspect of the femur, or the proximal aspect of the tibia was 127°, 97°, and 107°, respectively. The mean lengthening at the time of skeletal maturity was 4.5 cm, and the mean limb-length discrepancy was 0.7 cm. Forty-two percent of the patients experienced complications, with ten patients requiring prosthesis revision and two of these patients requiring amputation.

Conclusions.—Current technology does not offer a single best reconstruction option for children. Previous studies and the present series have indicated that physical and emotional functioning in patients treated with an expandable endoprosthesis are good but that complication rates remain high. Amputation and rotationplasty are alternative treatments if patients and their families are amenable to these procedures. The literature supports no single superior treatment among these three options with regard to physical or emotional health.

▶ These authors from the Moffitt Cancer Center report the largest North American experience to date with expandable prostheses for limb salvage in skeletally immature children. This is a retrospective review of 38 charts using 3 implant types between 1996 and 2009.

Results are both encouraging and sobering. The implants were generally successful in allowing function for children and lengthening with growth. However, at only a mean 48-month follow-up in the 26 surviving patients, the complication rate was 42%. I suspect the actuarial complication rate was higher than this because the article does not provide a clear time course to complications nor account for the changing number at risk as patients unfortunately succumbed to disease (12/38). As well, many outcome variables (functional data, leg-length equality, Pediatric Outcomes Data Collection Instrument) are collected in a variable and incomplete manner.

So where to put this article in the context of clinical care of children with bone sarcomas? These authors have reported a great experience that illustrates the potential of these implants but also their very real hazards. Readers are reminded of the excellent outcomes of rotationplasty and amputation for patients facing similar challenges.[1]

P. S. Rose, MD

Reference

1. Aboulafia AJ, Wilkerson J. Lower-limb preservation with an expandable endoprosthesis after tumor resection in children: is the cup half full or half empty?: commentary on an article by Eric R. Henderson, MD, et al.: "outcome of lower-limb preservation with an expandable endoprosthesis after bone tumor resection in children". *J Bone Joint Surg Am*. 2012;94:e391-e392.

Functional and Oncological Outcome Following Marginal Excision of Well-Differentiated Forearm Liposarcoma With Nerve Involvement

Kemp MA, Hinsley DE, Gwilym SE, et al (Nuffield Orthopaedic Centre, Oxford, UK)

J Hand Surg 36A:94-100, 2011

Purpose.—Liposarcoma is one of the most common soft tissue sarcomas in adults. It is often low-grade and can occasionally involve neurovascular structures. We present the functional and oncological outcome resulting from planned marginal excision of a series of forearm low-grade liposarcomas with nerve involvement.

Methods.—The Oxford tumor registry was used to identify cases of histologically proven, well-differentiated liposarcoma of the forearm, with nerve involvement, treated surgically between 1997 and 2006. Nerve involvement was identified clinically with symptoms or signs of nerve compression, or by images showing direct contact of the tumor with a nerve on magnetic resonance imaging. This was then further defined at the time of surgery as tumor abutting (capsular involvement) or encasing a peripheral nerve. Demographic and clinical data were collected and oncological outcome was assessed by noting local and distant recurrence during follow-up. Postoperative functional outcome was assessed using the Toronto Extremity Salvage Scores.

Results.—Eight cases were identified, 6 with preoperative neurological symptoms. The total group comprised 6 men and 2 women with a mean age of 61 (range, 30–71) years. At surgery, all had their tumors successfully excised, with preservation of the involved nerves. In those with preoperative neurological symptoms, complete recovery occurred by 18 months after surgery. The average follow-up was 5 years (range, 3–9 y). There were no cases of either local or distant recurrence of disease, with a mean Toronto Extremity Salvage Score of 99%.

Conclusions.—Planned marginal excision of a well-differentiated liposarcoma, arising in the forearm and involving nerve, can result in excellent functional and oncological outcome.

Type of Study/Level of Evidence.—Therapeutic IV.

▶ Lipomatous tumors exist along a spectrum, from purely benign and latent lipomas to high-grade liposarcomas. At the low end of this spectrum lie atypical lipomatous tumors, also known as *well-differentiated liposarcomas*. Contemporary practice favors the term *atypical lipomatous tumor* in recognition that these tumors have a propensity to recur locally if excised intralesionally but have no real metastatic potential unless they undergo dedifferentiation (a rare occurrence). Convention has shifted away from labeling an extremity tumor without metastatic potential a sarcoma.

I point this out because this article (both in its title and its text) refers to these tumors as *liposarcomas* in reporting a series of 8 cases with good outcomes following marginal excision. Although technically correct, this is not favored terminology.

That said, the authors report good outcome following function sparing marginal excision of these tumors. This remains the standard of care for these entities throughout the body.

P. S. Rose, MD

Survival after recurrent osteosarcoma: Data from 3 European Osteosarcoma Intergroup (EOI) randomized controlled trials

Gelderblom H, on behalf of the European Osteosarcoma Intergroup (Leiden Univ Med Ctr, The Netherlands; et al)

Eur J Cancer 47:895-902, 2011

Background.—Recurrence after osteosarcoma usually leads to death; thus prognostic factors for survival are of great importance.

Methods.—Between 1983 and 2002, the European Osteosarcoma Intergroup accrued 1067 patients to 3 randomized controlled trials of pre- and post-operative chemotherapy for patients with resectable non-metastatic high-grade osteosarcoma of the extremity. Control treatment in all trials was doxorubicin 75 mg/m^2 and cisplatin 100 mg/m^2. The comparators were additional high-dose methotrexate (BO02), T10-based multi-drug regimen (BO03) and G-CSF intensified-DC (BO06). Post-recurrence survival (PRS) was investigated on combined data with standard survival analysis methods.

Results.—Median recurrence-free survival was 31 months; 8 recurrences were reported more than 5 years after the diagnosis. In 564 patients with a recurrence (median 13 months post-randomisation), there was no difference in post-relapse survival between treatment arms. Patients whose disease recurred within 2 years after randomization had a worse prognosis than those recurring after 2 years. Patients with good initial histological response to pre-operative chemotherapy had a better overall survival after recurrence than poor responders. Local relapse was more often reported after limb-saving procedures (2 versus 8%; amputation versus limb-saving), independent of the primary tumour site. Site of first recurrence (local 20%, lung 62%, "other" 19%) affected survival, as patients recurring with non-lung distant metastases only or any combination of local relapse, lung metastases and non-lung metastases (=group "other") had significantly worse overall survival (local 39%, lung 19%, "other" 9% at 5 years).

Conclusions.—These data describing a large series of patients with recurrent extremity osteosarcoma confirm the relationship between early recurrence and poor survival. There was better PRS in patients after good histological response to pre-operative chemotherapy, or with local-only recurrence (Fig 2).

▶ Individual trials in the past have highlighted the very poor prognosis of patients with local or distant recurrence of osteosarcoma after surgery and radiotherapy. These authors bring together the largest study that I am aware of to date

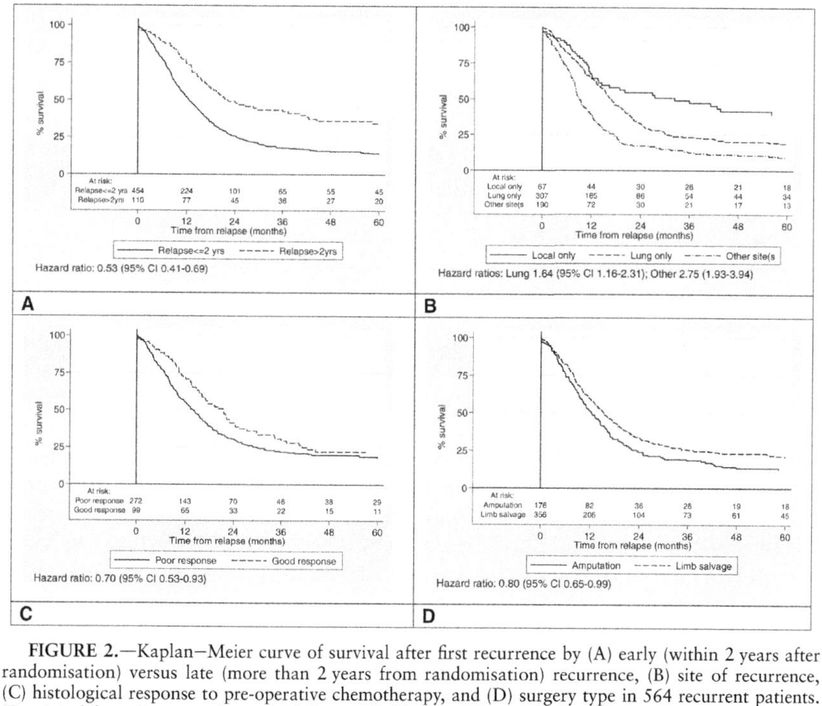

FIGURE 2.—Kaplan–Meier curve of survival after first recurrence by (A) early (within 2 years after randomisation) versus late (more than 2 years from randomisation) recurrence, (B) site of recurrence, (C) histological response to pre-operative chemotherapy, and (D) surgery type in 564 recurrent patients. (Reprinted from European Journal of Cancer. Gelderblom H, on behalf of the European Osteosarcoma Intergroup, Survival after recurrent osteosarcoma: data from 3 European Osteosarcoma Intergroup (EOI) randomized controlled trials. *Eur J Cancer.* 2011;47:895-902, Copyright 2011, with permission from Elsevier.)

to examine this subject combining 3 European randomized trials with high-quality data analysis. The title is slightly misleading in that they analyze both local and distant recurrence and, at first glance, one might think they were dealing with just local recurrence.

The article highlights how time to recurrence, anatomic sight of recurrence, and histologic response to the index chemotherapy treatment heavily influence patient outcomes. Patients with local-only recurrence had the best outcome in this series. Because we know that local recurrence is influenced by the surgical margin achieved as well as the response to preoperative chemotherapy, these results also influence our approach to these patients in an era in which closer and closer surgical margins are being commonly reported. Currently, we do not have a fully reliable mechanism to predict histologic response to chemotherapy before surgical intervention. The poor outcome of patients with local recurrence reported in this series shows the need to proceed with caution as new technologies (such as computerized navigation) allow us the ability to perform closer and closer tumor resections in the goal of improving patient function. We must temper our enthusiasm for this by acknowledging that our ultimate goal is patient survival. Again, the poor prognosis of patients with locally recurrent disease highlights the need to proceed with caution here.

Overall survival was influenced by the time and pattern of relapse as well as chemotherapy response as demonstrated in Fig 2. However, the overall survival rate in this cohort was less than 25%.

P. S. Rose, MD

Analysis of Prognostic Factors for Patients with Chordoma with Use of the California Cancer Registry

Lee J, Bhatia NN, Hoang BH, et al (Univ of California, Irvine)
J Bone Joint Surg Am 94:356-363, 2012

Background.—Chordoma is the most common primary malignant tumor of the spine. It is extremely rare and has been studied primarily in single-institution case series. Using data from a large, population-based cancer registry, we designed the present study to examine the outcome for patients with chordoma and to determine relevant prognostic factors.

Methods.—A retrospective analysis of the California Cancer Registry database was performed to identify patients with a diagnosis of chordoma in the years 1989 to 2007. Comparisons examined differences in demographics, disease characteristics, treatment, and survival. Survival analyses were performed with use of the Kaplan-Meier method with log-rank tests and Cox proportional hazards models.

Results.—Four hundred and nine patients with chordoma were identified; 257 (62.8%) were male and 152 (37.2%) were female. With regard to racial or ethnic distribution, 266 patients (65%) were white; ninety-three (22.7%), Hispanic; forty-three (10.5%), Asian or other; and seven (1.7%), black. The site of presentation was the head in 202 patients (49.4%), spine in 106 patients (25.9%), and pelvis and/or sacrum in 101 patients (24.7%). Hispanic race ($p = 0.0002$), younger age (less than forty years; $p < 0.0001$), and female sex ($p = 0.009$) were associated with cranial presentation, whereas older age (forty years or older; $p < 0.0001$) was associated with pelvic presentation. After adjustment for clinically relevant factors, a significantly decreased risk of death for chordoma-specific survival was seen for Hispanic race (hazard ratio = 0.51, 95% confidence interval [95% CI], 0.28 to 0.93; $p = 0.03$), high socioeconomic status (hazard ratio = 0.8, 95% CI, 0.67 to 0.95; $p = 0.01$), and local excision and/or debulking (hazard ratio = 0.38, 95% CI, 0.18 to 0.81; $p = 0.01$). Large tumor size was independently associated with an increased risk of death (hazard ratio = 2.05, 95% CI, 1.01 to 4.20; $p = 0.048$).

Conclusions.—In this study, the survival of patients with chordoma was significantly better for those who were Hispanic and had a small tumor, high socioeconomic status, and surgical intervention.

▶ These authors from the University of California at Irvine present data from the California Cancer Registry on 409 chordoma patients. In addition to its large size, this study is distinct from other registry studies (eg, the Surveillance, Epidemiology, and End Results database) in its analysis of prognostic factors and inclusion of other racial and socioeconomic data.

Chordomas are vexing tumors to treat, and this study is as notable for what it does not show as it is for its positive results. For rare, capricious tumors, one hopes that a large study will reveal a previously unrecognized factor that will aid in patient treatment. Unfortunately, no silver bullet emerged in this study. Large tumors and lack of surgery correlated with poor outcomes, and (not surprisingly) patients of higher socioeconomic status fared better. The primary treatment of chordoma remains surgery with a guarded prognosis.

P. S. Rose, MD

Living With Rotationplasty—Quality of Life in Rotationplasty Patients From Childhood to Adulthood

Forni C, Gaudenzi N, Zoli M, et al (Rizzoli Orthopedic Inst, Bologna, Italy; Bologna Hosp-Univ, Italy)

J Surg Oncol 105:331-336, 2012

Background.—Knowledge about the long-term sequelae of rotationplasty, in adults treated surgically in childhood for Osteosarcoma in the lower limb, mainly concerns function and performance; the aim of this study is to explore the experience and the Quality of Life (QoL) of the patients who underwent Rotationplasty from 1986 to 2006 in Italy.

Methods.—Quantitative test: Administration SF-36 questionnaire to 20 subjects aged ≥ 16 years. Qualitative test: Semi-structured interview recorded in 10 of these subjects.

Results.—Greater well-being was found in the Mental Component Summary (MCS) scale of subjects aged over 24 years, with a score mean

TABLE 2.—SF-36 Scores of Rotationplasty Patients and the General Italian Population[†]

	SF-36 Scores							
Subjects	Physical Functioning	Role-Physical	Bodily Pain	General Health	Vitality	Social Functioning	Role-Emotional	Mental Health
Rotationplasty patients n. 20	89.3* ± 8.8	81.3 ± 30.2	88.2 ± 19.7	83.6* ± 12.4	71.8 ± 13.7	81.3 ± 20.5	88.3 ± 22.4	80.8* ± 12.0
Italian population 18–34 years n. 560	95.5* ± 15.7	89.2 ± 42.0	83.0 ± 34.1	76.7* ± 23.4	68.2 ± 26.3	81.7 ± 32.3	83.4 ± 50.4	72.7* ± 25.9

[†]Values given are mean ± SD.
*$P < 0.05$ (rotationplasty patients vs. Italian population 18–34 years).

of 54.2 (±4.8), compared with that of those aged up to 24 years, with a mean score of 48.0 (±6.6), $P = 0.04$. Relational and emotional difficulty in adolescence, which had been partially overcome in adulthood, was revealed.

Conclusions.—The assessment of QoL by the SF-36 questionnaire was effective, and a correspondence was found between what emerged from the quantitative study and the contents of the interview. Knowing the strengths and weaknesses that were highlighted is indispensable for parents and operators when choosing among the various surgical options and to facilitate coming to terms with the injury and the "*scars*" (Table 2).

▶ These authors present both qualitative (assessed in structured interview) and quantitative (SF-36) results in 20 patients greater than 16 years old and more than 2 years from surgery who underwent rotationplasty as children for the treatment of bone tumors. Interestingly, SF-36 domain results were generally similar to population norms and, in fact, greater in the fields of mental and general health (Table II).

However, the difficulties of adolescence were apparent, with Mental Component Summary scores lower in patients younger than 24 years than in older patients. As well, bodily pain increased with time from surgery. The results of the structured interview highlight the day-to-day problems these patients may continue to face.

This is a great study for surgeons who treat children with bone tumors. It confirms the benefit of this surgery (objective quality of life equivalent to population norms) while highlighting some specific areas in which patients struggle. Despite the technologic advances in expandable prostheses, rotationplasty remains a valuable option in the treatment of patients. Studies of this nature confirm its value and continuing role in surgical oncology.

P. S. Rose, MD

Exposure to Ionizing Radiation and Development of Bone Sarcoma: New Insights Based on Atomic-Bomb Survivors of Hiroshima and Nagasaki

Samartzis D, Nishi N, Hayashi M, et al (Radiation Effects Res Foundation, Hiroshima and Nagasaki, Japan)

J Bone Joint Surg Am 93:1008-1015, 2011

Background.—Radiation-induced bone sarcoma has been associated with high doses of ionizing radiation from therapeutic or occupation-related exposures. However, the development of bone sarcoma following exposure to lower doses of ionizing radiation remains speculative.

Methods.—A cohort analysis based on the Life Span Study (n = 120,321) was performed to assess the development of bone sarcoma in atomic-bomb survivors of Hiroshima and Nagasaki followed from 1958 to 2001. The excess relative risk per gray of ionizing radiation absorbed by the bone marrow was estimated. Additional subject demographic, survival, and clinical factors were evaluated.

Results.—Nineteen cases of bone sarcoma (in eleven males and eight females) were identified among the 80,181 subjects who met the inclusion criteria, corresponding to an incidence of 0.9 per 100,000 person-years. The mean ages at the time of the bombing and at diagnosis were 32.4 and 61.6 years, respectively. The mean bone marrow dose was 0.43 Gy. Osteosarcoma was the most commonly identified bone sarcoma. The most common bone sarcoma site was the pelvis. The overall unadjusted five-year survival rate was 25%. A dose threshold was found at 0.85 Gy (95% confidence interval, 0.12 to 1.85 Gy), with a linear dose-response association above this threshold. The linear slope equaled an excess relative risk of 7.5 per Gy (95% confidence interval, 1.34 to 23.14 per Gy) in excess of 0.85 Gy.

Conclusions.—On the basis of what we believe is one of the longest and largest prospective studies assessing the development of bone sarcoma in individuals exposed to ionizing radiation, it appears that the development of radiation-induced bone sarcomamay be associated with exposure to much lower doses of ionizing radiation than have previously been reported. Such new insights may potentially improve bone sarcoma prevention measures and broaden our understanding of the role of ionizing radiation from various sources on the development of malignant tumors. This study stresses the need to become increasingly aware of the various health risks that may be attributable to even low levels of ionizing radiation exposure.

Level of Evidence.—Prognostic Level I. See Instructions to Authors for a complete description of levels of evidence.

▶ This article deals with the fascinating topic of the long-term risk of bone sarcoma in survivors of the World War II atomic bomb explosions in Japan. The authors draw from a longitudinal cohort study of more than 80 000 patients with known radiation exposures from the atomic blasts. They demonstrate an increased risk of bone sarcoma from a threshold dose of 0.85 Gy as well as a dose response curve for higher doses (Fig 3 in the original article).

The article is limited by small numbers—only 19 cases of bone sarcoma—and an inability to control for potential risk factors (eg, smoking, therapeutic radiotherapy); thus, the confidence intervals are broad. However, we are unlikely to ever see another study of this type in the near future.

The results of this study most interest me in their implication for the use of radiotherapy in children; firm conclusions are hard to draw, but data of this nature give pause to ready radiation of pediatric sarcomas if aggressive surgery can obtain good local control.

P. S. Rose, MD

Genotype-Phenotype Correlation Study in 529 Patients with Multiple Hereditary Exostoses: Identification of "Protective" and "Risk" Factors

Pedrini E, Jennes I, Tremosini M, et al (Rizzoli Orthopaedic Inst, Bologna, Italy)

J Bone Joint Surg Am 93:2294-2302, 2011

Background.—Multiple hereditary exostoses is an autosomal dominant skeletal disorder characterized by wide variation in clinical phenotype. The aim of this study was to evaluate whether the severity of the disease is linked with a specific genetic background.

Methods.—Five hundred and twenty-nine patients with multiple hereditary exostoses from two different European referral centers participated in the study. According to a new clinical classification based on the presence or absence of deformities and functional limitations, the phenotype of the patients was assessed as mild (the absence of both aspects), intermediate, or severe (the concurrent presence of both aspects). An identical molecular screening protocol with denaturing high-performance liquid chromatography and multiplex ligation-dependent probe amplification was performed in both institutions.

Results.—In our cohort of patients, variables such as female sex (odds ratio = 1.840; 95% confidence interval, 1.223 to 2.766), fewer than five skeletal sites with exostoses (odds ratio = 7.588; 95% confidence interval, 3.479 to 16.553), EXT2 mutations (odds ratio = 2.652; 95% confidence interval, 1.665 to 4.223), and absence of EXT1/2 mutations (odds ratio = 1.975; 95% confidence interval, 1.051 to 3.713) described patients with a mild phenotype; in contrast, a severe phenotype was associated with male sex (odds ratio = 2.431; 95% confidence interval, 1.544 to 3.826), EXT1 mutations (odds ratio = 6.817; 95% confidence interval, 1.003 to 46.348), and more than twenty affected skeletal sites (odds ratio = 2.413; 95% confidence interval, 1.144 to 5.091).Malignant transformation was observed in 5% of patients, and no evidence of association between chondrosarcoma onset and EXT mutation, sex, severity of disease, or number of lesions was detected.

Conclusions.—The identified "protective" and "risk" factors, as well as the proposed classification system, represent helpful tools for clinical management and follow-up of patients with multiple hereditary exostoses; moreover, homogeneous cohorts of patients, useful for studies on the pathogenesis of multiple hereditary exostoses, have been identified.

▶ This is a great study of more than 500 patients with multiple hereditary exostoses (MHE) from 2 European referral centers; the authors classified the clinical severity of patients and correlated this with mutation data. In nearly 10% of patients, no mutation was identified in the EXT gene loci.

Female sex, lesser skeletal involvement, and non-EXT1 mutations correlated with less severe phenotypes. Interestingly, sporadic mutations showed greater phenotype severity. However, a full spectrum of clinical severity was seen in individuals with identical mutations, in both related and unrelated individuals, highlighting our incomplete understanding of this disease process.

Studies of this nature will continue to improve our understanding of the molecular basis of our diseases. Unfortunately, the authors were not able to draw a genotype-phenotype correlation with malignant degeneration, the most clinically significant feature of MHE patients. This null result does not detract from the value of this study.

P. S. Rose, MD

Unicameral Bone Cysts: Comparison of Percutaneous Curettage, Steroid, and Autologous Bone Marrow Injections

Canavese F, Wright JG, Cole WG, et al (The Hosp for Sick Children, Toronto, Ontario, Canada)

J Pediatr Orthop 31:50-55, 2011

Background.—The purpose of this study was to compare the outcome of percutaneous curettage with intralesional injection of methylprednisolone and bone marrow for unicameral bone cysts (UBCs).

Methods.—This was a retrospective review of 46 children and adolescents with UBC treated with autologous bone marrow injection, methylprednisolone acetate injection or percutaneous curettage alone. Inclusion criteria were a radiological diagnosis of UBC and at least 24 months follow-up from the last procedure. Healing was determined using Neer/Cole 4-grades rating scale.

Results.—The 3 treatment groups were comparable with regard to age, sex, location of the cyst, and the number of procedures undertaken. At 2 years follow-up, the proportion of patients with satisfactory healing (Neer/Cole grades I and II) was greatest among those who underwent percutaneous curettage (70%) compared with bone marrow injection (21%) and methylprednisolone acetate injection (41%) ($P = 0.03$). We found no association between healing and age ($P = 0.80$) nor between healing and sex ($P = 0.61$).

Conclusions.—These results suggest that mechanical disruption of the cyst membrane may be helpful in healing of cysts and that this technique may be preferred to simple intralesional injections.

Level of Evidence.—Level III.

▶ Unicameral bone cysts are commonly seen in the pediatric population; management varies significantly among surgeons based on treatment biases. One thing that has been commonly observed is that cysts often heal reliably after pathologic fracture. However, it is clearly in the patient's interest if we can devise a treatment to allow healing without this.

These authors compared treatment with a percutaneous curettage procedure, steroid injection, and autologous bone marrow injection and found that the percutaneous curettage patients had a significantly improved rate of healing. They illustrate their treatment nicely in the article.

Although by no means a definitive study because of the modest number of patients and a retrospective methodology, this article helps to inform our treatment of patients of this nature. It casts doubt on the efficacy of simple bone marrow injection, which has at times had favor in some centers as a minimally invasive treatment for these conditions.

P. S. Rose, MD

Utility of CT-Guided Biopsy of Suspicious Skeletal Lesions in Patients With Known Primary Malignancies

Toomayan GA, Major NM (Duke Univ Med Ctr, Durham, NC; Hosp of the Univ of Pennsylvania, Philadelphia)

AJR Am J Roentgenol 196:416-423, 2011

Objective.—Patients with a known primary malignancy and one or more suspicious skeletal lesions are often assumed to have skeletal involvement by the known malignancy. We set out to determine how often one would be correct in making this assumption.

Materials and Methods.—All CT-guided bone biopsies performed at our institution between January 2006 and January 2009 in patients with a history of a single biopsy-proven malignancy were retrospectively reviewed. Pathology results were assigned to one of three outcomes: skeletal involvement by known malignancy, newly diagnosed malignancy, or no malignancy identified. Patients categorized as no malignancy identified required repeat biopsy or stability on follow-up imaging for confirmation.

Results.—Of 104 patients with a known primary malignancy, 11 were excluded. Of the 93 included patients, there was skeletal involvement by the known malignancy in 82 (88%), a newly diagnosed malignancy in seven (8%), and no malignancy identified in four (4%).

Conclusion.—Biopsy of a suspicious skeletal lesion in a patient with a solitary known malignancy reveals a newly diagnosed malignancy or no evidence of malignancy in 12% of patients, emphasizing the importance of biopsy.

▶ The appearance of metastatic lesions in a patient with an established diagnosis of cancer has tremendous clinical and emotional importance. From a clinical standpoint, the identification of metastatic disease in a patient with previously localized cancer changes treatment protocols and switches to an overall supportive and palliative care strategy in the vast majority of patients. From the patient's perspective, the diagnosis of metastatic cancer has a large emotional weight because patients must confront their own mortality. In many clinical situations, survival will be less than 1 year.

These authors retrospectively reviewed a series of 93 patients with a history of known malignancy undergoing biopsy to assess for skeletal metastases. Twelve percent of patients either had a second malignancy diagnosed or benign lesion identified. This is a useful article; it highlights that in a substantial minority of patients—1 in 8—the assumption that the lesion represents metastatic disease may be incorrect. The exact same clinical scenario occurred in my own clinic this week. These results highlight the need for clinicians to proceed with caution when assuming a metastatic process is directly tied to the previous known oncologic diagnosis. There are obvious treatment implications for the correct diagnosis of a secondary malignancy or in avoiding the diagnosis of metastatic disease in a patient with benign skeletal findings.

P. S. Rose, MD

Quality of Randomized Controlled Trials Reporting in the Treatment of Sarcomas

Toulmonde M, Bellera C, Mathoulin-Pelissier S, et al (Institut Bergonié, Bordeaux, France; Cancer Trials Data Ctr, Bordeaux, France)

J Clin Oncol 29:1204-1209, 2011

Purpose.—Randomized controlled trials (RCTs) represent the best evidence in oncology practice. The aim of this study was to assess the reporting quality of sarcoma RCTs and to identify significant predictors of quality.

Patients and Methods.—Two investigators searched MEDLINE for pediatric and adult bone and soft tissue sarcoma RCTs published between January 1988 and December 2008. The quality of each report was assessed by using a 15-point overall reporting quality score based on 15 items from the revised Consolidated Standards of Reporting Trials (CONSORT) statement (overall quality score [OQS] range, 0 to 15 points). Concealment of allocation, appropriate blinding, and analysis according to intention-to-treat principle were assessed separately because of their crucial methodologic importance by using a 3-point key methodologic index score (MIS; range, 0 to 3).

Results.—We retrieved 72 relevant RCTs that included 16,029 patients. The median OQS was 9.5. Allocation concealment, blinding, and analysis by intent to treat were reported only in 21 (29%), nine (12.5%), and 23 (32%) of the 72 RCTs, respectively. The median MIS was 1 with a minimum of 0 and a maximum of 2. On multivariate analysis, publication after 1996 and high impact factor remained independent and significant predictors of improved OQS. The sole variable associated with improved MIS was the publication of chemotherapy-only trials.

Conclusion.—Although the overall quality of sarcoma RCTs reporting has improved over time, reporting of key methodologic issues remains poor. This may lead to biased interpretation of sarcoma trial results.

▶ Orthopedic surgery unfortunately lags many other disciplines in performing high-quality prospective, randomized, controlled trials. In sarcoma treatment, trials may involve surgery, chemotherapy, and/or radiotherapy. These authors performed an analysis and standardized scoring to assess the methodologic quality of randomized trials reported in sarcomas.

Toulmonde et al did find real deficiencies in the methodology of many of our trials. Not all of their criticisms are justified. For example, appropriate blinding is not necessarily feasible for treatment such as radiotherapy and surgery in all cases. This is a weakness of this article, but its main message to call attention to deficiencies in our clinical investigations is sound and should be well received by all surgeons who care for these patients. Of note, publication after 1996 and publication in stronger journals were independent predictors of improved study quality. This offers hope that contemporary investigations published in our flagship journals represent high-quality evidence for the care of our patients.

P. S. Rose, MD

Tumor Reconstruction

Proximal Tibia Osteoarticular Allografts in Tumor Limb Salvage Surgery

Muscolo DL, Ayerza MA, Farfalli G, et al (Italian Hosp of Buenos Aires, Argentina)

Clin Orthop Relat Res 468:1396-1404, 2010

Background.—Resection of large tumors of the proximal tibia may be reconstructed with endoprostheses or allografts with fixation. Endoprosthetic replacement is associated with high failure rates and complications. Proximal tibia osteoarticular allografts after tumor resection allows restoration of bone stock and reconstruction of the extensor mechanism, but the long-term failure rates and complications are not known.

Questions/Purposes.—We therefore determined (1) the middle- and long-term survival of proximal tibia osteoarticular allografts, (2) their complications, and (3) functional (Musculoskeletal Tumor Society score) and radiographic (International Society of Limb Salvage) outcomes in patients treated with this reconstruction.

Patients and Methods.—We retrospectively reviewed 52 patients (58 reconstructions including six repeat reconstructions) who underwent osteoarticular proximal tibia allograft reconstructions after resection of a bone tumor. The minimum followup of the 46 surviving patients was 72 months (mean, 123 months; range, 10–250 months). Survival of the allograft was estimated using the Kaplan-Meier method. We documented outcomes using the Musculoskeletal Tumor Society functional scoring system and the International Society of Limb Salvage radiographic scoring system.

Results.—Six patients died from tumor-related causes without allograft failure before the 5-year radiographic followup. At last followup, 32 of the 52 remaining allografts were still in place; 20 failed owing to infections, local recurrences, or fractures. Overall allograft survival was 65% at 5 and 10 years, with an average Musculoskeletal Tumor Society functional score of 26 points and an average radiographic result of 87%.

Conclusions.—Based on these data we believe proximal tibia osteoarticular allograft is a valuable reconstructive procedure for large defects after resection of bone tumors.

Level of Evidence.—Level IV, therapeutic study. See the Guidelines for Authors for a complete description of levels of evidence.

▶ Many options are available to reconstruct the proximal tibia for musculoskeletal defects. Arthrodesis, endoprosthetic reconstruction, allograft prosthetic composite reconstruction, and osteoarticular allografts are the common choices.

Most commonly, allograft prosthetic composite and endoprosthetic reconstruction are used. Osteoarticular allografts have fallen out of favor because of a high complication rate. Osteoarticular allograft results are very much technique-dependent. The authors' institution has enormous experience with allograft reconstructions, and this is reflected in their results. Reconstruction of proximal tibial defects with allografts has some strong advantages. Notably, the femur is not violated with reimplantation of a prosthesis. In the absence of complications, osteoarticular allografts do well. It is important to maintain this reconstructive option in the repertoire of surgical capabilities.

C. P. Beauchamp, MD

Proximal and Total Humerus Reconstruction With the Use of an Aortograft Mesh

Marulanda GA, Henderson E, Cheong D, et al (Univ of South Florida, Tampa, FL; H. Lee Moffitt Cancer Ctr & Res Inst, Tampa, FL)

Clin Orthop Relat Res 468:2896-2903, 2010

Background.—The shoulder is commonly affected by primary and metastatic tumors. Current surgical techniques for complex shoulder reconstruction frequently result in functional deficits and instability. A synthetic mesh used in vascular surgery has the biological properties to provide mechanical constraint and improve stability after tumor related shoulder reconstruction.

Questions/Purposes.—We describe (1) surgical technique using a synthetic mesh during humerus reconstructions; (2) functional level defined as shoulder ROM of patients undergoing the procedure; (3) incidence of postoperative

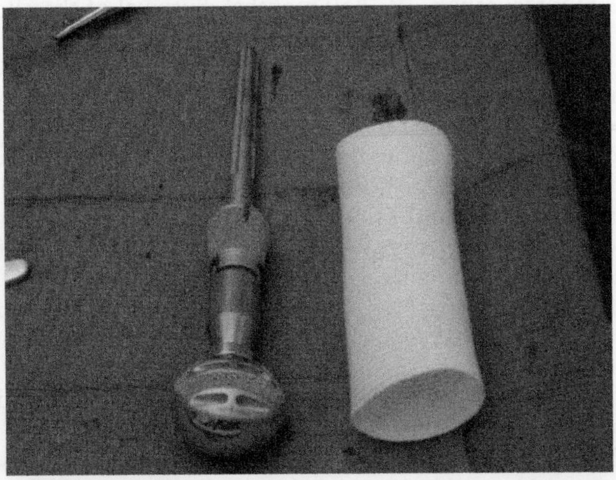

FIGURE 1.—Aortograft mesh with proximal humerus replacement is shown. (Reprinted from Marulanda GA, Henderson E, Cheong D, et al. Proximal and total humerus reconstruction with the use of an aortograft mesh. *Clin Orthop Relat Res.* 2010;468:2896-2903, with kind permission from Springer Science+Business Media.)

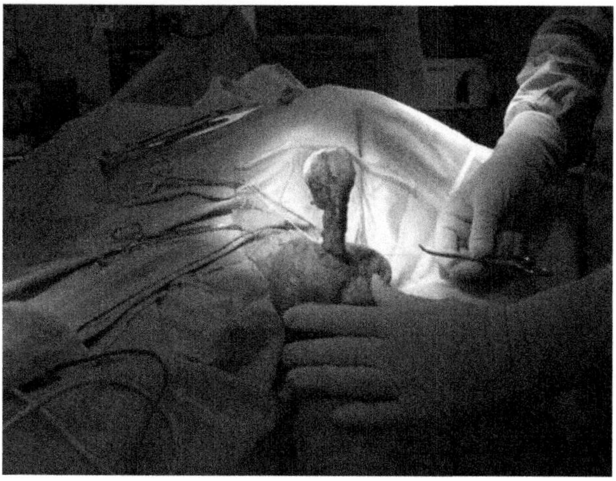

FIGURE 2.—Identification of the level of resection of proximal humerus is shown. (Reprinted from Marulanda GA, Henderson E, Cheong D, et al. Proximal and total humerus reconstruction with the use of an aortograft mesh. *Clin Orthop Relat Res.* 2010;468:2896-2903, with kind permission from Springer Science+Business Media.)

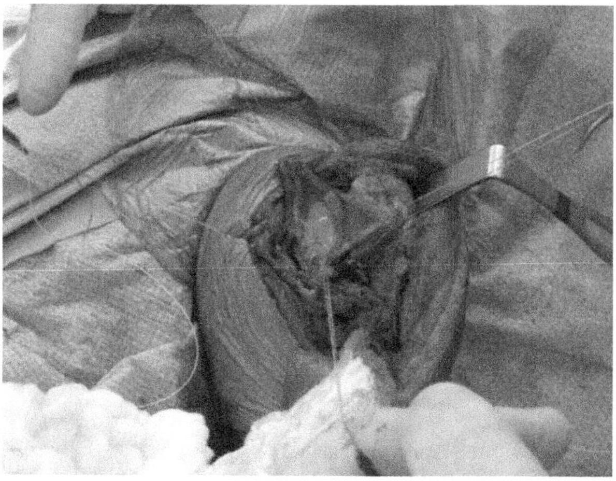

FIGURE 3.—Soft tissue structures, capsule and rotator cuff muscles are tagged and identified for repair. (Reprinted from Marulanda GA, Henderson E, Cheong D, et al. Proximal and total humerus reconstruction with the use of an aortograft mesh. *Clin Orthop Relat Res.* 2010;468:2896-2903, with kind permission from Springer Science+Business Media.)

dislocation and shoulder instability; and (4) complications associated with the use of the device.

Methods.—We retrospectively reviewed 16 patients with proximal humerus replacements reconstructed with a synthetic mesh from February 2006 to July 2008. Patients were followed clinically and radiographically for a minimum of 13 months (mean, 26 months; range, 13–43 months).

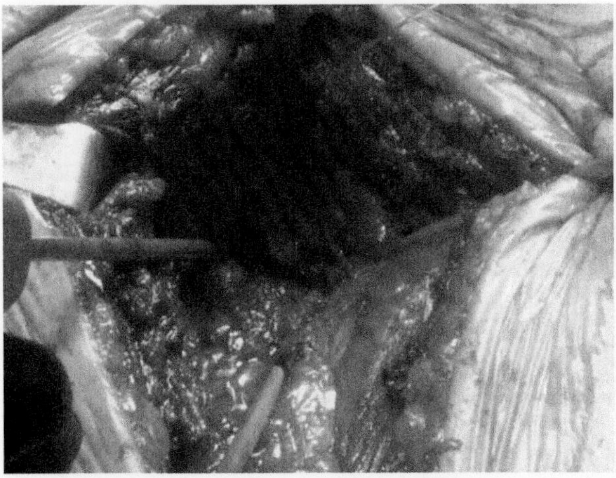

FIGURE 4.—The glenoid is visualized for anchoring of the aortograft mesh. (Reprinted from Marulanda GA, Henderson E, Cheong D, et al. Proximal and total humerus reconstruction with the use of an aortograft mesh. *Clin Orthop Relat Res.* 2010;468:2896-2903, with kind permission from Springer Science+Business Media.)

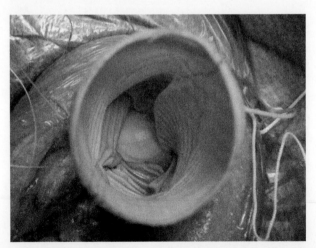

FIGURE 5.—The glenoid view with the aortograft secured in place is shown. (Reprinted from Marulanda GA, Henderson E, Cheong D, et al. Proximal and total humerus reconstruction with the use of an aortograft mesh. *Clin Orthop Relat Res.* 2010;468:2896-2903, with kind permission from Springer Science+Business Media.)

Results.—There were no shoulder dislocations at the latest followup. The mean shoulder flexion was 43° (range, 15°–170°) and mean shoulder abduction of 38 (range, 15°–110°). The mean operative time was 121 minutes (range, 80–170 minutes) and the mean blood loss was 220 mL (range, 50–750 mL). One patient had a superficial wound infection and none a deep infection requiring removal of the graft or prosthesis.

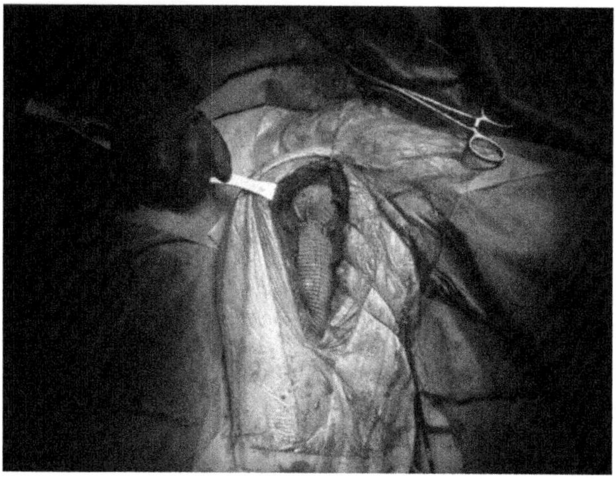

FIGURE 6.—A pursestring suture on the aortograft securing the neck of the prosthesis is shown. (Reprinted from Marulanda GA, Henderson E, Cheong D, et al. Proximal and total humerus reconstruction with the use of an aortograft mesh. *Clin Orthop Relat Res.* 2010;468:2896-2903, with kind permission from Springer Science+Business Media.)

Conclusions.—The data suggest the use of a synthetic vascular mesh for proximal humerus reconstruction may reduce dislocations and facilitate soft tissue attachment and reconstruction after tumor resection (Figs 1-6).

▶ The main problems we encounter when using an endoprosthesis to replace the proximal humerus are instability and poor function, primarily because of our inability to predictably reconstruct the soft tissue envelope around the implant. There is little hope of any biologic fixation to the metal. The use of synthetic fabric materials has been described to achieve stability around the prosthesis. This article describes a technique that is particularly effective in improving the major issues we have with this form of skeletal reconstruction. It is commendable that they did not have any patients with dislocations. This is a readily available solution to the major problem of proximal humeral replacement.

C. P. Beauchamp, MD

What is the Emotional Acceptance After Limb Salvage with an Expandable Prosthesis?

Henderson ER, Pepper AM, Marulanda GA, et al (USF Laurel Drive, Tampa, FL; et al)

Clin Orthop Relat Res 468:2933-2938, 2010

Background.—Limb preservation surgery for extremity sarcomas offers the promise of improved function and cosmesis over amputation. Application of limb salvage surgery for pediatric patients with expandable metallic endoprostheses is gaining acceptance. The few studies reporting these devices have focused on functional outcomes; one has addressed quality of life.

Questions/Purposes.—We asked the following questions: (1) how happy are these patients; (2) how do these patients perceive their bodies; (3) do these children have difficulty with social interactions; and (4) how satisfied are patients and their parents with their outcomes?

Methods.—We retrospectively identified and contacted 26 living patients who underwent limb salvage with an expandable device. The Pediatric Outcomes Data Collection Instrument was administered to 15 of the 26 families. Attention was paid to the happiness domain of the Pediatric Outcomes Data Collection Instrument and specific answers within this domain were reported.

Results.—Children who received limb salvage with an expandable endoprosthesis showed high emotional satisfaction with their outcome. Overall patients reported excellent perceptions of body image and physical attractiveness. Most patients reported frequent social interactions with their peers and no difficulty with making new friends.

Conclusions.—Although this study has a limited number of subjects and no control group, the data correlate with previously scores and indicate a high degree of emotional acceptance after limb salvage with an expandable endoprosthesis in a pediatric population.

▶ Limb preservation surgery for extremity sarcomas in the pediatric population has many challenges. There are a number of treatment options, ranging from amputation to limb preservation using some form of a growing or expandable prosthesis. Some of these treatments involve numerous surgical interventions. More modern devices allow for implant expansion without surgery. No matter which device or technique is used, numerous interventions are required to ultimately achieve skeletal maturity. The concern with all of these treatments is the effect this has on a growing child's psychological development. Children have been found to be remarkably resilient to surgical intervention and illness. Their ability to adapt to limb preservation surgery with expandable implants has been confirmed by this study. Although the size of the study group is small, this article provides reassuring support for the continued use of expandable endoprostheses in a pediatric population.

C. P. Beauchamp, MD

Non-invasive extendible endoprostheses for limb reconstruction in skeletally-mature patients

Sewell MD, Spiegelberg BGI, Hanna SA, et al (The Royal Natl Orthopaedic Hosp, Stanmore, England)

J Bone Joint Surg [Br] 91-B:1360-1365, 2009

We describe the application of a non-invasive extendible endoprosthetic replacement in skeletally-mature patients undergoing revision for failed joint replacement with resultant limb-length inequality after malignant or non-malignant disease. This prosthesis was developed for tumour surgery in skeletally-immature patients but has now been adapted for use in revision procedures to reconstruct the joint or facilitate an arthrodesis, replace bony defects and allow limb length to be restored gradually in the post-operative period.

We record the short-term results in nine patients who have had this procedure after multiple previous reconstructive operations. In six, the initial reconstruction had been performed with either allograft or endoprosthetic replacement for neoplastic disease and in three for non-neoplastic disease. The essential components of the prosthesis are a magnetic disc, a gearbox and a drive screw which allows painless lengthening of the prosthesis using the principle of electromagnetic induction. The mean age of the patients was 37 years (18 to 68) with a mean follow-up of 34 months (12 to 62). They had previously undergone a mean of six (2 to 14) open procedures on the affected limb before revision with the non-invasive extendible endoprosthesis.

The mean length gained was 56 mm (19 to 107) requiring a mean of nine (3 to 20) lengthening episodes performed in the outpatient department. There was one case of recurrent infection after revision of a previously infected implant and one fracture of the prosthesis after a fall. No amputations were performed. Planned exchange of the prosthesis was required in three patients after attainment of the maximum lengthening capacity of the implant. There was no failure of the lengthening mechanism. The Mean Musculoskeletal Tumour Society rating score was 22 of 30 available points (18 to 28).

The use of a non-invasive extendible endoprosthesis in this manner provided patients with good functional results and restoration of leg-length equality, without the need for multiple open lengthening procedures.

▶ We continue to make advances with expandable prostheses. It is clear that closed lengthening devices work and are becoming more reliable. The next task is to make an expandable device that is durable and can achieve the goal of being implanted without the need for future revision. This small series shows the potential of expandable devices in the revision situation. In many situations with a failed prosthetic reconstruction, a major limb length deficiency is part of the problem. The use of this device provides another tool to the reconstructive surgeon. The need for an expandable option with permanent reliable fixation and durable bearings is the next step.

C. P. Beauchamp, MD

The use of osteo-articular allografts for reconstruction after resection of the distal radius for tumour

Scoccianti G, Campanacci DA, Beltrami G, et al (Careggi Univ Hosp, Firenze, Italy)

J Bone Joint Surg [Br] 92-B:1690-1694, 2010

Several techniques have been described to reconstruct a mobile wrist joint after resection of the distal radius for tumour. We reviewed our experience of using an osteo-articular allograft to do this in 17 patients with a mean follow-up of 58.9 months (28 to 119).

The mean range of movement at the wrist was 56° flexion, 58° extension, 84° supination and 80° pronation. The mean ISOLS-MSTS score was 86% (63% to 97%) and the mean patient-rated wrist evaluation score was 16.5 (3 to 34). There was no local recurrence or distant metastases. The procedure failed in one patient with a fracture of the graft and an arthrodesis was finally required. Union was achieved at the host-graft interface in all except two cases. No patient reported more than modest non-disabling pain and six reported no pain at all. Radiographs showed early degenerative changes at the radiocarpal joint in every patient.

A functional pain-free wrist can be restored with an osteo-articular allograft after resection of the distal radius for bone tumour, thereby avoiding the donor site morbidity associated with an autograft. These results may deteriorate with time.

▶ Distal radius skeletal defects can be reconstructed in a variety of ways. An osteoarticular allograft offers the benefits of no donor morbidity as one would have using an autograft fibula and usually a good outcome. The authors have shown again the advantages of an osteoarticular graft in this series of patients. They have had extensive experience with the use of allografts, and their results emphasize again that experienced centers that use allografts frequently have the best results.

C. P. Beauchamp, MD

Tumor Treatment

Single Ray Amputation for Tumors of the Hand

Puhaindran ME, Healey JH, Athanasian EA (Memorial Sloan-Kettering Cancer Ctr, NY)

Clin Orthop Relat Res 468:1390-1395, 2010

Single ray amputation after hand trauma or infection can result in good aesthetic and functional outcomes. The role of this procedure in the management of aggressive benign or malignant hand tumors has been described only in case reports and small case series. We retrospectively reviewed the records of all 25 patients who underwent single ray amputations at our center during a 10-year period; there were seven index, five middle, six ring, and seven small ray amputations performed. The minimum followup was 2 months (mean, 36 months; range, 2–120 months), with four patients having a followup of 1 year or less. No patients had local recurrences, although two patients had positive resection margins. One underwent repeat resection followed by radiotherapy. The other was treated with radiotherapy alone, as local tumor control would have required a hand amputation. Functional assessment based on the Musculoskeletal Tumor Society staging system showed an average of 27.5 (range, 21–30). Patients who underwent perioperative radiotherapy experienced a decrease in functional ability. Grip strength was an average of 66% (range, 38%–100%) of the contralateral side. Our study suggests single ray amputation for hand tumors has a low local recurrence rate and high functional scores. However, function can be compromised by radiotherapy and a decrease in grip strength by a mean of 34% is to be expected.

Level of Evidence.—Level IV, case series. See Guidelines for Authors for a complete description of levels of evidence.

▶ This study includes a large group of patients who underwent a single ray amputation for a hand neoplasm. It has been shown that a single ray hand amputation results in minimal disruption to hand function. With careful planning and careful attention to details in the evaluation workup and biopsy of soft tissue tumors of the hand, excellent functional results can be obtained. The oncologic outcomes of this group of patients also reflects the careful treatment they received.

C. P. Beauchamp, MD

Staged Lengthening Arthroplasty for Pediatric Osteosarcoma around the Knee

Kong C-B, Lee S-Y, Jeon D-G (Korea Cancer Ctr Hosp, Seoul)
Clin Orthop Relat Res 468:1660-1668, 2010

Background.—Orthopaedic oncologists often must address leg-length discrepancy after resection of tumors in growing patients with osteosarcoma. There are various alternatives to address this problem. We describe a three-stage procedure: (1) temporary arthrodesis, (2) lengthening by Ilizarov apparatus, and (3) tumor prosthesis.

Questions/Purposes.—We asked (1) to what extent are affected limbs actually lengthened; (2) how many of the patients who undergo a lengthening procedure eventually achieve joint arthroplasty; and (3) can the three-stage procedure give patients a functioning joint with equalization of limb length?

Patients and Methods.—We reviewed 56 patients (younger than 14 years) with osteosarcoma who had staged lengthening arthroplasty between 1991 and 2004.

Results.—Thirty-five of the 56 patients (63%) underwent soft tissue lengthening, and of these 35, 28 (50% of the original group of 56) had implantation of a mobile joint. Three of the 28 prostheses were later removed owing to infection after arthroplasty. The overall average length gained was 7.8 cm (range, 4–14 cm), and 25 (71%) of the 35 patients had a mobile joint at final followup. The average Musculoskeletal Tumor Society functional score was 23.2 (range, 15–28) and limb-length discrepancy at final followup was 2.6 cm (range, 0–6.5 cm). Although most mobile joints had an acceptable ROM (average, 74.2°; range, 35°–110°), extension lag was frequent.

Conclusions.—Our approach is one option for skeletally immature patients, especially in situations where an expandable prosthesis is not available. However, this technique requires multiple stages and would be inappropriate for patients who cannot accept prolonged functional deficit owing to a limited lifespan or other reasons.

Level of Evidence.—Level IV, therapeutic study. See Guidelines for Authors for a complete description of levels of evidence (Fig 1).

▶ We have struggled for years to find the best method to care for patients who have skeletal defects with an immature skeleton. Tremendous advances have

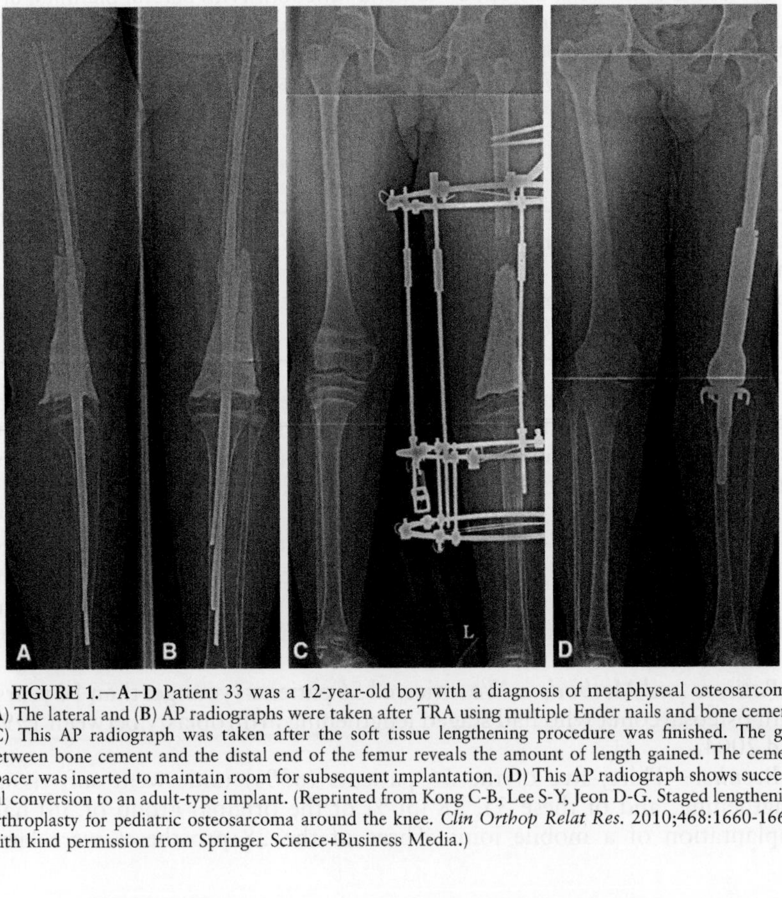

FIGURE 1.—A–D Patient 33 was a 12-year-old boy with a diagnosis of metaphyseal osteosarcoma. (A) The lateral and (B) AP radiographs were taken after TRA using multiple Ender nails and bone cement. (C) This AP radiograph was taken after the soft tissue lengthening procedure was finished. The gap between bone cement and the distal end of the femur reveals the amount of length gained. The cement spacer was inserted to maintain room for subsequent implantation. (D) This AP radiograph shows successful conversion to an adult-type implant. (Reprinted from Kong C-B, Lee S-Y, Jeon D-G. Staged lengthening arthroplasty for pediatric osteosarcoma around the knee. *Clin Orthop Relat Res.* 2010;468:1660-1668, with kind permission from Springer Science+Business Media.)

been made recently with expandable or growing endoprostheses. These devices are not available everywhere, and innovative techniques as described in this article further our surgical capabilities, allowing limb-sparing procedures to be offered to patients whose only alternative option is amputation. The surgical technique described is challenging, and with the use of an external fixator, the risk of infection is a concern. Nonetheless, this is an alternative method that can achieve limb preservation with equal leg lengths.

C. P. Beauchamp, MD

No Recurrences in Selected Patients after Curettage with Cryotherapy for Grade I Chondrosarcomas

Souna BS, Belot N, Duval H, et al (Centre Hospitalier Universitaire de Rennes, France)

Clin Orthop Relat Res 468:1956-1962, 2010

Background.—The low aggressiveness of Grade I chondrosarcomas is compatible with conservative surgical treatment.

Questions/Purpose.—We asked whether combined curettage and cryotherapy would yield low rates of recurrence and whether supplemental internal fixation would retain function with low rates of complications in patients with Grade I central chondrosarcomas of the proximal humerus or distal femur.

Methods.—We retrospectively reviewed 15 patients: nine women and six men with a mean age of 45 years (range, 26–70 years). All patients underwent curettage and cryosurgery through a cortical window; we replaced the window and plated the region with at least three screws beyond the curetted area. None of the patients was lost to followup, and 14 patients (93%) were reexamined by us after a minimum of 5 years (mean, 8 years; range, 5–11 years).

Results.—There were no perioperative anesthetic, neurologic, hardware, or healing complications. None of the patients had local recurrence or metastases develop. At last followup, the Musculoskeletal Tumor Society score was 27.9 (range, 22–30) and all patients had resumed their previous activities. No complications were associated with this simplified cryotherapy technique.

Conclusions.—The data confirm the appropriateness of conservative surgery for central low-grade chondrosarcomas of the proximal humerus and distal femur based on a combination of intralesional curettage and cryogenic parietal sterilization. Candidates for this approach should be chosen on the basis of the affected bone site, local extension staging, and clinicopathologic grading. We recommend supplementary internal fixation.

Level of Evidence.—Level IV, therapeutic study. See Guidelines for Authors for a complete description of levels of evidence.

▶ It has become evident over the past few years that the treatment for grade 1 chondrosarcoma of bone is intralesional resection. Many publications support this treatment. Low rates of local recurrence have been reported. Clearly, the morbidity of an intralesional curettage is much less than that of a resection. It is difficult, however, to clearly define those patients with a true grade 1 chondrosarcoma. In most serious cases, there must exist patients who have only enchondromas. It would be helpful in reports of this nature to have a scoring system for the radiographic appearance of the cartilaginous lesion. The images used in this article resemble a benign enchondroma, a lesion I would observe rather than treat surgically. If it is included in the category of a grade 1 chondrosarcoma—and by the histologic description of the lesion it is—I would expect a good result with an intralesional procedure.

C. P. Beauchamp, MD

Radiofrequency Ablation of Osteoid Osteoma in Atypical Locations: A Case Series

Akhlaghpoor S, Ahari AA, Shabestari AA, et al (Noor Med Imaging Ctr, Tehran, Iran; Tehran Univ of Med Sciences, Iran)
Clin Orthop Relat Res 468:1963-1970, 2010

Background.—Osteoid osteoma has a nidus surrounded by sclerotic bone with a size usually less than 20 mm. Its diagnosis is made on typical presentation of nocturnal pain and imaging findings. Excision of the niduses, which are often small and difficult to precisely identify, sometimes may result in resection of surrounding normal bone. Minimally invasive percutaneous treatments have been used to try to minimize resection of normal bone. Although minimally invasive radiofrequency ablation generally relieves pain, its ability to relieve pain is less well known in locations other than lower extremity long bones.

Questions/Purposes.—We determined the pain relief and complication rates after radiofrequency ablation of osteoid osteomas presenting in atypical locations and followed patients to assess possible recurrence or late complications.

Patients and Methods.—We retrospectively reviewed 21 patients with osteoid osteomas in unusual locations (eg, hip, radioulnar joint, and proximal phalanx) in whom we used radiofrequency ablation. Postoperative activities were not restricted for any of the patients. We assessed the time for patients to become symptom free, their activity status, and possible recurrence or complications. The minimum clinical followup was 12 months (mean, 27.8 months; range, 12–37 months).

Results.—All patients became symptom free within 24 hours to 1 week. During followup, none of the patients experienced recurrence or any major complications.

Conclusions.—Radiofrequency ablation for osteoid osteomas in unusual locations reliably relieves pain with few complications and recurrences at short-term followup.

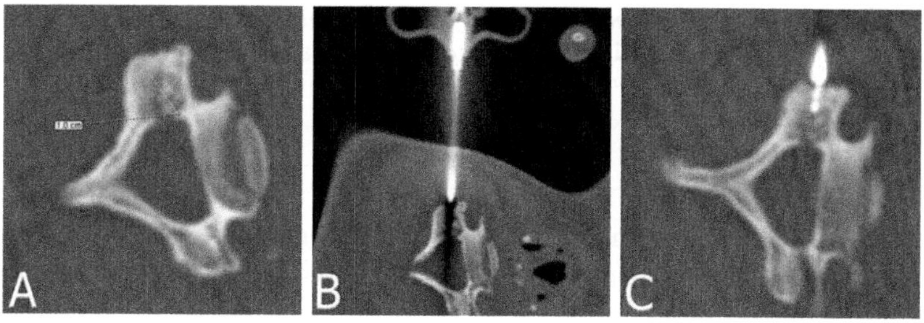

FIGURE 3.—**A–C** RFA for a 10-mm-diameter OO of C6 in a 17-year-old girl is shown. (**A**) Because of the risky position, drilling was not performed, and (**B**) the coaxial guide provided the track for the radiofrequency needle. (**C**) The radiofrequency needle is shown in the nidus. (Reprinted from Akhlaghpoor S, Ahari AA, Shabestari AA, et al. Radiofrequency ablation of osteoid osteoma in atypical locations: a case series. *Clin Orthop Relat Res.* 2010;468:1963-1970, with kind permission from Springer Science+Business Media.)

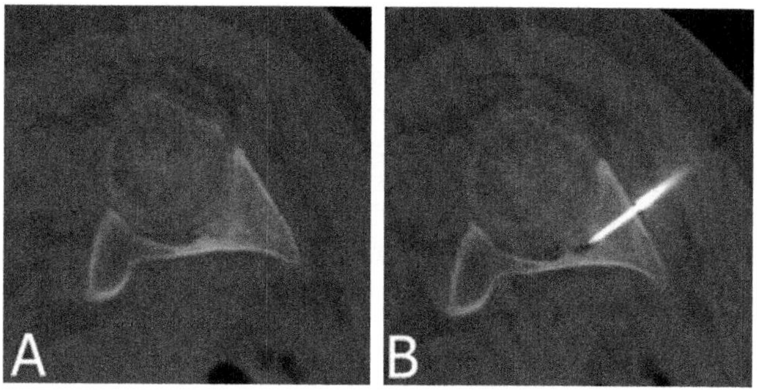

FIGURE 4.—**A–B** (**A**) An intraarticular OO of the acetabulum with an 11-mm-diameter nidus and (**B**) the radiofrequency needle placed in its nidus are shown. Surgical treatment of this lesion is difficult with possible major disabilities. (Reprinted from Akhlaghpoor S, Ahari AA, Shabestari AA, et al. Radiofrequency ablation of osteoid osteoma in atypical locations: a case series. *Clin Orthop Relat Res.* 2010;468:1963-1970, with kind permission from Springer Science+Business Media.)

Level of Evidence.—Level IV, case series. See Guidelines for Authors for a complete description of level of evidence (Figs 3 and 4).

▶ Percutaneous radiofrequency ablation has become the treatment of choice for osteoid osteomas. It has a low morbidity and complication rates and a high rate of cure. It is perhaps one of the greatest recent advances in tumor care when one considers the impact on the patient. As the authors have shown, this technique can be used almost anywhere in the body. Close proximity to major nervous structures and articular surfaces challenge the interventional radiologist. This can result in variable application of this technique in such locations. Until we have a method of monitoring collateral damage (MRI ablation), this will be the limitation of CT-guided radiofrequency ablation.

C. P. Beauchamp, MD

Multiplanar Osteotomy with Limited Wide Margins: A Tissue Preserving Surgical Technique for High-Grade Bone Sarcomas

Avedian RS, Haydon RC, Peabody TD (Stanford Univ Med Ctr, Redwood City, CA; Univ of Chicago Pritzker School of Medicine, IL)

Clin Orthop Relat Res 468:2754-2764, 2010

Background.—Limb-salvage surgery has been used during the last several decades to treat patients with high-grade bone sarcomas. In the short- and intermediate-term these surgeries have been associated with relatively good function and low revision rates. However, long-term studies show a high rate of soft tissue, implant, and bone-related complications. Multiplanar osteotomy with limited wide margins uses angled bone cuts to resect bone tumors with the goal of complete tumor removal while sparing host tissue although its impact on local recurrence is not known.

Questions/Purposes.—We determined whether multiplanar osteotomy was associated with local recurrences, reconstruction failures, and allograft nonunions.

Patients and Methods.—We retrospectively reviewed the charts of six patients. Four patients had an osteosarcoma, one had a Ewing's sarcoma, and one had a chondrosarcoma. Patient and treatment factors such as age, diagnosis, percent of tumor necrosis (if applicable), margin status, and time to allograft union were recorded. In all patients, reconstruction was performed with an intercalary allograft cut to fit the residual defect. The minimum followup was 25 months (average, 39 months; range, 24–66 months).

Results.—No patient experienced a local recurrence or metastasis, and all patients were alive and disease-free at the most recent followup. All allografts healed during the study period.

Conclusion.—With careful patient selection, the multiplanar osteotomy resection technique may be considered an option for treating patients with high-grade bone sarcomas, and, when compared with traditional surgical techniques, may lead to improved healing and function of the involved extremity.

Level of Evidence.—Level IV, therapeutic study. See the guidelines online for a complete description of levels of evidence (Fig 1).

▶ Improvements in radiographic imaging have had a great impact on the treatment of patients with musculoskeletal tumors. This is particularly so with bone tumors. Our ability to do joint-sparing resections with extremely narrow margins would not have been possible in the past. Such imaging permits us to preserve bone with other forms of resections. This study describes the outcomes of patients who had bone tumor resections with osteotomies that in the past would have removed more bone than necessary. In our quest to preserve more bone, we risk the possibility of increasing the chance of local recurrence. This study, although with small numbers, describes the use of a multiplanar osteotomy. This has the advantage of providing a greater surface area for bone healing

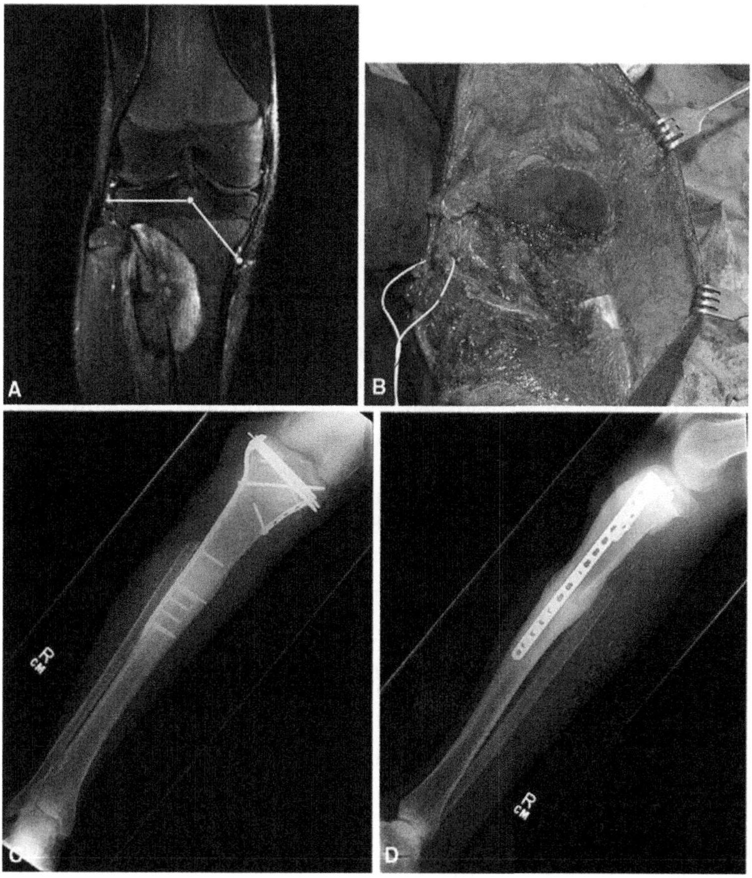

FIGURE 1.—Patient 4 was a 14-year-old boy with a high-grade osteosarcoma. (**A**) An example of preoperative planning on a coronal T2 MR image is shown. The yellow lines represent proposed osteotomy planes. Similar planning was completed on sagittal and axial images. The osteotomy spares a portion of the medial collateral ligament that provides stability to the final reconstruction. (**B**) An intraoperative photograph shows residual host bone after the multiplanar osteotomy making it possible to perform a joint-sparing intercalary osteotomy. (**C**) Anteroposterior and (**D**) lateral radiographs obtained 18 months after surgery show united allograft to host bone. For interpretation of the references to color in this figure legend, the reader is referred to web version of this article. (Reprinted from Avedian RS, Haydon RC, Peabody TD. Multiplanar osteotomy with limited wide margins: a tissue preserving surgical technique for high-grade bone sarcomas. *Clin Orthop Relat Res.* 2010;468:2754-2764, with kind permission from Springer Science+Business Media.)

and improving the options for skeletal fixation. This did not come at an increased risk of local recurrence in this small group of patients.

C. P. Beauchamp, MD

Revision of Broken Knee Megaprostheses: New Solution to Old Problems

Agarwal M, Gulia A, Ravi B, et al (PD Hinduja Natl Hosp & Med Res Centre, Mumbai, India; Tata Memorial Centre, Mumbai, India; Indian Inst of Technology, Powai, India)

Clin Orthop Relat Res 468:2904-2913, 2010

Background.—Low-cost indigenous megaprostheses used in the developing world are prone to mechanical failure but the frequency and causes are not well established.

Questions/Purposes.—We retrospectively analyzed the causes of failure, particularly design, and suggest changes to reduce the breakage. We also report our experience with revision surgery.

Methods.—We identified 28 breakages in 266 megaprosthetic knee arthroplasties performed between January 2000 and December 2006. Twenty-six breakages were revised to another prosthesis. The complications were studied and the function was evaluated. Prostheses were studied for failure by the computer-aided design program SolidWorks® and Hyperworks® for finite element analysis (FEA). Design improvements were performed based on these results.

Results.—In 21 cases, the failure occurred at the stem-collar junction, the point of maximum stress predicted by FEA. Stainless steel implants were prone to failure. There was one early and one late infection. Three patients died of metastatic disease. The most difficult surgical step involved the removal of the well-cemented broken stem from the intramedullary canal. Musculoskeletal Tumor Society scores varied from 27 to 29 after revision. FEA revealed stress could be reduced by filleting the stem-collar junction and by two-piece stems.

Conclusions.—Revisions of broken total knee megaprostheses, though technically difficult, have allowed patients reasonable function. We recommend design analysis for custom prostheses to point to areas of weakness. Breakages can be reduced by using titanium stems and filleting the junction or by having two-piece inserted stems. Incorporating these changes has reduced the failures in our experience.

▶ I selected this article because it demonstrates the capabilities of musculoskeletal oncologic surgeons throughout the world. There are many challenges to basic health care, let alone complex reconstructive procedures, in many countries in the world. The development and use of an endoprosthetic system that is both inexpensive and durable is a challenge. This article describes the evolution and ongoing improvements in the design and manufacturer of such an implant. It is a testament to the spread of medical and surgical education.

C. P. Beauchamp, MD

Site-dependent Replacement or Internal Fixation for Postradiation Femur Fractures After Soft Tissue Sarcoma Resection

Kim HJ, Healey JH, Morris CD, et al (Hosp for Special Surgery, NY; Memorial Sloan-Kettering Cancer Ctr, NY)

Clin Orthop Relat Res 468:3035-3040, 2010

Background.—High-dose radiation retards bone healing, compromising the surgical results of radiation-induced fractures. Prosthetic replacement has traditionally been reserved as a salvage option but may best achieve the clinical goals of eliminating pain, restoring function and avoiding complications.

Questions/Purposes.—We asked whether patients undergoing prosthetic replacement at index surgery for radiation-related subtrochanteric or diaphyseal fractures of the femur had fewer complications than those undergoing open reduction internal fixation at index operation.

Methods.—We retrospectively reviewed records from 1045 patients with soft tissue sarcomas treated with surgical resection and high-dose radiation therapy between 1982 and 2009 and identified 37 patients with 39 fractures. We recorded patient demographics, diagnosis, type of surgical resection, total radiation dose, fracture location and pattern, years after radiation the fracture occurred, type of surgical fixation, and associated complications.

Results.—Patients undergoing prosthetic replacement at index surgery had a lower number of major complications and revision surgeries than those undergoing index open reduction internal fixation. Patients undergoing open reduction internal fixation at index surgery had a nonunion rate of 63% (19 of 30). Fractures located in the metaphysis were more likely to heal than those located in the subtrochanteric or diaphyseal regions.

Conclusions.—Radiation-induced fractures have poor healing potential. Our data suggest an aggressive approach to fracture treatment with a prosthetic replacement can minimize complications and the need for revision surgery (Table 4).

► A radiation-associated fracture of the femur is a major problem and is completely different than a conventional femoral fracture. Unfortunately, the standard fracture management for this problem is fraught with complications. This fracture has a predictable nonunion outcome, and, unless the circumstances

TABLE 4.—Nonunion Rates Seen in Our Study and in Other Studies

Study	Nonunion Rate	Total Number of Patients in the Study	Overall Complication Rate (All Types)
Donati et al. [5]	57%	113	75%
Helmstedter et al. [10]	45%	20	65%
Lin et al. [13]	75%	12	75%
Kim et al. [current study]	63%	39	58%

Editor's Note: Please refer to original journal article for full references.

are favorable for healing (good soft tissues and a metaphyseal location), you can expect the fracture to not heal. It is difficult to make the decision to opt for endoprosthetic replacement as an index procedure, but the authors have demonstrated that in most cases it is the best choice. Persistent attempts to achieve fracture healing only contribute to a more difficult situation with increased scarring, infection risk, and the prospects of wound healing problems. The management of this problem should include the advice of surgeons familiar with radiation therapy and its consequences.

C. P. Beauchamp, MD

Recurrence After and Complications Associated With Adjuvant Treatments for Sacral Giant Cell Tumor

Ruggieri P, Mavrogenis AF, Ussia G, et al (Univ of Bologna, Italy; Athens Univ Med School, Greece)

Clin Orthop Relat Res 468:2954-2961, 2010

Background.—The best treatment of giant cell tumor of the sacrum is controversial. It is unclear whether adjuvant treatment with intralesional surgery reduces recurrences or increases morbidity.

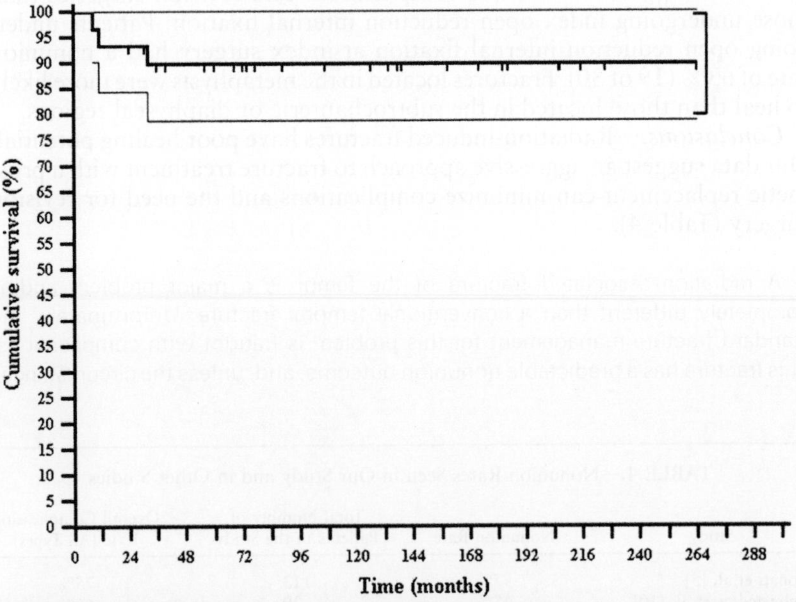

FIGURE 1.—A graph showing the overall survival to local recurrence. The overall survival to local recurrence was 90% at 60 and 120 months. (Reprinted from Ruggieri P, Mavrogenis AF, Ussia G, et al. Recurrence after and complications associated with adjuvant treatments for sacral giant cell tumor. *Clin Orthop Relat Res.* 2010;468:2954-2961, with kind permission from Springer Science+Business Media.)

Questions/Purposes.—We therefore asked whether adjuvants altered recurrence rates and complications after intralesional surgery for sacral giant cell tumors.

Methods.—We retrospectively studied 31 patients with sacral giant cell tumors treated with intralesional surgery with and without adjuvants. Survival to local recurrence was evaluated using Kaplan-Meier analysis. The differences in survival to local recurrence with and without adjuvants were evaluated using multivariate Cox regression analysis. Complications were recorded from clinical records and images. The minimum followup was 36 months (median, 108 months; range, 36–276 months).

Results.—Overall survival to local recurrence was 90% at 60 and 120 months. Survival to local recurrence with and without radiation was 91% and 89%, with and without embolization was 91% and 86%, and with and without local adjuvants was 88% and 92%, respectively. Adjuvants had no influence on local recurrence. Mortality was 6%: one patient died at 14 days postoperatively from a massive pulmonary embolism and another patient had radiation and died of a high-grade sarcoma. Fifteen of the 31 patients (48%) had one or more complications: eight patients (26%) had wound complications and seven patients (23%) had massive bleeding during curettage with hemodynamic instability. L5-S2

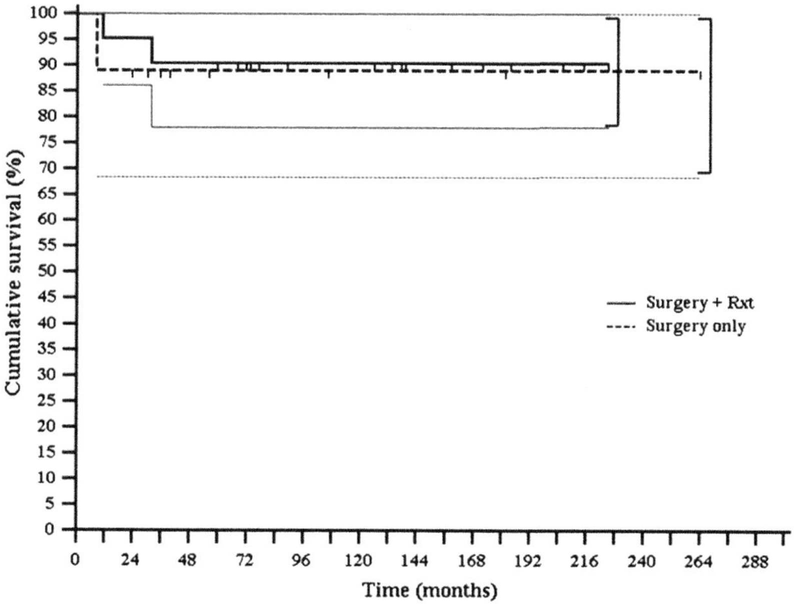

FIGURE 2.—A graph showing the survival to local recurrence with and without radiation therapy. The survival to local recurrence with and without radiation therapy was 91% and 89%, respectively, at 60 and 120 months (95% confidence interval: 0.064–8.605). (Reprinted from Ruggieri P, Mavrogenis AF, Ussia G, et al. Recurrence after and complications associated with adjuvant treatments for sacral giant cell tumor. *Clin Orthop Relat Res.* 2010;468:2954-2961, with kind permission from Springer Science+Business Media.)

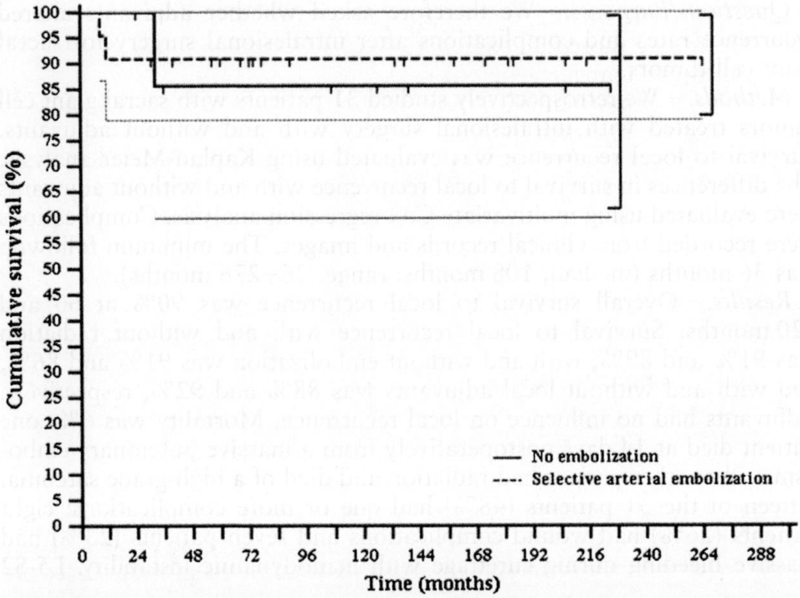

FIGURE 3.—A graph showing the survival to local recurrence with and without preoperative selective arterial embolization. The survival to local recurrence with and without preoperative selective arterial embolization was 91% and 86% at 60 and 120 months, respectively (95% confidence interval: 0.068–8.449). (Reprinted from Ruggieri P, Mavrogenis AF, Ussia G, et al. Recurrence after and complications associated with adjuvant treatments for sacral giant cell tumor. *Clin Orthop Relat Res.* 2010;468:2954-2961, with kind permission from Springer Science+Business Media.)

neurologic deficits decreased from 23% preoperatively to 13% postoperatively; S3-S4 deficits increased from 16% to 33%.

Conclusions.—Adjuvants did not change the likelihood of local recurrence when combined with intralesional surgery but the complication rate was high (Figs 1-3).

▶ Giant cell tumors (GCTs) arising in the sacrum are difficult to manage. The use of adjuvant treatment is heavily relied on. Topical or intralesional adjuvants such as thermal or chemical treatments are limited in their use because of their potential neurotoxicity. Global adjuvants such as embolization or radiation therapy are more universally applied, yet we have few data to support their effectiveness. This article with admitted limitations supports that fact. The authors have not shown any advantage to adjuvant treatment of patients with GCTs of the sacrum. It is unlikely that we will ever have a controlled study of this problem, and we will be left to wrestle with the issue of adjuvant treatment for local control every time we care for a patient with a sacral GCTs.

C. P. Beauchamp, MD

Surgical Management of 121 Benign Proximal Fibula Tumors

Abdel MP, Papagelopoulos PJ, Morrey ME, et al (Mayo Clinic, Rochester, MN; Athens Univ Med School, Greece)

Clin Orthop Relat Res 468:3056-3062, 2010

Background.—Tumors of the fibula comprise only 2.5% of primary bone lesions. Patients with aggressive benign tumors in the proximal fibula may require en bloc resection. Peroneal nerve function, knee stability, and recurrence are substantial concerns with these resections. The incidence and fate of these complications is not well-known owing to the small numbers of patients in previous reports.

Questions/Purposes.—We therefore analyzed the incidence of peroneal nerve palsy, knee stability, and local recurrence following surgical treatment of benign proximal fibula tumors.

Methods.—We retrospectively reviewed the charts of 120 patients (121 tumors) with histologically confirmed aggressive benign tumors of the proximal fibula. There were 56 males and 64 females with an average age of 24 years (range, 2–64 years). The most common diagnosis was osteochondroma (38%) followed by giant cell tumor (19%). Pain (94%), palpable mass (39%), and peroneal nerve symptoms (12%) were the most common presenting symptoms. Of the 121 tumors, 56 (46%) underwent en bloc resection. The minimum followup was 2 years (mean, 9 years; range 2 to 49 years; median, 7.4 years).

Results.—Postoperative complications included nine peroneal nerve palsies (six transient, three permanent), one deep venous thrombosis, and one wound dehiscence. No long-term knee instability was seen with repair of the lateral collateral ligament. Ten patients had recurrences, with 70% of local recurrences occurring in patients who underwent intralesional excision.

Conclusions.—Given the higher recurrence rate with curettage, patients with aggressive proximal fibula tumors benefit from en bloc resection.

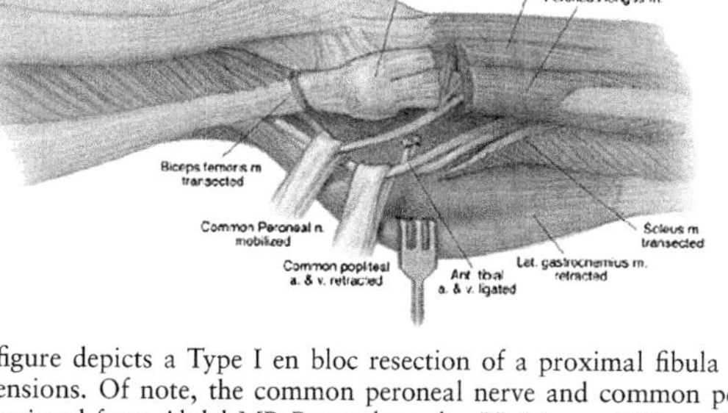

FIGURE 3.—This figure depicts a Type I en bloc resection of a proximal fibula tumor with a thin muscle cuff in all dimensions. Of note, the common peroneal nerve and common popliteal artery and vein are preserved. (Reprinted from Abdel MP, Papagelopoulos PJ, Morrey ME, et al. Surgical management of 121 benign proximal fibula tumors. *Clin Orthop Relat Res.* 2010;468:3056-3062, with kind permission from Springer Science+Business Media.)

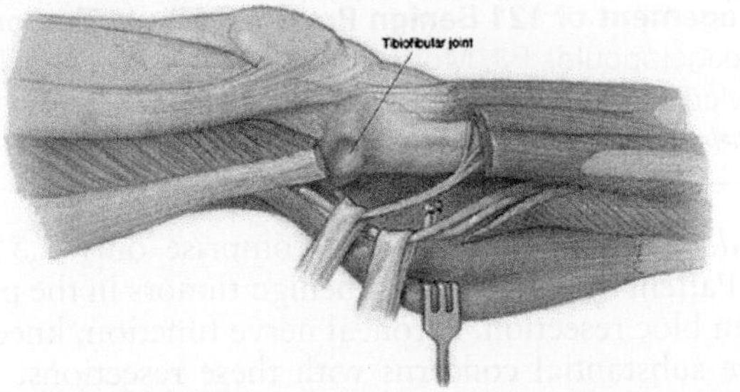

FIGURE 4.—Type I en bloc proximal fibula resections require detachment of the lateral collateral ligament and biceps femoris tendon. After the resection, the tibiofibular joint is exposed. (Reprinted from Abdel MP, Papagelopoulos PJ, Morrey ME, et al. Surgical management of 121 benign proximal fibula tumors. *Clin Orthop Relat Res*. 2010;468:3056-3062, with kind permission from Springer Science+ Business Media.)

The overall morbidity is low, but postoperative permanent peroneal palsy remains a concern (3%) (Figs 3 and 4).

▶ Benign tumors of the proximal fibula are rare. This study includes a large group of patients with this condition. The treatment options for this group are either intralesional curettage or proximal fibular resection. The authors have demonstrated that resecting the proximal fibula carries with it a low risk of complications. Local control is improved, and knee stability is not an issue. Ligamentous reconstruction is relatively straightforward, and because stability is not a significant problem postoperatively, it may not be crucial. Nerve injury, however, is a problem. The peroneal nerve is unpredictable in its sensitivity to surgical dissection. Nonetheless, for those lesions that have a propensity to local recurrence, a proximal fibular resection is preferable to intralesional curettage.

C. P. Beauchamp, MD

Surgical Margins and Local Control in Resection of Sacral Chordomas

Ruggieri P, Angelini A, Ussia G, et al (Univ of Bologna, Italy)
Clin Orthop Relat Res 468:2939-2947, 2010

Background.—The treatment of choice in sacral chordoma is surgical resection, although the risk of local recurrence and metastasis remains high. The quality of surgical margins obtained at initial surgery is the primary factor to improve survival reducing the risk of local recurrence, but proximal sacral resections are associated with substantial perioperative morbidity.

Questions/Purposes.—We considered survivorship related to local recurrence in terms of surgical margins, level of resection, and previous surgery.

Methods.—We retrospectively reviewed 56 patients with sacral chordomas treated with surgical resection. Thirty-seven were resected above S3 by a combined anterior and posterior approach and 19 at or below S3 by a posterior approach. Nine of these had had previous intralesional

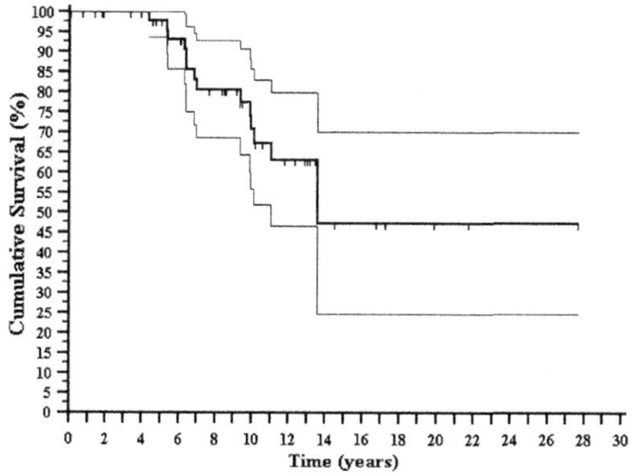

FIGURE 1.—Survival was 97% at 5 years, 71% at 10 years, and 47% at 15 years. (Reprinted from Ruggieri P, Angelini A, Ussia G, et al. Surgical margins and local control in resection of sacral chordomas. *Clin Orthop Relat Res.* 2010;468:2939-2947, with kind permission from Springer Science+Business Media.)

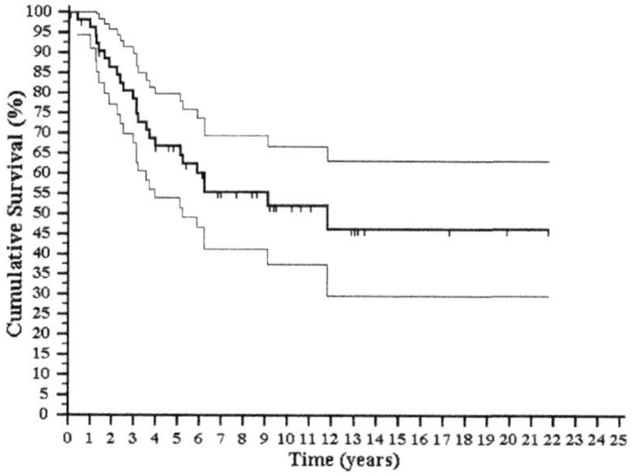

FIGURE 2.—Survivorship to local recurrence was 65% at 5 years and 52% at 10 years. (Reprinted from Ruggieri P, Angelini A, Ussia G, et al. Surgical margins and local control in resection of sacral chordomas. *Clin Orthop Relat Res.* 2010;468:2939-2947, with kind permission from Springer Science+Business Media.)

surgery elsewhere. The minimum followup was 3 years (mean, 9.5 years; range, 3–28 years).

Results.—Overall survival was 97% at 5 years, 71% at 10 years, and 47% at 15 years. Survivorship to local recurrence was 65% at 5 years and 52% at 10 years. Thirty percent of patients developed metastases. Wide margins were associated with increased survivorship to local recurrence. We found no differences in local recurrence between wide and wide-contaminated margins (that is, if the tumor or its pseudocapsule was exposed intraoperatively, but further tissue was removed to achieve wide margins). Previous intralesional surgery was associated with an increased local recurrence rate. We observed no differences in the recurrence rate in resections above S3 or at and below S3.

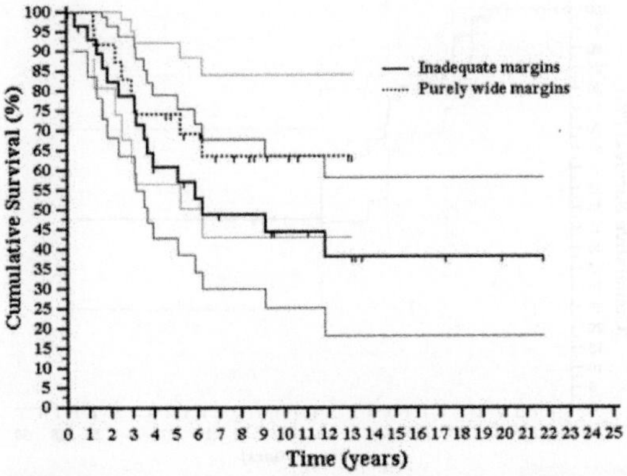

FIGURE 3.—Survivorship to local recurrence was increased (p = 0.045) in patients with wide compared with inadequate margins. (Reprinted from Ruggieri P, Angelini A, Ussia G, et al. Surgical margins and local control in resection of sacral chordomas. *Clin Orthop Relat Res*. 2010;468:2939-2947, with kind permission from Springer Science+Business Media.)

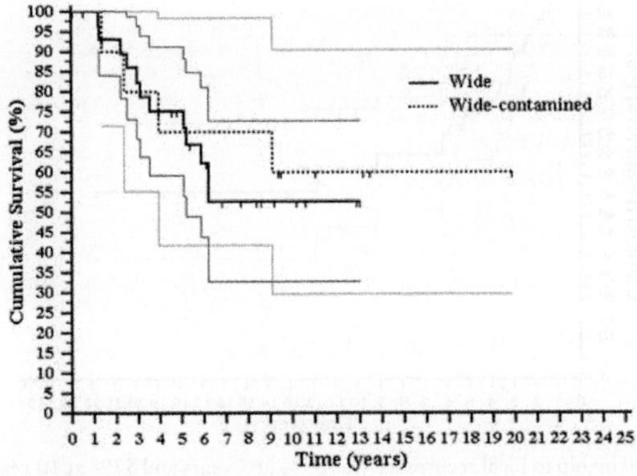

FIGURE 4.—Survivorship to local recurrence was not increased (p = 0.677) in patients with wide compared with wide-contaminated margins. (Reprinted from Ruggieri P, Angelini A, Ussia G, et al. Surgical margins and local control in resection of sacral chordomas. *Clin Orthop Relat Res*. 2010;468:2939-2947, with kind permission from Springer Science+Business Media.)

Conclusions.—Surgical margins affect the risk of local recurrence. Previous intralesional surgery was associated with a higher rate of local recurrence. Intraoperative contamination did not affect the risk of local recurrence when wide margins were subsequently attained (Figs 1-6).

▶ Chordomas are rare, low-grade, slow-growing, primary bone tumors. Surgery is the primary method of management. Because adjuvant treatments are not available for this disease, proper surgical management is crucial to patient survival. This article is from one of the most experienced oncologic groups in the world. The surgical management of chordomas is one of the more challenging orthopedic oncologic procedures. They have demonstrated that there

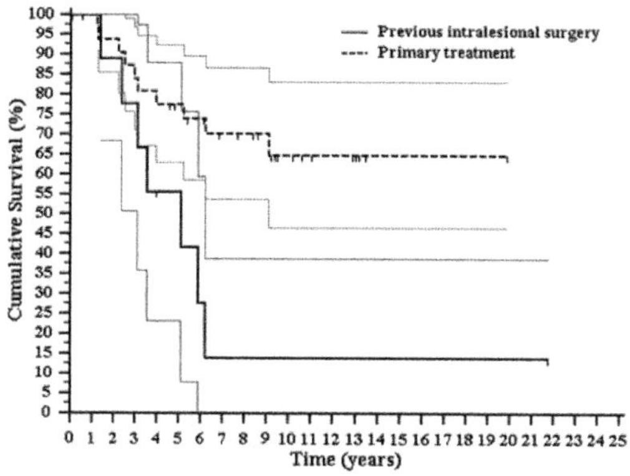

FIGURE 5.—Survivorship to local recurrence was decreased (p = 0.010) in patients with previous intralesional surgery compared with patients with primary surgical treatment at our institution. (Reprinted from Ruggieri P, Angelini A, Ussia G, et al. Surgical margins and local control in resection of sacral chordomas. *Clin Orthop Relat Res.* 2010;468:2939-2947, with kind permission from Springer Science+Business Media.)

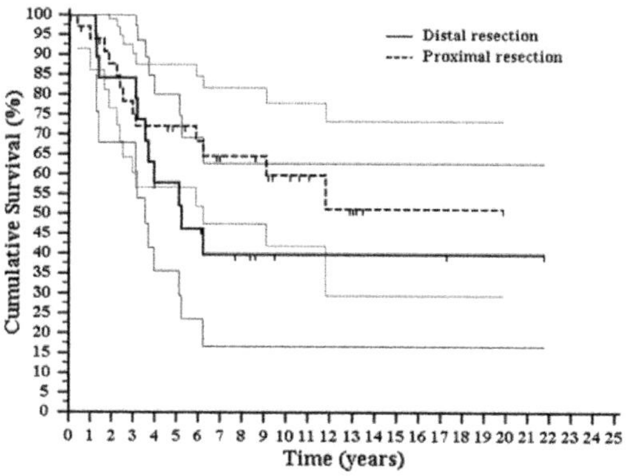

FIGURE 6.—No differences (p = 0.224) between proximal and distal sacral resection were observed. (Reprinted from Ruggieri P, Angelini A, Ussia G, et al. Surgical margins and local control in resection of sacral chordomas. *Clin Orthop Relat Res.* 2010;468:2939-2947, with kind permission from Springer Science+Business Media.)

is no difference between wide and wide contaminated margins. This emphasizes the importance of careful surgical technique, as they were able to recover a contaminated margin with further tissue removal. Previous interlesional surgery implies a poorly planned surgical intervention. Understandably, even with further surgery, this carries a higher risk of local recurrence. Above all else, chordomas require adequate surgery.

C. P. Beauchamp, MD

The Role of Surgery and Adjuvants to Survival in Pagetic Osteosarcoma

Ruggieri P, Calabrò T, Montalti M, et al (Univ of Bologna, Italy)

Clin Orthop Relat Res 468:2962-2968, 2010

Background.—Osteosarcoma is a rare complication of Paget's disease with a very poor prognosis. Treatment is controversial: the older age of the patients affected by Paget's disease may limit the use of chemotherapy and axial involvement may limit the practicality of surgery.

Questions/Purposes.—The purposes of this study are (1) to report the survival in patients treated for osteosarcoma in Paget's disease; (2) to identify correlations between type of treatment and survival comparing our data with those in the literature; (3) to determine if the extent of Paget's disease and risk of malignant transformation are associated; (4) to assess if prognosis is related with site; and (5) to identify the variations of histologic subtypes of these osteosarcomas.

Methods.—We retrospectively reviewed the medical records of 26 patients treated between 1961 and 2006 who had bone sarcoma arising from a site of Paget's disease. Twenty two of the 26 patients had surgery. In six surgery only was performed; three had surgery, adjuvant chemotherapy, and radiotherapy; one surgery and radiotherapy; 12 underwent surgery and chemotherapy, adjuvant in 10 patients and neoadjuvant in two; two had only radiotherapy and two had only chemotherapy. We performed survival analyses between various combinations of treatment.

Results.—At last followup four patients had no evidence of disease (NED) at a minimum followup of 42.6 months (mean, 139 months; range, 42.6–257.4 months) and 22 died with disease (DWD) at a minimum time of 1 month (mean, 20.2 months; range, 1–84 months). One of the six patients (11%) treated with surgery only had NED at 10 years; the other five died from disease at a mean of 30 months. Three of 12 patients (25%) treated with surgery and chemotherapy are NED at a mean followup

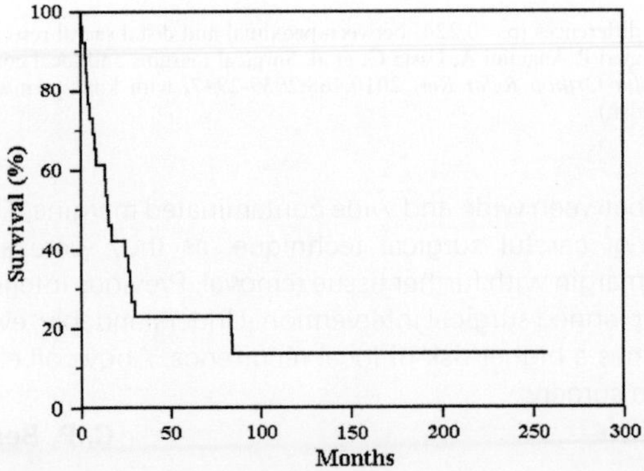

FIGURE 3.—Kaplan-Meier curve of all 26 patients shows a 5-year survival rate less than 25%. There is a higher mortality rate in the first 2 years after treatment. (Reprinted from Ruggieri P, Calabrò T, Montalti M, et al. The role of surgery and adjuvants to survival in pagetic osteosarcoma. *Clin Orthop Relat Res.* 2010;468:2962-2968, with kind permission from Springer Science+Business Media.)

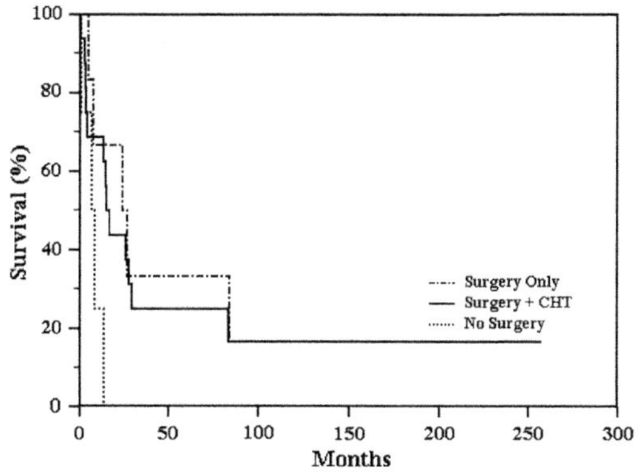

FIGURE 4.—Kaplan-Meier curve reporting the type of treatment outlines the high mortality in patients treated without surgery. The curve shows a better trend ($p = 0.1057$) in patients treated with surgery only or with surgery plus chemotherapy (CHT). (Reprinted from Ruggieri P, Calabrò T, Montalti M, et al. The role of surgery and adjuvants to survival in pagetic osteosarcoma. *Clin Orthop Relat Res.* 2010;468:2962-2968, with kind permission from Springer Science+Business Media.)

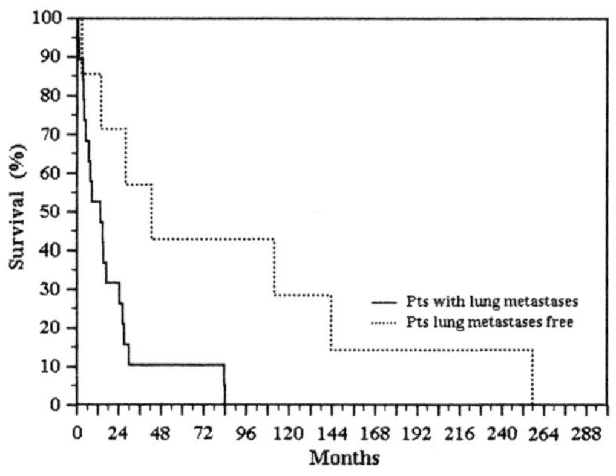

FIGURE 5.—Kaplan-Meier curve compares survival of patients with pulmonary metastatic disease with survival of patients who are lung tumor-free. Patients with pulmonary metastatic disease at the time of diagnosis had worse survival ($p = 0.013$) than those who did not. (Reprinted from Ruggieri P, Calabrò T, Montalti M, et al. The role of surgery and adjuvants to survival in pagetic osteosarcoma. *Clin Orthop Relat Res.* 2010;468:2962-2968, with kind permission from Springer Science+Business Media.)

of 12 years; nine died of disease at a mean of 24 months. All patients treated without surgery died at a mean of 7.5 months (range, 1–13.7 months).

Conclusions.—Despite improvements in surgery and medical treatments the prognosis remains poor in patients with Paget's sarcoma (Figs 3-5).

► Osteosarcomas are a rare complication of Paget's disease. Typically, this occurs in an older age population. Standard treatment for osteogenic sarcoma includes aggressive high-dose chemotherapy, something that this age group cannot tolerate well. Historically, osteosarcoma in Paget's disease has a poor prognosis. This report comes from a large and very experienced sarcoma group. Despite advances in diagnosis, staging, and treatment, both medically and surgically, the prognosis remains dismal for this group of patients. The overall 5-year survival rate was less than 25%.

C. P. Beauchamp, MD

Morbidity and Functional Status of Patients With Pelvic Neurogenic Tumors After Wide Excision

Alderete J, Novais EN, Dozois EJ, et al (Mayo Clinic, Rochester, MN)
Clin Orthop Relat Res 468:2948-2953, 2010

Background.—We previously reported that over the last 10 years our practice has evolved in the treatment of neurogenic tumors of the pelvis to include a multispecialty team of surgeons, a factor that might decrease morbidity and improve recurrence, survival, and function.

Questions/Purposes.—Therefore, we (1) assessed the morbidity associated with surgical excision in patients with neurogenic tumors of the pelvis; (2) determined the function of these patients; and (3) determined the rates of local recurrence, metastasis, and overall survival with this new approach.

Methods.—We reviewed the records of all 38 patients who had surgery for a pelvic plexus tumor between 1994 and 2005. Twenty one were male. The mean age of all patients was 38 years and median follow up was 2.1 years. Twelve patients had a malignant tumor. We recorded demographic data, postoperative complications, tumor-specific recurrence, and determined survival.

Results.—Postoperative complications occurred in nine of the 38 patients (23%): hematoma (n = 3), wound infection or deep abscess (n = 3), and deep venous thrombosis (n = 3). Surgical complications occurred more frequently in patients with malignant disease. Patients with benign tumors had a mean MSTS score of 94%, while survivors of malignant disease had a mean of 57%. For malignant tumors, the 5-year rate of local recurrence was 40%, the estimated 5-year rate of metastasis was 67% and 5-year survival rate was 50%.

Conclusion.—Using a team approach, surgical excision provided high functional scores for patients with benign disease with a low rate of complications. In patients with malignant tumors, intentional wide resection is associated with higher morbidity but yields acceptable functional scores.

▶ Musculoskeletal tumors can occur in any location in the body. Sometimes these locations can be extremely challenging to get to. In these situations, it is extremely important to get help in removing tumors from locations rarely seen surgically. Often, these locations are on the boundaries of surgical areas commonly seen by other surgical specialties. An example of this would be the side wall of the pelvis or the lumbosacral plexus. Putting together a surgical team to address these lesions in difficult locations is crucial for their successful removal. The group reporting these results has had decades of experience managing such situations.

Using a multidisciplinary approach greatly facilitates the surgical care of this challenging group of patients.

C. P. Beauchamp, MD

Pathological fractures of the proximal humerus treated with a proximal humeral locking plate and bone cement

Siegel HJ, Lopez-Ben R, Mann JP, et al (Univ of Alabama at Birmingham Med Centre)

J Bone Joint Surg [Br] 92-B:707-712, 2010

Bone loss secondary to primary or metastatic lesions of the proximal humerus remains a challenging surgical problem. Options include preservation of the joint with stabilisation using internal fixation or resection of the tumour with prosthetic replacement. Resection of the proximal humerus often includes the greater tuberosity and adjacent diaphysis, which may result in poor function secondary to loss of the rotator cuff and/or deltoid function. Preservation of the joint with internal fixation may reduce the time in hospital and peri-operative morbidity compared

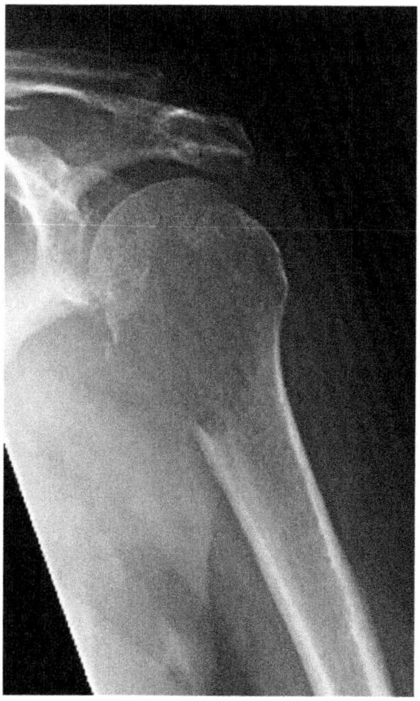

FIGURE 1.—Pre-operative radiograph of a pathological fracture involving the proximal humerus. The patient was diagnosed with multiple myeloma. A large lytic lesion is seen replacing the surgical neck, with extension to the articular surface. (Reprinted from Siegel HJ, Lopez-Ben R, Mann JP, et al. Pathological fractures of the proximal humerus treated with a proximal humeral locking plate and bone cement. *J Bone Joint Surg [Br]*. 2010;92-B:707-712, Copyright 2010 of the British Editorial Society of Bone and Joint Surgery.)

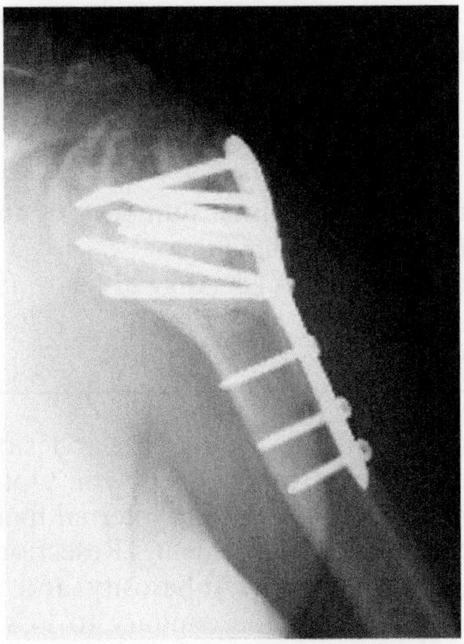

FIGURE 2.—Post-operative radiograph of the patient from Figure 1 two years after surgery. The patient has returned to full activities, with no restrictions and no pain. The reconstruction remains stable, without evidence of recurrence. (Reprinted from Siegel HJ, Lopez-Ben R, Mann JP, et al. Pathological fractures of the proximal humerus treated with a proximal humeral locking plate and bone cement. *J Bone Joint Surg [Br]*. 2010;92-B:707-712, Copyright 2010 of the British Editorial Society of Bone and Joint Surgery.)

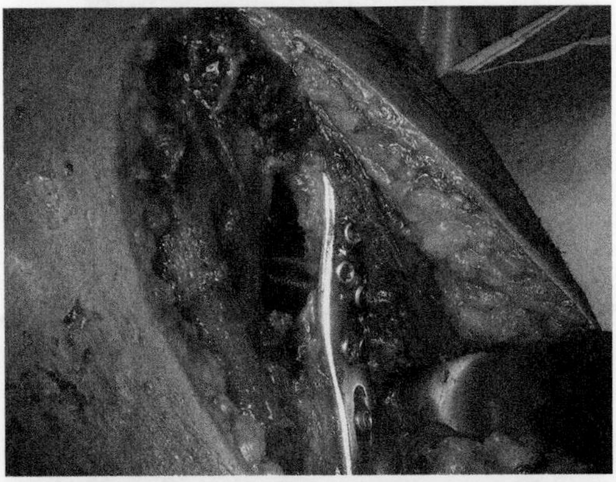

FIGURE 3.—Intra-operative photograph demonstrating multiple locking screws placed in the bone defect just prior to cementation. The locking screws will act as a reinforcing bar to enhance stability. Cement will be placed through this bone window. (Reprinted from Siegel HJ, Lopez-Ben R, Mann JP, et al. Pathological fractures of the proximal humerus treated with a proximal humeral locking plate and bone cement. *J Bone Joint Surg [Br]*. 2010;92-B:707-712, Copyright 2010 of the British Editorial Society of Bone and Joint Surgery.)

with joint replacement, and result in a better functional outcome. We included 32 patients with pathological fractures of the proximal humerus in this study. Functional and radiological assessments were performed. At a mean follow-up of 17.6 months (8 to 61) there was no radiological evidence of failure of fixation. The mean revised musculoskeletal Tumour Society functional score was 94.6% (86% to 99%). There was recurrent tumour requiring further surgery in four patients (12.5%). Of the 22 patients who were employed prior to presentation all returned to work without restrictions.

The use of a locking plate combined with augmentation with cement extends the indications for salvage of the proximal humerus with good function in patients with pathological and impending pathological fractures (Figs 1-3).

▶ The proximal humerus is a common location for both primary and secondary bone neoplasms. Various treatment options to achieve skeletal stability exist for intralesional curettage to proximal humeral replacement. Achievement of durable skeletal fixation has been difficult to predictably achieve until the fairly recent introduction of locking periarticular plates. Previously, intralesional curettage and cementation supplemented with a conventional plate and screws provided adequate fixation in most cases, but a locked plate supplemented with cement has taken this method to the next level. There is no question that preservation of the joint is a far superior choice to an endoprosthesis. The authors have shown that in most cases this can be achieved, and an endoprosthesis is needed only if there is not enough tissue left to support cement and a locking plate.

C. P. Beauchamp, MD

The prognosis for patients with osteosarcoma who have received prior manipulative therapy

Wu P-K, Chen W-M, Lee OK, et al (Taipei Veterans General Hosp, Taiwan; Natl Yang-Ming Univ, Taipei, Taiwan)

J Bone Joint Surg [Br] 92-B:1580-1585, 2010

We evaluated the long-term outcome of patients with an osteosarcoma who had undergone prior manipulative therapy, a popular treatment in Asia, and investigated its effects on several prognostic factors. Of the 134 patients in this study, 70 (52%) patients had manipulative therapy and 64 (48%) did not. The age, location, and size of tumour were not significantly different between the groups. The five-year overall survival rate was 58% and 92% in the groups with and without manipulative therapy ($p = 0.004$). Both the primary and overall rates of lung metastasis were significantly higher in the manipulative group (primary: 32% *vs* 3%, $p = 0.003$; overall lung metastasis rate: 51.4% *vs* 18.8%, $p < 0.001$). Patients who had manipulative therapy had higher local recurrence rates in comparison to patients who did not (29% *vs* 6%, $p = 0.011$). The prognosis for patients with osteosarcoma who had manipulative therapy was significantly poorer than those who had not. Manipulative therapy was an independent factor for survival.

This form of therapy may serve as a mechanism to accelerate the spread of tumour cells, and therefore must be avoided in order to improve the outcome for patients with an osteosarcoma.

▶ This important article is a must read. The authors have shown in this prospective study the extremely harmful effects traditional Chinese manipulation therapy can have on the prognosis of osteosarcomas. It indicates that physical contact has a biological effect on tumor behavior and that association is strong. The North American equivalent of this would be massage therapy and should be avoided when someone presents with a lump. Manipulation during surgery could potentially be more harmful or important than we imagined it to be.

C. P. Beauchamp, MD

Twenty Years of Follow-Up of Survivors of Childhood Osteosarcoma: A Report From the Childhood Cancer Survivor Study

Nagarajan R, Kamruzzaman A, Ness KK, et al (Cincinnati Children's Hosp Med Ctr, OH; Univ of Alberta, Edmonton, Canada; St Jude Children's Res Hosp, Memphis, TN; et al)

Cancer 117:625-634, 2011

Background.—Osteosarcoma survivors have received significant chemotherapy and have undergone substantial surgeries. Their very long-term outcomes (20 year) are reported here.

Methods.—The authors assessed the long-term outcomes of 733 5-year survivors of childhood osteosarcoma diagnosed from 1970 to 1986 to provide a comprehensive evaluation of medical and psychosocial outcomes for survivors enrolled in the Childhood Cancer Survivor Study (CCSS). Outcomes evaluated included overall survival, second malignant neoplasms (SMNs), recurrent osteosarcoma, chronic health conditions, health status (general and mental health and functional limitations), and psychosocial factors. Outcomes of osteosarcoma survivors were compared with general-population statistics, other CCSS survivors, and CCSS siblings.

Results.—Survivors had a mean follow-up of 21.6 years. The overall survival of children diagnosed with osteosarcoma who survived 5 years at 20 years from original diagnosis was 88.6% (95% confidence interval [CI], 86.6%-90.5%). The cumulative incidence of SMNs at 25 years was 5.4%, with a standardized incidence ratio of 4.79 (95% CI, 3.54-6.33; $P<.01$). Overall, 86.9% of osteosarcoma survivors experienced at least 1 chronic medical condition, and >50% experienced ≥2 conditions. Compared with survivors of other cancers, osteosarcoma survivors did not differ in their reported general health status (odds ratio [OR], 0.9; 95% CI, 0.7-1.2), but were more likely to report an adverse health status in at least 1 domain (OR, 1.9; 95% CI, 1.6-2.2), with activity limitations (29.1%) being the most common.

Conclusions.—Childhood osteosarcoma survivors in this cohort did relatively well, considering their extensive treatment, but are at risk of

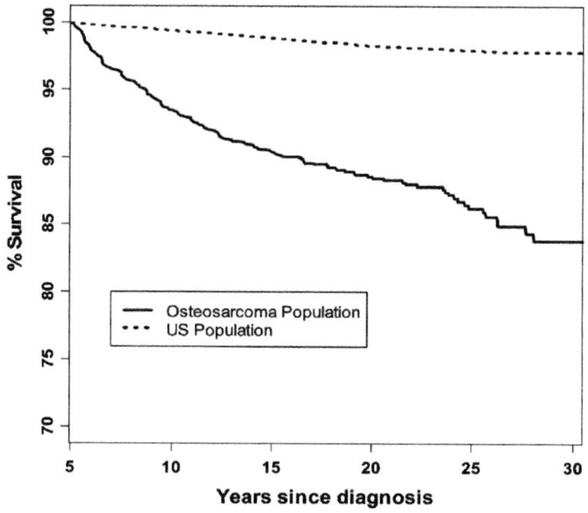

FIGURE 1.—The survival curve of Childhood Cancer Survivor Study osteosarcoma survivors versus US population is shown. (Reprinted from Nagarajan R, Kamruzzaman A, Ness KK, et al. Twenty years of follow-up of survivors of childhood osteosarcoma: a report from the childhood cancer survivor study. *Cancer.* 2011;117:625-634, Copyright 2011 American Cancer Society, with permission of Wiley-Liss, Inc., a subsidiary of John Wiley & Sons, Inc.)

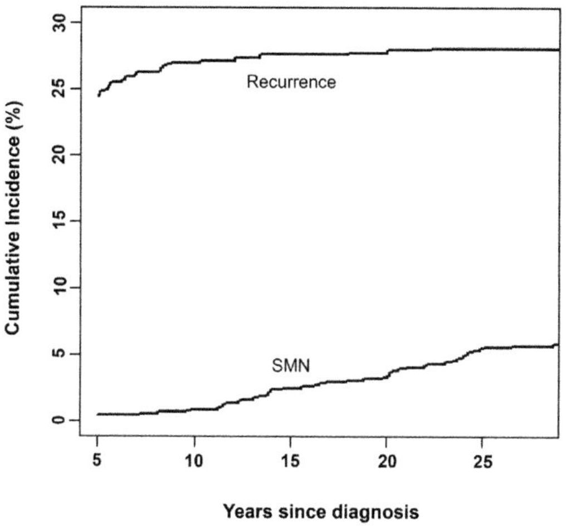

FIGURE 2.—Cumulative incidence curves of second malignant neoplasm (SMN) and recurrence are shown. (Reprinted from Nagarajan R, Kamruzzaman A, Ness KK, et al. Twenty years of follow-up of survivors of childhood osteosarcoma: a report from the childhood cancer survivor study. *Cancer.* 2011;117:625-634, Copyright 2011 American Cancer Society, with permission of Wiley-Liss, Inc., a subsidiary of John Wiley & Sons, Inc.)

experiencing chronic medical conditions and adverse health status. Survivors warrant life-long follow-up (Figs 1 and 2).

▶ We continue to get updates on the long-term consequences of our treatment for childhood malignancies. While strides have been made in patient survival, this group is not normal in terms of their ongoing health-related problems. As a group, there is a higher risk of second malignancies as well as other treatment- and disease-related medical problems, in addition to the consequences of their musculoskeletal reconstructions. These children require ongoing long-term follow-up. The usual transition from childhood to adult health care can be challenging but is particularly important for this group. Clinics are being designed to specifically address this issue.

C. P. Beauchamp, MD

Surgery for skeletal metastases in lung cancer: Complications and survival in 98 patients

Weiss RJ, Wedin R (Karolinska Univ Hosp, Stockholm, Sweden)
Acta Orthop 82:96-101, 2011

Background and Purpose.—Most lung cancer patients with skeletal metastases have a short survival and it is difficult to identify those patients who will benefit from palliative surgery. We report complication and survival rates in a consecutive series of lung cancer patients who were operated for symptomatic skeletal metastases.

Methods.—This study was based on data recorded in the Karolinska Skeletal Metastasis Register. The study period was 1987–2006. We identified 98 lung cancer patients (52 females). The median age at surgery was 62 (34–88) years. 78 lesions were located in the femur or spine.

Results.—The median survival time after surgery was 3 (0–127) months. The cumulative 12-month survival after surgery was 13% (95% CI: 6–20). There was a difference between the survival after spinal surgery (2 months) and after extremity surgery (4 months) ($p = 0.03$). Complete pathological fracture in non-spinal metastases (50 patients) was an independent negative predictor of survival (hazard ratio (HR) = 1.8, 95% CI: 1–3). 16 of 31 patients with spinal metastases experienced a considerable improvement in their neurological function after surgery. The overall complication rate was 20%, including a reoperation rate of 15%.

Interpretation.—Bone metastases and their subsequent surgical treatment in lung cancer patients are associated with high morbidity and

TABLE 2.—Pre- and Postoperative Neurological Function in 31 Patients With Spine Metastasis Graded According to Frankel

	Preop.	Follow-Up
A. Complete paraplegia	2	1
B. No motor function	6	2
C. Motor function useless	14	7
D. Slight motor deficit	6	16
E. No motor deficit	3	5

mortality. Our findings will help to set appropriate expectations for these patients, their families, and surgeons (Table 2).

▶ Decision making in the management of patient with metastatic lung cancer can be difficult, especially if the reconstructive option is highly complex and carries with it a high complication rate. A good example is metastatic disease of the acetabulum. As the life expectancy of this diagnosis is especially grim, it is important to try not to have the patient spend the majority of his or her remaining time on a surgical ward instead of at home or in hospice care. This article is important reading for those who manage the skeletal manifestations of lung cancer.

C. P. Beauchamp, MD

Physeal Distraction for Joint Preservation in Malignant Metaphyseal Bone Tumors in Children

Betz M, Dumont CE, Fuchs B, et al (Univ of Zurich, Switzerland; Orthopädie Zentrum Zürich, Switzerland)

Clin Orthop Relat Res 470:1749-1754, 2012

Background.—Physeal distraction facilitates metaphyseal bone tumor resection in children and preserves the adjacent joint. The technique was first described by Cañadell. Tumor resection procedures allowing limb-sparing reconstruction have been used increasingly in recent years without compromising oncologic principles.

Questions/Purposes.—We report our results with Cañadell's technique by assessing tumor control, functional outcome, and complications.

Methods.—Six consecutive children with primary malignant metaphyseal bone tumors underwent physeal distraction as a part of tumor resection. Tumor location was the distal femur in four patients, the proximal humerus in one patient, and the proximal tibia in one patient. The functional outcome was evaluated after a minimum of 18 months (median, 62 months; range, 18–136 months) using the Musculoskeletal Tumor Society (MSTS) score and the Toronto Extremity Salvage Score (TESS).

Results.—At latest followup, five patients were alive and disease-free and one had died from metastatic disease. All tumor resections resulted in local control; there were no local recurrencies. The mean MSTS score was 79% (range, 53%–97%) and corresponding mean TESS was 83% (range, 71%–92%). In one case, postoperative infection required amputation of the proximal lower leg. All physeal distractions were successful except for one patient in whom distraction resulted in rupturing into the tumor. This situation was salvaged by transepiphyseal resection.

Conclusions.—We consider Cañadell's technique a useful tool in the armamentarium to treat children with malignant tumors that are in close proximity to an open physis.

Level of Evidence.—Level IV, therapeutic study. See Guidelines for Authors for a complete description of levels of evidence.

▶ Physeal distraction to promote limb salvage resections in metaphyseal tumors of skeletally immature patients was first introduced in 1994. However, the procedure has seen very limited application, and published reports are from the originator of the technique. Thus, this series of 6 patients from Zurich is a welcome addition to the literature from a separate center.

These authors nicely illustrate the technique with both a successful and an unsuccessful case to introduce points of discussion. The complexity of this procedure is highlighted by the fact that patients underwent an average of 2.2 additional operations to manage complications (including 1 amputation).

Where to place this technique in our surgical armamentarium? This procedure bears consideration in cases where surgeons would otherwise be considering a complex multiplanar osteotomy for a transphyseal or transepiphyseal resection. In such settings, physeal separation may provide a greater degree of safety. The high complication rate illustrated by an experienced surgical team and the close margins these resections require will limit the applicability of this technique. That said, this is a valuable report and treatment option for metaphyseal pediatric malignancies.

P. S. Rose, MD

Reirradiation of metastatic spinal cord compression: Definitive results of two randomized trials

Maranzano E, Trippa F, Casale M, et al ("S. Maria" Hosp, Terni, Italy)
Radiother Oncol 98:234-237, 2011

Purpose.—Incidence, outcome and prognostic factors of metastatic spinal cord compression (MSCC) patients reirradiated for in-field recurrence were analyzed. Radiation therapists' attitude in reirradiate spinal cord relapses, doses adopted and incidence of myelopathy were also examined.

Materials and Methods.—Data deriving from 579 evaluable patients entered two randomized trials on radiotherapy (RT) for MSCC were revised.

Results.—Twenty-four (4.15%) patients had an in-field recurrence and 12 (50%) were reirradiated. At the time of analysis all reirradiated patients had died. Median time from first and second RT was 5 months (range, 2–31). Six patients received an 8 Gy single-dose, 2 patients 5×3 Gy and remaining four patients 2×8, 5×4, or a single dose of 7 and 4 Gy, respectively. The median cumulative Biologically Effective Dose (BED) calculated was 114.5 Gy_2 (range, 80–120 Gy_2). Six of seven (85.7%) ambulant patients maintained walking ability, whereas none of five not ambulant patients recovered the function. Median duration of response was 4.5 months (range, 1–24). The effect of reirradiation on motor function was significantly associated with walking capacity before reirradiation. Myelopathy was never recorded.

Conclusions.—In MSCC reirradiation was safe and effective. Patient walking capacity before reirradiation was the strongest prognostic factor

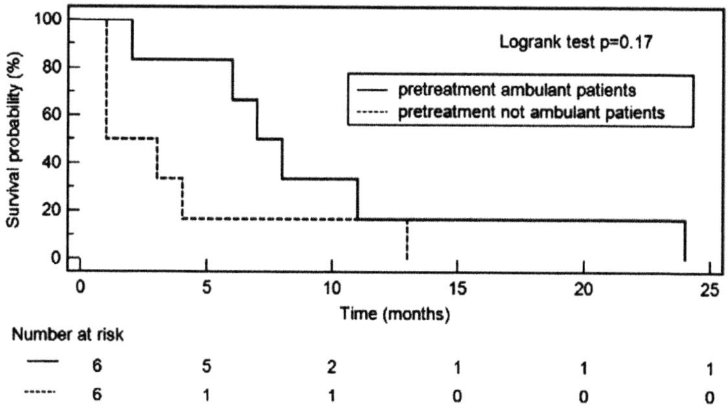

FIGURE 1.—Kaplan–Meier plot of overall survival probability as a function of prereirradiation walking capacity. The number of patients at risk and *p*-value are presented as well. (Reprinted from Maranzano E, Trippa F, Casale M, et al. Reirradiation of metastatic spinal cord compression: definitive results of two randomized trials. *Radiother Oncol.* 2011;98:234-237, Copyright 2011, with permission from Elsevier.)

for functional outcome. Reirradiation was given in about one-half of patients with in-field recurrence and different doses and fractionations were used, even though cumulative BED was in all cases $\leq$120 Gy_2 (Fig 1).

► Symptomatic tumor recurrence or progression following radiotherapy is unfortunately seen in a large number of patients with cancer. These patients pose a very difficult clinical problem because they often are in the later stages of their disease; surgical management is very unattractive because of overall poor medical fitness as well as a higher risk of complication with surgery following previous radiotherapy. As such, consideration of reirradiation often comes into play.

However, many physicians are hesitant to recommend reirradiation of a previously radiated spine because of concerns of inducing radiation myelopathy. Radiation myelopathy is most likely to occur after a biologic dose of more than 5000 cGy (risk estimated at 5% of patients in 5-year follow-up). The median life expectancy of patients with recurrent metastatic disease to the spine rarely achieves this; however, the risk of myelopathy from reirradiation in this clinical setting is poorly defined and often serves as a barrier to further radiation treatment.

The authors of this study have performed previous landmark studies in radiation oncology and thankfully saw no evidence of radiation-induced myelopathy with reirradiation. As in many studies with metastatic disease, pretreatment ambulatory status was the strongest predictor of functional outcome. The overall oncologic prognosis for these patients (either walking or not walking) was unfortunately poor as shown in Fig 1.

This is a study that confirms the clinical viability of a treatment option that is sometimes neglected because of concerns of long-term toxicity in a patient population with short to intermediate life expectancy. I think this is a valuable article to give us confidence in discussing the role of reirradiation with our oncology colleagues when other treatment options are less attractive. The adverse prognostic factor of oncologic paraplegia, already well established, was seen again in this study.

P. S. Rose, MD

Similar Survival but Better Function for Patients after Limb Salvage versus Amputation for Distal Tibia Osteosarcoma

Mavrogenis AF, Abati CN, Romagnoli C, et al (Univ of Bologna, Italy)
Clin Orthop Relat Res 470:1735-1748, 2012

Background.—Amputation has been the standard surgical treatment for distal tibia osteosarcoma. Advances in surgery and chemotherapy have made limb salvage possible. However, it is unclear whether limb salvage offers any improvement in function without compromising survival.

Questions/Purposes.—We therefore compared the survival, local recurrence, function, and complications of patients with distal tibia osteosarcoma treated with limb salvage or amputation.

Methods.—We retrospectively reviewed 42 patients with distal tibia osteosarcoma treated from 1985 to 2010. Nineteen patients had amputations and 23 had limb salvage and allograft reconstructions. We graded the histology using Broders classification, and staged patients using the Musculoskeletal Tumor Society (MSTS) and American Joint Committee on Cancer (AJCC) systems. The tumor grades tended to be higher in the group of patients who had amputations. We determined survival, local recurrence, MSTS function, and complications. The minimum followup was 8 months (median, 60 months; range, 8–288 months).

Results.—The survival of patients who had limb salvage was similar to that of patients who had amputations: 84% at 120 and 240 months versus 74%, respectively. The incidence of local recurrence was similar: three of 23 patients who had limb salvage versus no patients who had amputations. The mean MSTS functional score tended to be higher in patients who had limb salvage compared with those who had amputations: 76% (range, 30%–93%) versus 71% (range, 50%–87%), respectively. The incidence of complications was similar.

Conclusion.—Patients treated with either limb salvage or amputation experience similar survival, local recurrence, and complications, but better function is achievable for patients treated with limb salvage versus amputation. Local recurrence and complications are more common in patients with limb salvage.

Level of Evidence.—Level III, retrospective comparative study. See the Guidelines for Authors for a complete description of levels of evidence.

▶ These authors from the Rizzoli Institute present an intriguing analysis of patients with osteosarcoma of the distal tibia who underwent limb salvage (n = 19 with intercalary, osteoarticular, or allograft arthrodesis techniques) and compare it with a cohort of patients treated with amputation (n = 23), the traditional treatment for tumors in this location. Readers should note that this is a retrospective study and that patients in the amputation group had more high-grade tumors than those in the limb salvage group.

Surprisingly, patients in the limb salvage group had equivalent outcomes for survival and function. Although the authors report a barely statistically significant improvement in Musculoskeletal Tumor Society outcome scores in the limb salvage group, the difference is not likely to be clinically relevant (76% vs 71%) and within the variability of this arbitrary rating system. Three patients in the limb salvage group required secondary amputation for local recurrence; interestingly, all 3 had above average outcome scores that were credited to the limb salvage group, a potential source of confounding. Had these patients been dropped from the outcome analysis or summed with the amputation group, no statistical difference in outcome is seen.

This article demonstrates that limb salvage in select osteosarcomas of the distal tibia is a reasonable treatment option. The overall outcomes in this report are similar between groups (acknowledging the larger number of higher-grade tumors in the amputation group). Despite the title and article assertions, I do not see this report as demonstrating superior functional outcomes with limb salvage. Surgical oncologists will need to continue to weigh the achievable margins of resection and anticipated functional outcome in selecting the best oncologic resection for these tumors.

P. S. Rose, MD

Predictors of Survival After Surgical Treatment of Spinal Metastasis

Arrigo RT, Kalanithi P, Cheng I, et al (Stanford Univ School of Medicine, CA; Stanford Univ Med Ctr, Palo Alto, CA; et al)

Neurosurgery 68:674-681, 2011

Background.—Surgery for spinal metastasis is a palliative treatment aimed at improving patient quality of life by alleviating pain and reversing or delaying neurologic dysfunction, but with a mean survival time of less than 1 year and significant complication rates, appropriate patient selection is crucial.

Objective.—To identify the most significant prognostic variables of survival after surgery for spinal metastasis.

Methods.—Chart review was performed on 200 surgically treated spinal metastasis patients at Stanford Hospital between 1999 and 2009. Survival analysis was performed and variables entered into a Cox proportional hazards model to determine their significance.

Results.—Median overall survival was 8.0 months, with a 30-day mortality rate of 3.0% and a 30-day complication rate of 34.0%. A Cox proportional hazards model showed radiosensitivity of the tumor (hazard ratio: 2.557, $P < .001$), preoperative ambulatory status (hazard ratio: 2.355, $P = .0001$), and Charlson Comorbidity Index (hazard ratio: 2.955, $P < .01$) to be significant predictors of survival. Breast cancer had the best prognosis (median survival, 27.1 months), whereas gastrointestinal tumors had the worst (median survival, 2.66 months).

TABLE 6.—One-, Three-, and Five-Year Survival Rates

	Percentage Surviving 1 Year	3 Years	5 Years
Overall	38.3	21.1	9.41
Ambulatory status			
Ambulatory	47.7	27.5	12.2
Nonambulatory	11.1	0.0[a]	0.0[a]
Charlson Comorbidity Index score			
0 or 1	40.1	22.1	9.85
≥2	0.0	0.0	0.0
Primary tumor type			
Breast (best survival)	59.0	20.2	0.0
Other gastrointestinal[b] (worst survival)	45.0	0.0	0.0
Radiosensitivity of tumor			
Radiosensitive	53.6	29.4	25.7
Radioresistant	39.5	10.2	0.0

[a]At 18 months, the only surviving patient was lost to follow-up.
[b]Other gastrointestinal is all noncolon gastrointestinal cancers.

Conclusion.—We identified the Charlson Comorbidity Index score as one of the strongest predictors of survival after surgery for spinal metastasis. We confirmed previous findings that radiosensitivity of the tumor and ambulatory status are significant predictors of survival (Table 6).

▶ The majority of patients who die of cancer have spinal metastases present on autopsy; although only a minority are symptomatic before death, the sheer numbers involved imply that at least 20 000 patients per year in the United States are treated for metastatic epidural spinal cord compression. These authors report the largest study to date (except registry studies) that have looked at predictors of survival after surgical treatment of spinal metastasis. Their patients were selected over a decade between 1999 and 2009 at a modern tertiary treatment center. This distinguishes this study from others that have looked at similar topics by the large number of patients involved and the relatively tight timeframe (a decade in which there have been relatively few changes in our overall treatment protocols). Readers should know that this is a retrospective study but drawn from a high-quality institutional database.

This report highlights the guarded survival in this patient population and the high complication rate (seen in one-third of patients at 30 days). The authors were able to identify the ambulatory status, Charleston Comorbidity Index, tumor histology, and radiosensitivity to be very strong predictors of survival as outlined in their Table 6 reproduced below. These results confirm what has been seen in other studies in a larger and more tightly controlled patient population.

Studies of this nature influence our counseling of patients with metastatic spine disease and our decision to pursue surgical rather than less aggressive and invasive treatments. As well, the authors have identified the Charleston Comorbidity Index as a strong factor in predicting survival which (if not accounted for) poses a large confounding factor in future studies and trials of this subject.

P. S. Rose, MD

Treatment of Unicameral Bone Cyst: Surgical Technique

Hou H-Y, Wu K, Wang C-T, et al (Natl Taiwan Univ Hosp, Taipei)

J Bone Joint Surg Am 93:92-99, 2011

Background.—There is a variety of treatment modalities for unicameral bone cysts, with variable outcomes reported in the literature. Although good initial outcomes have been reported, the success rate has often changed with longer-term follow-up. We introduce a novel, minimally invasive treatment method and compare its clinical outcomes with those of other methods of treatment of this lesion.

Methods.—From February 1994 to April 2008, forty patients with a unicameral bone cyst were treated with one of four techniques: serial percutaneous steroid and autogenous bone-marrow injection (Group 1, nine patients); open curettage and grafting with a calcium sulfate bone substitute either without instrumentation (Group 2, twelve patients) or with internal instrumentation (Group 3, seven patients); or minimally invasive curettage, ethanol cauterization, disruption of the cystic boundary, insertion of a synthetic calcium sulfate bone-graft substitute, and placement of a cannulated screw to provide drainage (Group 4, twelve patients). Success was defined as radiographic evidence of a healed cyst or of a healed cyst with some defect according to the modified Neer classification, and failure was defined as a persistent or recurrent cyst that needed additional treatment. Patients who sustained a fracture during treatment were also considered to have had a failure. The outcome parameters included the radiographically determined healing rate, the time to solid union, and the total number of procedures needed.

Results.—The follow-up time ranged from eighteen to eighty-four months. Group-4 patients had the highest radiographically determined healing rate. Healing was seen in eleven of the twelve patients in that group compared with three of the nine in Group 1, eight of the twelve in Group 2, and six of the seven in Group 3. Group-4 patients also had the shortest mean time to union: 3.7 ± 2.3 months compared with 23.4 ± 14.9, 12.2 ± 8.5, and 6.6 ± 4.3 months in Groups 1, 2, and 3, respectively.

Conclusions.—This new minimally invasive method achieved a favorable outcome, with a higher radiographically determined healing rate and a shorter time to union. Thus, it can be considered an option for initial treatment of unicameral bone cysts.

▶ Unicameral bone cysts are commonly encountered in clinical practice; a variety of treatment options have been proposed and executed; their efficacy roughly parallels their invasiveness.

Hou and colleagues present a well-illustrated percutaneous treatment algorithm for unicameral cysts, which showed rapid healing in 11 of 12 patients. The technique includes curettage, ethanol lavage, cyst boundary disruption, calcium sulfate grafting, and percutaneous screw placement (Fig 8 in the original article). These authors also compared this technique against serial steroid and bone marrow aspirate injection and open curettage and grafting with or without instrumentation and found both a higher success rate and more rapid healing.

The treatment of these lesions will always vary with surgeon and patient/parent preferences as well as unique factors of each lesion. This article nicely illustrates a successful technique for surgeons to consider in their treatment of unicameral bone cysts.

P. S. Rose, MD

Factors Associated with Recurrence of Primary Aneurysmal Bone Cysts: Is Argon Beam Coagulation an Effective Adjuvant Treatment?

Steffner RJ, Liao C, Stacy G, et al (Univ of Chicago Med Ctr, IL)
J Bone Joint Surg Am 93:e1221-e1229, 2011

Background.—Our goal was to assess the effectiveness and safety of argon beam coagulation as an adjuvant treatment for primary aneurysmal bone cysts, to reevaluate the adjuvant effectiveness of the use of a high-speed burr alone, and, secondarily, to identify predictors of aneurysmal bone cyst recurrence.

Methods.—We retrospectively reviewed the records of ninety-six patients with primary aneurysmal bone cysts who were managed at our institution from January 1, 1983, to December 31, 2008. Forty patients were managed with curettage, a high-speed burr, and argon beam coagulation; thirty-four were managed with curettage and a high-speed burr without argon beam coagulation; and the remaining twenty-two were managed with curettage with argon beam coagulation alone, curettage with no adjuvant treatment, or resection of the entire lesion. Demographic, clinical, and radiographic data were viewed comparatively for possible predictors of recurrence. Kaplan-Meier survival analysis with a log-rank test was performed to measure association and effectiveness.

Results.—The median age at the time of diagnosis was fifteen years (range, one to sixty-two years). The median duration of follow-up was 29.5 months (range, zero to 300 months). The overall rate of recurrence of aneurysmal bone cyst after surgical treatment was 11.5%. The rate of recurrence was 20.6% after curettage and high-speed-burr treatment alone and 7.5% after curettage and high-speed-burr treatment plus argon beam coagulation. The five-year Kaplan-Meier survival estimate was 92% for patients managed with curettage and adjuvant treatment with a high-speed burr and argon beam coagulation, compared with 73% for patients managed with curettage and a high-speed burr only ($p = 0.060$).

Conclusions.—Surgical treatment of aneurysmal bone cyst with curettage and adjuvant argon beam coagulation is effective. Postoperative fracture appears to be a common complication of this treatment and needs to be studied further. Treatment with curettage and high-speed burr alone may not reduce recurrence.

Level of Evidence.—Therapeutic Level III. See Instructions for Authors for a complete description of levels of evidence.

▶ Aneurysmal bone cysts can be vexing benign bone tumors to treat; the high rate of recurrence following simple curettage has led surgeons to try a number of surgical adjuvants—embolization, phenol, liquid nitrogen, and methylmethacrylate, to name a few. These adjuvants may be classified as mechanical (eg, high-speed burr), chemical (phenol, alcohol, peroxide), and thermal (traditionally liquid nitrogen) adjuvants. Steffner and colleagues add a large series to the literature using argon beam coagulation as an alternative thermal adjuvant to extend the local zone of necrosis in aneurysmal bone cysts.

This technique has previously been shown to be effective in the treatment of giant cell tumor of bone;[1] the current article demonstrates a significant decrease in the local recurrence rate of aneurysmal bone cysts with the use of the argon beam coagulator in an admittedly retrospective study (Fig 5 in the original article).

This is a useful technique for surgeons to be familiar with—the equipment is available in any large hospital and easily and precisely applied to bone tumor work. Nothing is without drawbacks, however, and the authors do note higher fracture and other complication rates in patients treated with the argon beam coagulator.

P. S. Rose, MD

Reference

1. Lewis VO, Wei A, Mendoza T, Primus F, Peabody T, Simon MA. Argon beam coagulation as an adjuvant for local control of giant cell tumor. *Clin Orthop Relat Res*. 2007;454:192-197.

Palliative radiotherapy for bone metastases: An ASTRO evidence-based guideline

Lutz S, Berk L, Chang E, et al (Blanchard Valley Regional Cancer Ctr, Findlay, OH; Moffitt Cancer Ctr, Tampa, FL; Univ of Texas M.D. Anderson Cancer Ctr, Houston; et al)

Int J Radiat Oncol Biol Phys 79:965-976, 2011

Purpose.—To present guidance for patients and physicians regarding the use of radiotherapy in the treatment of bone metastases according to current published evidence and complemented by expert opinion.

Methods and Materials.—A systematic search of the National Library of Medicine's PubMed database between 1998 and 2009 yielded 4,287 candidate original research articles potentially applicable to radiotherapy for bone metastases. A Task Force composed of all authors synthesized the published evidence and reached a consensus regarding the recommendations contained herein.

Results.—The Task Force concluded that external beam radiotherapy continues to be the mainstay for the treatment of pain and/or prevention of the morbidity caused by bone metastases. Various fractionation schedules can provide significant palliation of symptoms and/or prevent the morbidity of bone metastases. The evidence for the safety and efficacy of repeat treatment to previously irradiated areas of peripheral bone metastases for pain was derived from both prospective studies and retrospective data, and it can be safe and effective. The use of stereotactic body radiotherapy holds theoretical promise in the treatment of new or recurrent spine lesions, although the Task Force recommended that its use be limited to highly selected patients and preferably within a prospective trial. Surgical decompression and postoperative radiotherapy is recommended for spinal cord compression or spinal instability in highly selected patients with sufficient performance status and life expectancy. The use of bisphosphonates, radionuclides, vertebroplasty, and kyphoplasty for the treatment or prevention of cancer-related symptoms does not obviate the need for external beam radiotherapy in appropriate patients.

Conclusions.—Radiotherapy is a successful and time efficient method by which to palliate pain and/or prevent the morbidity of bone metastases. This Guideline reviews the available data to define its proper use and provide consensus views concerning contemporary controversies or unanswered questions that warrant prospective trial evaluation.

▶ Lutz et al present the evidence-based treatment guidelines for skeletal metastases from the American Society of Radiation Oncology developed by a multidisciplinary working group including input from orthopedic surgery. This article is a contemporary and excellent review of different radiotherapy options based on the available evidence in the literature. The article includes a thorough discussion and presentation of evidence for radiotherapy in the spine, index treatment and reirradiation of extremity lesions, and the use of radionucleotides. As such, it is a succinct work covering a large area of clinical practice, well referenced with conclusions supported by the literature. As surgeons who evaluate and treat patients with bony metastases, a full understanding of the radiation oncology options is critical to make the best treatment decisions for them. This article provides a nice, solid reference in that direction.

P. S. Rose, MD

Article Index

Chapter 1: Basic Science

Chapter 2: General Orthopedics

Chapter 3: Trauma and Amputation

Chapter 4: Forearm, Wrist, and Hand

Chapter 5: Shoulder and Elbow

Chapter 6: Total Hip Arthroplasty

Chapter 7: Total Knee Arthroplasty

Chapter 8: Sports Medicine

Chapter 9: Foot and Ankle

Chapter 10: Spine

Chapter 11: Orthopedic Oncology

Author Index

E

F

G

H

I

J

K

L

M

T

U

V

W

Y

Z

Printed and bound by CPI Group (UK) Ltd, Croydon, CR0 4YY
08/05/2025
01864678-0012